W0106092

Clinical Use of Calcium Channel Antagonist Drugs

Clinical Use of Calcium Channel Antagonist Drugs

by:

Lionel H. Opie, MD, PhD, FRCP
Professor of Medicine
University of Cape Town
Cape Town, South Africa;
Consultant Professor
Division of Cardiology
Stanford University Medical Center
Stanford, California

With a chapter by:

William A. Coetzee, DSc
Principal Scientific Investigator
Heart Research Unit
University of Cape Town
South Africa

KLUWER ACADEMIC PUBLISHERS
BOSTON   DORDRECHT   LONDON

Distributors for North America:
Kluwer Academic Publishers
101 Philip Drive
Assinippi Park
Norwell, Massachusetts 02061 USA

Distributors for all other countries:
Kluwer Academic Publishers Group
Distribution Centre
Post Office Box 322
3300 AH Dordrecht, THE NETHERLANDS

Library of Congress Cataloging-in-Publication Data

Opie, Lionel H.
  Clinical use of calcium channel antagonist drugs /
  by Lionel H. Opie ; with a chapter by William A.
  Coetzee.
      p.   cm.
  Chapters 1-5 previously published in Cardiovascular
  drugs and therapy as parts I-V.
  Includes index.
  ISBN-13: 978-1-4612-8208-2   e-ISBN-13: 978-1-4613-0863-8
  DOI: 10.1007/ 978-1-4613-0863-8

  1. Calcium—Antagonists.   2. Heart—Diseases—
  Chemotherapy.
I. Coetzee, William A. II. Cardiovascular drugs and
therapy.
III. Title.
  [DNLM: 1.Calcium Channel Blockers—therapeutic
  use—collected works. 150 061c]
RC684.C34C55 1989
616.1'2061—dc19
DNLM/DLC   89-2543
for Library of Congress   CIP

CONTENTS

AUTHOR'S PREFACE

Calcium antagonists are now regarded as the most important advance in cardiac drug therapy since the advent of beta-adrenergic blocking agents. Acting basically as vasodilators—though with many other complex mechanisms especially in the case of the anti-arrhythmic calcium antagonists, these agents have grown in importance to become among the therapeutic agents of first choice for angina pectoris and hypertension.

The major aim of the present book is to present the clinician with the information needed for the *practical use of calcium antagonists*. What do all the numerous and often conflicting trials say? Do these agents really work? If so, which agent and in what dose? How do the three front runners, verapamil, nifedipine and diltiazem compare in the efficacy and side-effects with each other? How do the new second generation agents, now entering the North American market, slot in and compare with the three first-liners? When the gloss is taken away from the advertisements, what is really left?

The strong clinical bias of the present book should be complimented by further reading of books slanted towards fundamentals. One of the most important and recent of these is that by Dr Winifred Nayler (Calcium Antagonists, Academic Press, 1988). That book should be basic for essential background knowledge in the area of calcium antagonists. The important basic contributions of Fleckenstein deserve emphasis. A particularly important article outlining the basic myocardial properties of the calcium antagonists was that published by Fleckenstein in "Calcium and the Heart" (eds. P Harris, L Opie), Academic Press, London, 1971, pp 135-138. His more recent concepts are fully discussed in "Calcium Antagonism in Heart and Smooth Muscle", Wiley, New York, 1983. Another important recent edition is that edited by Godfraind and others on "Calcium Entry Blockers and Tissue Protection" (Raven Press, New York, 1985) which covers some novel aspects of calcium antagonism including the use in cerebrovascular conditions. These books by masters in the area of basic research will provide the background knowledge required to fully understand the clinical effects of these agents.

Finally, a word on terminology. I prefer the term 'calcium antagonists', used by Fleckenstein and recommended by the recent International Committee of the International Society and Federation of Cardiology (see Opie et al, Am J Cardiol 60: 630-632,.1987). Next most popular is probably the term 'calcium entry blocker' or simply 'calcium blocker'. Scientifically most correct is probably the term 'calcium channel antagonist'. All these terms have the same meaning. These agents unequivocally act on the calcium channel to decrease the slow inward calcium current, described by my electrophysiological colleague, Dr W Coetzee DSc, in his opening chapter. Remarkably specific, yet remarkably diverse when one compound is compared with another, the calcium channel antagonists have revolutionized cardiovascular therapy.

This book aims to simplify the revolution and to fortify the clinician with the information needed to use calcium channel antagonists with complete confidence that the best principles of treatment and the best compound can be applied to the therapy of the individual patient.

L H Opie

FOREWORD

The development of the calcium channel angatonists represents one of the major advances in cardiovascular therapeutics of the latter half of the twentieth century. In contrast to other cardioactive agents such as antihypertensive, antiarrhythmic, antiischemic, and positive inotropic agents, calcium antagonists are unique in that they play an important role in the treatment of a wide variety of cardiovascular disorders. They are effective and useful in the treatment of conditions as diverse as hypertension, supraventricular tachyarrhythmias, angina pectoris and hypertrophic cardiomyopathy and are usually well tolerated. The effectiveness and low toxicity of calcium channel antagonists has rapidly led to their very wide adoption in clinical medicine. In the United States alone, the sales of these drugs in 1988 exceeded one billion dollars. The drugs are prescribed widely not only by cardiovascular specialists but increasingly by internists and family physicians as well.

Many patients with mild to moderate essential hypertension and angina pectoris can be treated with only a calcium channel antagonist, greatly simplifying therapy for this enormous number of patients. However, in many patients, calcium antagonists must be used together with other drugs active on the cardiovascular system and the physician must be cognizant of their potential interactions. Another important challenge in dealing with these agents is raised by the fact that there are at least three distinct families of calcium antagonists. The patriarchs (or matriarchs if you prefer) of these three families are verapamil, nifedipine and diltiazem. Each of these now has a rapidly expanding number of progeny whose actions, side effects and pharmacokinetics differ from and, in many instances offer some advantages over the parent compounds.

Professor Lionel Opie's book offers scholarly physicians, regardless of their clinical specialty, as well as investigators, teachers and advanced students of cardiology and pharmacology, the most authoritative, comprehensive, and up-to-date information available about calcium channel antagonists and it does so with clarity and lucidity. After a review of the role of the channel-mediated calcium current in the heart, it moves on to the actions and pharmacokinetics of the primary classes of antagonists, to a description of second and third generation drugs, as well as to the interaction of calcium antagonists with other drugs, particularly cardiovascular agents. Despite the enormous quantity of material covered in this book, it is readable, easily understandable and not intimidating; the diagrams and tables are especially well planned and useful.

Professor Opie, a distinguished cardiovascular scientist and a gifted author and teacher, should be congratulated for preparing this definitive book on calcium channel antagonists, drugs which contribute so uniquely and importantly to the care of so many patients with a wide variety of cardiovascular disorders.

Eugene Braunwald, M.D.
Boston, Mass., USA

Clinical Use of Calcium Channel Antagonist Drugs

INTRODUCTION

CHANNEL-MEDIATED CALCIUM CURRENT IN THE HEART

William A. Coetzee

SUMMARY. Calcium ions play an important role in the regulation of cardiac functions. Calcium ions may enter or leave the myocardial cell through various mechanisms, including several exhange mechanisms and pumps. This review concentrates on the influx of calcium ions through channels in the sarcolemma, resulting in an electric current flow. The calcium current plays an important role in the maintenance of the action potential duration, in the generation of pacemaker activity, and in the initiation of contraction.

The calcium current displays both activation and a subsequent inactivation when the membrane potential is changed in a stepwise fashion. Previously, the activation was thought to occur rather slowly, hence the name "slow inward current." Recent evidence suggests that the calcium current occurs much faster and that two types of calcium currents might exist, differing in their selectivity to other ions and in their sensitivity to membrane potential and to drugs.

It is not quite clear how the calcium current is changed during myocardial ischemia. Factors that may reduce the calcium current during ischemia are the increased extracellular potassium concentration, metabolic inhibition and a decreased ATP level, and acidosis. Raised levels of intracellular cAMP, however, should lead to an increased calcium current.

The calcium current is modulated by several drugs. Beta-adrenergic stimulation increases the calcium current by increasing the opening probability of the calcium channel. The effects of acetylcholine are less well described. There also exists a class of drugs, called calcium channel blockers (or calcium antagonists) that decrease the flow of calcium ions through calcium channels.

The concentration of free intracellular calcium ions ($[Ca^{2+}]_i$) is now widley recognized as a major intracellular messenger for physiologic and pathophysiologic cellular function.

Various mechanisms exist in the cell membrane to regulate cytosolic calcium (Figure 1). They include the influx of calcium into the cell via 1) the calcium current, 2) the Na^+-Ca^{2+} exchange mechanism, and 3) the passive leakage of calcium into the cell. Mechanisms must also exist for the extrusion of calcium from the cell interior, to avoid the accumulation of cytosolic calcium. The two main mechanisms are 1) efflux of Ca^{2+} through the Na^+-Ca^{2+} exchange mechanism (a reversible reaction, depending on the concentration gradients and the membrane potential): 2) an active adenosine triphosphate (ATP)-dependent calcium pump in the membrane. For normal cellular function to occur, there must be a fine balance among all these mechanisms.

For the purpose of this review, we will examine only one of these mechanisms, namely, the influx of calcium ions through channels in the cell membrane. Because the calcium ion is positively charged, the influx of calcium ions occurs as an electronic current, hence the name "the calcium current" (Figure 2).

History of the Calcium Current

In 1952, the classical description of the action potential of nerve cells was that it consisted mainly of two time-dependent currents—an inward sodium current and an outward potassium current [1]. During these early electrophysiologic studies a logical conclusion was that all electrical phenomena could be explained by these two current systems. An exception was crustacean muscle fibers in which calcium-mediated action potentials with a long plateau could be evoked [2]. The cardiac action potential, which has a different shape and a much longer duration than that of the nerve, was not thought to be caused by a calcium current—mainly because of the obscure observation that

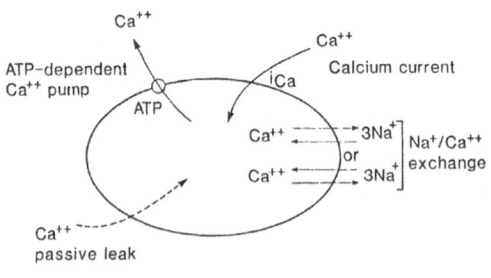

Fig. 1. A schematic diagram of a myocardial cell showing the various possible entry/exit pathways for calcium ions under normal physiologic conditions.

the action potential duration paradoxically *increased* when the $[Ca^{2+}]_0$ was decreased [3]. Even as late as 1962, the cardiac action potential was explained solely by two time-dependent currents—the sodium current and the potassium current [4]. The long duration (and even pacemaker activity) was explained by the same sodium and potassium currents, but they were assumed to exhibit slower kinetics.

In the following few years, the possibility that calcium ions might also play a role in the maintenance of the cardiac action potential was proposed [5-7]. However it was only when the more sophisticated technique of voltage clamping was applied to heart tissue [8] that final proof of the involvement of calcium during the action potential was obtained [9] (see Figure 2).

Physiologic Role of Calcium Current

The calcium current plays an important role in general cardiac function, ranging from the initiation of excitation and maintenance of the regular beating of the heart, to the correct timing between the contractions of the atria and the ventricles, and contraction.

Role of the Calcium Current in
Pacemaker Activity

The heart exhibits intrinsic automaticity, even when isolated from the rest of the body. This rhythmic activity is governed by the sinoatrial (SA) node, which is located in the right atrium.

The pacemaker activity of the SA node is a direct result of the membrane potential spontaneously decreasing to a less negative potential, until the threshold potential is reached, causing the firing of a new action potential. This process occurs repeatedly following each action potential.

Theoretically, the gradual decline in membrane potential during diastolic depolarization can be caused by a gradual increase of an inward current, or by a decrease of an outward current. It was found that both processes play a role in pacemaker activity, and that the change in membrane potential is a result of a fine balance between an outward (potassium) current, and an inward (calcium) current [10,11]. The potassium component is a result of a slow decline of an outward potassium current that was switched on during the action potential plateau. The calcium current,

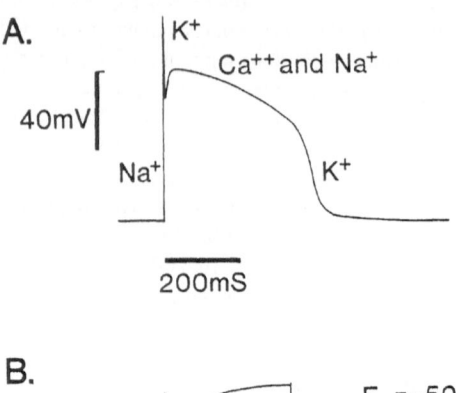

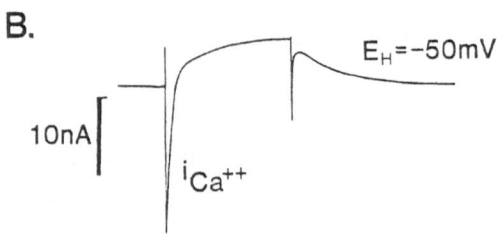

Fig. 2. A, An action potential recorded from the Purkinje
fiber of a rabbit heart. The sudden change of the membrane
potential from a resting value of -76 to $+34mV$ is mostly
caused by the influx of sodium ions (the sodium current).
The initial rapid repolarization is caused by (1) the inactivation of the sodium current and (2) an increase in potassium
conductance. The calcium current is thought to contribute to
the plateau of the action potential, and in this fiber even pro-
duces a secondary "hump" depolarization. Final repolarization to the resting membrane potential is caused by the inactivation of the calcium current and by the activation of a
potassium current. The relative role of the electrogenic Na-
Ca exchange current in this sequence of events is not clear.
B, An example of the calcium current as recorded from a
sheep Purkinje fiber. The membrane potential was changed
in a stepwise fashion using the voltage clamp technique from
a holding potential of -50 mV (where most of the sodium
current is inactivated) to -10 mV for a duration of 500 msec.
The resulting current flow is depicted in the figure. On depolarization of the membrane, a small capacitive spike can
be observed, which is followed by the activation of the inward
calcium current (downward deflection of the current trace).
The calcium current peaks, after which it becomes smaller
(inactivation). The current during the later phases of
the clamp step, as well as the "tail" current following the
clamp step, is caused by the outward flow of potassium ions.

however, also plays a major role in pacemaker activity
of nodal tissue, and is slowly activated to help cause
the spontaneous diastolic depolarization. The spontaneous diastolic depolarization of Purkinje fibers oc-

curs in a different range of membrane potential (-70 to -90 mV), and is caused by a special pacemaker current (i_f), which is carried by Na^+ and K^+ [12]. i_f also occurs in nodal tissue [10], but its contribution to pacemaker activity is small, because of the different potential range where pacemaker activity occurs in this tissue (-60 to -40 mV).

Role of the Calcium Current in Impulse Propagation

Another important function of the calcium current is in the conduction of the electrical impulse across the atria and atrioventricular (AV) node.

The cable theory predicts that conduction velocity is proportional to the upstroke velocity of the action potential (V_{max}). The calcium current contributes significantly to the upstroke of the atrial action potential [13]. Atrial muscle and nodal tissue thus have a lower V_{max} than the action potential of Purkinje fibers, where mainly the sodium current is responsible for the upstroke of the action potential. Several physiologic implications arise. First, the conduction velocity of atria is much lower than that of Purkinje fibers or ventricular muscle. In the AV node, the calcium current plays an even larger role in the upstroke of the action potential, and the AV node has an even smaller conduction velocity [13]. The implication is that there is a delay in conduction from the atria to the ventricle. The delay gives the atria enough time to empty before the impulse is conducted to the ventricles and ventricular contraction occurs.

Maintenance of the Action Potential Duration and Contraction

The action potential of cardiac muscle differs from that of nerve tissue, in that it exhibits a much longer duration (see Figure 2). Following the initial rapid depolarization, there is a delay before final repolarization occurs during which the membrane potential remains depolarized; this is called the *action potential plateau*. The net current flow during repolarization is very small, and is a result of a fine balance between small inward and outward currents [14]. The inward current responsible for the action potential plateau is partly carried by calcium (i_{Ca}) [15], by a residual sodium "window" current [16], and by a slowly inactivating component of the sodium current [17]. The contribution of the electrogenic Na^+-Ca^{2+} exchange should also be considered [18]. Beyond a certain time, the net current during repolarization changes in the outward direction, to cause the membrane potential to return to the maximum diastolic potential. This net outward current is caused by 1) an inward calcium current decreasing as a function of time (inactivation), and 2) and outward potassium current that increases (activates).

During the action potential plateau, calcium ions enter the cell as the calcium current, which eventually triggers contraction [19]. When cardiac cells are injected with a protein (called aequorin) that emits light when it binds to calcium, it can be shown that the cytosolic calcium activity increases transiently, even before contraction takes place [20,21]. This rise in intracellular calcium concentration is due to the calcium current, and to a calcium-induced calcium release from the sarcoplasmic reticulum [22]. Thus, the calcium current supplies calcium ions for the activation of contraction, in conjunction with the sarcoplasmic reticulum and other transport mechanisms.

Description of the Calcium Current

The Calcium Channel in the Membrane

By definition, the movement of positively charged ions into the cell causes an inward electrical current. Since the intracellular calcium concentration is much lower (around 3×10^{-7} M) than the extracellular concentration (around 1.5 to 2×10^{-3} M), there exists a large diffusion gradient for calcium ions into the cell. The membrane is, however, relatively impermeable to calcium ions, and calcium only enters the cell when pores or channels in the membrane open. The channels are membrane proteins which probably span the membrane, and this allows a very selective pathway into the cell for calcium ions when changing from a closed to an open state. Along the lines of a simplified model developed for nerve muscle by Hodgkin and Huxley [1], each channel in the membrane has two "gates" which control the opening of the channel. Calcium ions can only pass when both gates are in the open position. The movement of the gates is dependent on 1) membrane voltage and 2) time. Furthermore, the two gates in the membrane differ from each other (Figure 3). The one gate normally is in a open position at the resting membrane potential (also called the f or inactivation gate), while at the same potential, the other (called the d or activation gate) is in a closed position. The result is that no calcium current flows through the calcium channel at the resting membrane potential.

Activation and Inactivation

For calcium ions to pass through the channel, both gates need to be open. When the membrane potential

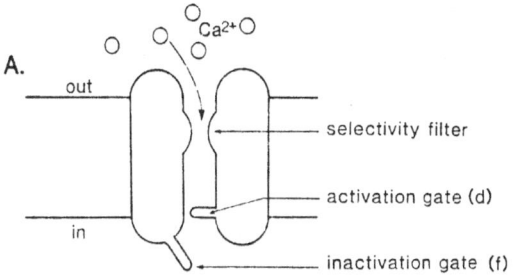

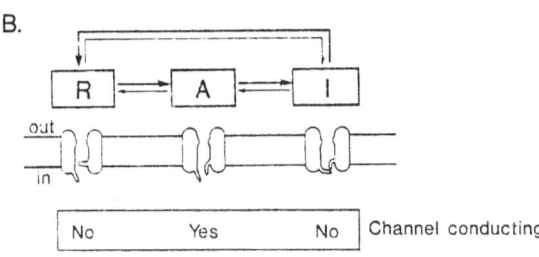

Fig. 3. A, A representation of a calcium channel in the membrane, after the model proposed by Hodgkin and Huxley [1]. The channel is thought to be a protein molecule extending through the membrane. In the channel molecule there is a d- or activation gate and a f- or inactivation gate. The selectivity of the channel for calcium is determined by the selectivity filter. B, The channel only allows calcium ions to pass when both the gates are open. When the membrane is depolarized, the activation gate opens (A); normally this gate is closed in the resting (R) state. With sustained depolarization, the activation gate remains opened, but the inactivation gate closes, stopping the current flow. The channel is now said to be inactivated (I).

suddenly changes to a more positive value (e.g., -10 mV), as during the upstroke of the action potential or during voltage clamping, the two gates change their individual states, because they are voltage dependent. However, the speed at which they change differs. First, the activation gate opens very rapidly, and the calcium current is said to be activated. Since both gates are open, current can now flow through the channel. Next, the inactivation gate closes at a slower rate, and the channel is said to be inactivated, with the result that current stops flowing.

If one looks at all the calcium channels on the membrane rather than a single channel, one can call the proportion of channels in the activated state "d." Likewise, one can refer to the proportion of channels in the inactivated state as "f." Since both these proportions are a function of time, one needs to observe these proportions at steady state (d_∞ or f_∞). For the calcium

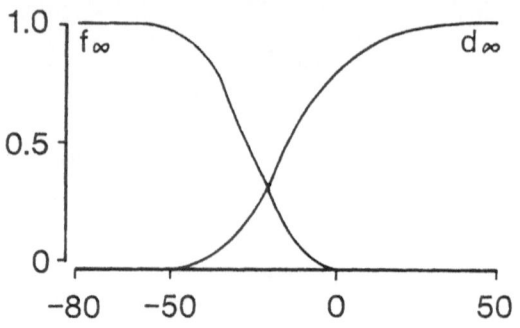

Fig. 4. A schematic diagram depicting the steady-state activation (d_∞) and steady-state inactivation (f_∞) relationships
as a function of membrane potential (E_m). The calcium current begins to activate at about −60mV, and is fully activated at about +10mV. The steady state inactivation parameter (f) starts to decrease at about −40 mV, and is fully
inactivated at about 10mV. Note that this graph is for the
steady state (time infinity), and do not take into account the
effect of time on these parameters. Normally, the d parameter will change much faster than the f parameter as a result
of a sudden change of the membrane potential.

current, it can be shown that the channels start to activate around −50 mV, and start to inactivate around
the same potential (Figure 4).

Kinetics of the Calcium Current

Compared to the sodium current of heart muscle, the
calcium current occurs much slower, and was for long
known as the "slow inward current." The time constant of activation ranges between 20 and 50 msec at
membrane potentials of −60 to −40 mV. Inactivation
usually occurs slower, and has a time constant of 60 to
180 msec at −40 mV [23–32].

Experiments with voltage clamping on single, isolated myocytes suggest that the calcium current is
much faster than was previously thought [33–36]. The
activation time constant is around 1 msec at threshold
potential, while the calcium current peaks in 2–3
msec. The inactivation time constant is 5–80 msec.
The discrepancy is attributed to artifacts in multicellular preparations during voltage clamping, where
the high series resistance normally caused by endothelium and extracellular cleft spaces causes a slowing
of the observed transients.

Selectivity of the Calcium Channel

The calcium channel is very selective for calcium ions,
and the selectivity of the calcium channel is governed
by the so-called selectivity filter (see Figure 3).

The reversal potential of any current (E_{rev}) can be determined experimentally, and is usually indicative of the specific selectivity of a channel. Thus, if E_{rev} is equal to the equilibrium potential[1] for any given ion, one can assume that the current under study is only carried by that particular ion. However, if other ions contribute to the current, E_{rev} will be somewhere between the calculated equilibrium potentials for the individual ions. The individual contributions of the different ionic species can be calculated using the constant field equation.

The measurement of the reversal potential for the calcium current (E_{Ca}) is complicated by a number of factors in heart tissue. First, outward currents often develop in the depolarized tissue, which interferes with the measurement of the calcium current. Second, in multicellular preparations, accumulation or depletion of ions occur in the clefts between the cells on strong depolarization of the membrane [37], causing the concentration, and thus the driving force for an ion, to change. Third, blockers of the calcium current are not very specific for the calcium current (see below), and cannot be used to estimate the calcium current.

In spite of these problems, estimations of E_{Ca} range between +33 and +80 mV for an extracellular calcium concentration of about 2 mM [23, 24, 30, 32, 38-40]. These values are far lower than the estimated E_{Ca} of 120 mV [32]. The latter authors assumed that E_{Ca} was so low because other ions (Na^+ and K^+) can pass through the calcium channel, as later confirmed with single-cell voltage clamping [34]. In spite of the seeming "nonselectivity" of the calcium channel for calcium ions, it should be kept in mind that the calcium ion is vastly outnumbered by other cations (both inside the cell and out). In fact, the calcium channel is far more specific for calcium ions than the sodium channel is for sodium ions [41].

Some cations can replace Ca^{2+} as a charge carrier for the calcium current, while others act as a blocker of the flow of calcium ions through the calcium channels. As mentioned previously, Na^+ ions can permeate through the calcium channel, although the permeability ratio is quite low (100:1 for Ca:Na) [32]. Ba^{2+} and Sr^{2+} can both not only replace Ca^{2+}, but are preferred to Ca^{2+} ions [42,43]. Although Mn^{2+} ions are often used as a blocker of the calcium conductance [2,44], Mn^{2+} can also permeate the calcium channels

---

[1]The equilibrium potential of an ion x (E_x) is given by the equation $E_x = RT/zF.\ln ([x]_o/[x]_i)$, where R stands for the gas constant, T the absolute temperature, z the ion valence, and F the Faraday constant. Therefore, at 35°C, $E_{Ca} = 30.5 \log ([Ca]_o/[Ca]_i)$. A value of around +120 mV is predicted for a 10,000-fold concentration gradient.

to a certain extent, so that Mn-dependent action potential can be evoked in the absence of Na^+, Mg^{2+}, and Ca^{2+} [45]. Other cations that can block the calcium current are Ni^{2+}, La^{3+}, Cd^{2+}, and Co^{2+} [44,46]. Li^+ ions, which can pass through the Na^+ channel [47], seem not to act as a charge carrier for the calcium current [48]. Potassium ions can also permeate the calcium channel—especially as an outward current at levels of membrane potential beyond E_{rev} [32,34].

Patch Clamping—Recent Evidence

A new technique in electrophysiology, called patch clamping, allows the study of current flowing through one individual channel at the molecular level [49]. A piece of cell membrane containing the channel under study (the patch) is detached from the rest of the cell by means of a microelectrode. Every time the channel opens and closes, a square pulse of current is observed (Figure 5), also called the *unitary or single channel current*.

The unitary calcium current. The patch clamp technique has also been applied to cardiac muscle in the study of calcium channels [50,51]. Because the unitary calcium current is too small to detect and because barium passes more easily through the calcium channel, these investigators used very high concentration gradients of barium and calcium. The first interesting observation was that the calcium channel opens in bursts (groups of channel openings). The probability of channel opening increased with a depolarization of the membrane (as expected for activation) and decreased as a function of time at any given

Fig. 5. *An example of currents obtained with the patch clamp technique with only one potassium channel in the patch of membrane (Holding potential 0 mV in top trace, −50 mV bottom trace; calibrations are 1 second and 5 pA.) Every time the channel opens, a square pulse of current is observed. The channel opens in a random manner, with the individual channel openings ranging from milliseconds to several seconds. The amplitude of the single channel current is always the same for any given membrane potential, and is referred to as the* unitary channel current. *For the calcium channel, openings are described to occur in groups, or bursts. (JCJ Saunders and LC Isaacson, with permission.)*

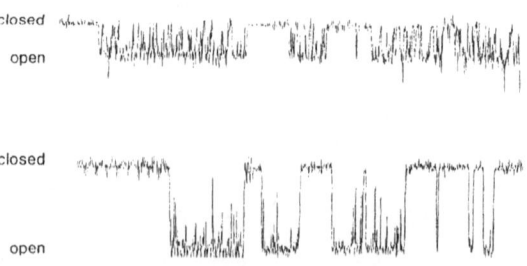

Table 1. Calcium current of cardiac muscle as studied using multicellular and single-cell voltage clamping and with the patch clamping technique

Multicellular voltage clamping

Current	Kinetics	Blockers	Authors
i_{si}	Slow	Various blockers	See text

Single-cell voltage clamping

Current	Kinetics	Blockers	Authors
$i_{Ca,f}$	Fast/large	Cd^{2+}	Lee et al [99, 100]
I_{fast}	Fast/large	Co^{2+}, less by nitrendipine	Bean [98]
$i_{Ca,s}$	Slow/small	Cd^{2+}, no effect	Lee et al [99, 100]
I_{slow}	Slow/small	Co^{2+}, nitrendipine	Bean [98]

Patch Clamping (Nilius et al [52])

Channel	Kinetics	Conductance	Blockers	Selectivity
T-type	Fast	8 pS	Not blocked	Ba = Ca
L-type	Slow	25 pS	Cd^{2+}	Ba > Ca

membrane potential (as expected for inactivation). Neither group was able to detect any clear reversal of current through the calcium channel.

L- and T-type channels. The first reports of the existence of different calcium currents was made for nerve tissue. Recent evidence suggests that there might be more than one type of calcium channel in cardiac tissue [52] (Table 1). The latter authors identified a new calcium channel with a faster kinetics, called the T-type calcium channel. They named the "conventional" calcium channel (as described above) the L-type channel. The first (L-type) channel to be described exhibits quite slow kinetics, is blocked by calcium channel blockers, and has an increased activity with catecholamines. It conducts Ba^{2+} better than Ca^{2+}, and has a single channel conductance of around 25 pS^2 in 100 mM Ba^{2+}. The more recent type of calcium channel to be described (T-type) has much faster kinetics, is not blocked by calcium channel blockers, has equal sensitivity to Ba^{2+} and Ca^{2+}, and has a much smaller single channel conductance of around 8 pS in 100 mM Ba^{2+}. Also, it appears to be activated at much more negative potentials (around -50 mV) than the L-type. Because the T-type channel is so fast, it is thought that it might play a bigger role in pacemaker activity of nodal tissue (and perhaps contribute to the upstroke of the action potential), while the function of the L-type is restricted to maintenance of the action potential plateau.

Factors Affecting the Calcium Current

The calcium current in heart muscle is affected by a variety of factors including ions, neurotransmitters, and blockers.

Beta-Adrenoceptor Neurotransmitters

The function of the heart is continuously modulated by neurotransmitters. Adrenaline, for example, has a positive chronotropic effect (faster heart rate) and a positive inotropic effect (stronger contractions).

Calcium current is increased by beta-adrenoceptor agonists. The finding that adrenaline leads to an increased ^{45}Ca influx in stimulated, but not in quies-

---

[2] The *Siemens* (S) is a unit of measuring conductance, which in turn is the inverse of resistance. One Siemens is equal to 1 V $\times$ 1 A.

cent, heart muscle [53,54] suggested that the calcium current might be increased by adrenaline. Adrenaline leads to an elevated action potential plateau [55] which suggests that an inward plateau current may be increased [9]. Furthermore, action potentials [56] and contractions [57] can be induced by catecholamines in preparations rendered inexcitable by an elevated extracellular potassium concentration. These action potentials are called "slow response" action potentials, and are thought to be caused by the calcium current [56]. Final proof that the calcium current is increased by beta-adrenergic neurotransmitter stimulation came with the voltage clamp technique where it was found that the size of the calcium current increased by adrenaline (Figure 6), while the kinetics remained largely unchanged [9,56,58–60].

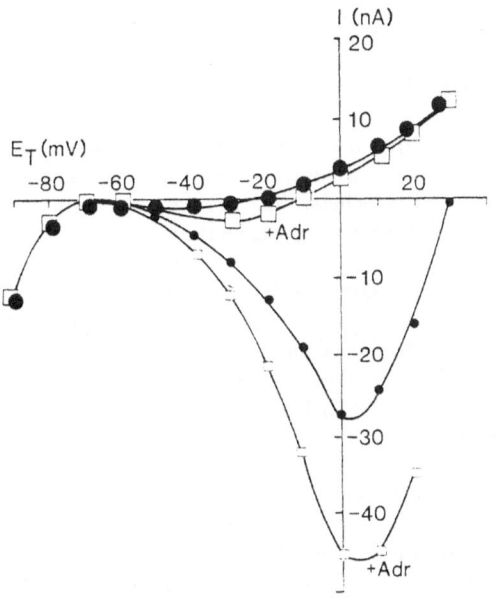

Fig. 6. The effect of adrenaline $(6 \times 10^{-7}M)$ on the current-voltage relation of a rabbit Purkinje fiber where the sodium current was blocked using tetrodotoxin (Coetzee WA: unpublished observations). Rectangular voltage clamp steps with a duration of 1,000 msec were applied from a holding potential of -70 mM to different test potentials (E_T). The currents at the beginning (small symbols) and at the end of the individual clamp steps were plotted as a function of E_T. During control conditions (solid symbols), the current at the beginning of the clamp step became inward for potentials beyond -50 mV, indicative of the activation of the calcium current. At the end of the clamp step, the current was less inward, indicating that the calcium current was inactivated. Adrenaline (open symbols) markedly increased the peak of the calcium current.

Mechanism of the increase in the calcium current. The exact mechanism for the increase in the calcium current by adrenaline [59,60] could occur through four possible mechanisms: 1) An increase in the driving force was largely excluded, since the apparent E_{Ca} remained unchanged. 2) A change in the kinetics of the calcium current was also excluded from the voltage clamp data. 3) A possible increased current through each individual calcium channel, or 4) a possible increase in the total number of open calcium channels, could equally well have led to the increase in maximal calcium conductance found by Reuter [59]. He could not distinguish between these last two possibilities on the basis of the voltage clamp data alone, and the "best guess" at the time was that the number of functional calcium channels was increased. Recent patch clamp experiments show that the catecholamines do indeed lead to an increased opening probability upon depolarization of the membrane, while the single-channel conductance remains unchanged—thus leading to an increased overall calcium current [61].

The effects of beta-adrenoceptor agonists are mediated by intracellular cAMP. The intracellular effects of catecholamines are normally mediated via beta-adrenergic receptors on the outside surface of the cell membrane, and secondary via intracellular cAMP. The same mechanism operates in heart muscle: 1) Catecholamines operate from the outside of the cell membrane as demonstrated by a positive inotropic effect by isoproterenol even when covalently linked to glass beads [62]. 2) The increase of the calcium current by catecholamines is blocked by beta- but unaffected by alpha-adrenoceptor antagonists [56,59,63]. 3) A role for intracellular cAMP is suggested by the ability of phosphodiesterase inhibitors to mimic the effects of catecholamines [56,64], and confirmed by the findings that 4) dBcAMP, a membrane-permeable analog of cAMP, has the same effects on the calcium current as catecholamines [59]. 5) Finally, the injection of cAMP into heart cells [65] or the catalytic, but not the regulatory subunit of cAMP-dependent protein kinase [66] also leads to an increased calcium current. These observations led to the hypothesis, which developed independently in two laboratories [32,59,60,67], that the calcium channel needs to be phosphorylated in order to open.

Cholinergic Modulation of the Calcium Current

The overall effect of vagal stimulation and the application of acetylcholine is a slowing of the heart rate and a negative inotropic effect [68].

The electrophysiologic effects of acetylcholine in atrial tissue are mainly due to an increased potassium conductance, which in turn causes a membrane hyperpolarization and action potential shortening [13,69]. The severe shortening of the action potential might be sufficient to decrease the calcium current in atrial tissue. Nevertheless, a direct inhibitory effect of acetylcholine on the calcium current of atrial muscle is well documented [70–72], and may contribute to the negative inotropic effect of this neurotransmitter. However, recent evidence suggests that this decrease of the calcium current seen with acetylcholine might be purely due to a "masking" effect of an increased potassium conductance [73].

For conducting tissue and for ventricular muscle, the effects of acetylcholine appear to be species-dependent. Acetylcholine causes a lengthening of the action potential duration in sheep Purkinje fibers and cat papillary muscle, does not affect cow Purkinje fibers, and causes a shortening in rabbit Purkinje fibers [74]. In sheep Purkinje fibers, acetylcholine decreases the calcium current [75], but in rabbit Purkinje fibers and frog ventricles, the calcium current is unchanged by acetylcholine [73,76]. However, when the calcium current has been increased by catecholamines, acetylcholine is very effective in reducing this catecholamine-mediated increase in the calcium current [76,77].

The electrophysiologic effects of acetylcholine are probably due to a stimulation of muscarinic, and not nicotinic, receptors. The actions of acetylcholine are blocked by the muscarinic receptor antagonist, atropine, but not by alpha- or beta-adrenoceptor antagonists [78].

Other transmitters that may also affect the calcium current are histamine [79] dopamine and tryptamine [80] and angiotensin II [81].

Calcium Antagonist Drugs (Organic Blockers of the Calcium Current)

We have already seen that the calcium current can be blocked by some other cations than Ca^{2+} (e.g., La, Mn, etc). There are, however, a group of pharmaceutical compounds designed to exert a powerful blocking effect on the calcium current, which are normally referred to as (organic) calcium channel blockers or calcium channel antagonists. These drugs are widely used in the treatment of angina, hypertension, and ischemic or reperfusion arrhythmias [82]. The calcium channel blockers mostly used in cardiovascular disease include verapamil (and related compound D600), diltiazem, and the dihydropyridine group (nifedipine, nisoldipine, nitrendipine, and others).

The action of calcium channel blockers on the calcium current is well characterized. These drugs both block slow response action potentials and the calcium current [83–87]. Voltage clamp data suggest that this decrease is not only due to a decrease in the maximal slope conductance, but also to a slowing by up to seven times of the activation of the calcium current [84]. Such a slowing of activation was not observed in more recent experiments using single cardiac myocytes [88]. None of these drugs are, however, truly specific for the calcium channel, and potassium currents [83] and sodium channels [89] are also affected. Nisoldipine is one of the most selective calcium channel blockers [86].

At the level of the single channel (with patch clamping) the effect of calcium channel blockers is evident as an increased probability that a channel will occur in the closed state, so that the likelihood of channel opening on depolarization of the membrane will be less [90].

The action of calcium channel blockers is dependent on the membrane potential (voltage dependence) and on the rate at which the tissue is stimulated (use dependence). The potency of the blocking effect is increased by depolarization of the membrane and during rapid stimulation [91–94]. At slow heart rates, the blocking effect of nitrendipine will be much more than with D-600 or diltiazem [88].

Different Types of Calcium Currents in the Heart?

Different Cardiac Tissue Types

In the heart, there exist different types of tissue that together ensure general heart function. There does not seem to be large differences in the calcium current when comparing the different myocardial tissue types. The calcium current was studied in atrial muscle [58], ventricular muscle [24,28], conduction tissue [31, 95, 96], and smooth muscle cells [97]. In all cases, the calcium current showed activation and inactivation within roughly the same potential ranges, while the kinetics were comparable.

Macroscopic Calcium Current

The macroscopic calcium current of the heart (irrespective of tissue type) is more complex than it appears at first sight (see Table 1) [18,98]. Using multicellular preparations, chiefly Purkinje fibers, the calcium current was described as occurring much slower than the sodium current, and was therefore called the slow inward current (i_{si}). The calcium current was even more selective for Ba^{2+} than for Ca^{2+} ions. The current could also be blocked by calcium channel blockers. However, several observations complicate this simplistic view. 1) The calcium current of single cell preparations ($i_{Ca,f}$) occurs an order of magnitude faster than its counterpart in multicellular preparations, which might [33] or might not totally [18] be attributable to the high series resistance of the latter preparation. 2) In the presence of tetrodotoxin (a sodium channel blocker) and Cd^{2+} (an inorganic calcium channel blocker) a small inward current still flows, big enough to support a slow response action potential. This residual inward current has a very slow time course, and is inhibited by the further removal of calcium from the bathing solution [99,100]. These observations suggested that the calcium current partly consists of two components. Recently, two kinds of calcium current have been demonstrated in atrial cells [98]. The fast type (I_{fast}) 1) activated at negative potentials (about -50 mV), 2) occurred fast (in the millisecond range), 3) did not discriminate between Ba^{2+} and Ca^{2+} as charge carriers, and 4) was blocked by Co^{2+} and nitrendipine. The slow type (I_{slow}) 1) was activated at about -30 mV, 2) occurred slower, 3) was bigger when Ba^{2+} was the charge carrier, and 4) was less sensitive to nitrendipine. These data are complemented by patch clamp data, where two types of calcium channels were found—the T-type (fast) and L-type slow) channels [50–52,101]. (See Table 1; see "Patch clamping—recent evidence, above). Since I_{slow} has a differential sensitivity to calcium channel blockers than the slow component of the calcium current as described by Lee et al [99,100] there might even be more than two types of calcium current in the heart.

Calcium Current During Myocardial Ischemia

During myocardial ischemia, the blood supply is reduced, and the myocardial tissue suffers from a lack of oxygen and nutrients, while waste products accumulate [102].

There is increasing evidence that cellular damage, and eventual necrosis, is mediated by an excess of intracellular calcium [103–105]. Furthermore, during myocardial ischemia, lethal arrhythmias may develop, which might hypothetically be mediated by the influx of calcium across the cell membrane, or perhaps by an increased intracellular calcium concentration [106,107]. For these reasons, it is important to know how the calcium current is changed during myocardial ischemia. The possible change of the calcium current during myocardial ischemia has never been resolved—mainly because of a lack of an in vitro model of true ischemia [108]. However, it is possible that the calcium current decreases during ischemia, and that the putative increased cytosolic calcium concentration may mainly develop through 1) an enhanced sarcolemmal influx of calcium (e.g., the Na/Ca or a nonspecific "leak"), 2) a reduced sarcolemmal efflux of calcium, or 3) a release of calcium by intracellular organelles. Reasons for a possible decrease in the calcium current during ischemia may include the following:

1. During myocardial ischemia, potassium accumulates in the intercellular spaces and reaches concentrations of almost 15 mM after 15 minutes after the onset of ischemia, with a resulting membrane depolarization to around −50 mV [109]. Theoretically, the effect of such a depolarization is to diminish the calcium current, provided the membrane potential moves into the region where steady-state inactivation of the calcium current occurs. Under these conditions, the T-channel might be affected more than the L-channel.

2. During myocardial ischemia, energy metabolism is inhibited. Metabolic inhibition causes the action potential to shorten, mainly because of an increase in a potassium conductance [110–112]. A decrease of the calcium current, however, has also been reported under these conditions [110,113]. Both these phenomena might explain the decrease of slow response action potentials by metabolic inhibition [114].

3. Another major component of ischemia, namely, intracellular acidosis, might cause the calcium current to decrease during ischemia. A reduced extracellular pH decreases the calcium current [48,115,116], and even abolishes the slow response action potential [114]. Intracellular acidosis, by the injection of protons intracellularly, leads to similar results [117].

There are additional factors that might change the amplitude of the calcium current during ischemia. First, during myocardial ischemia, cAMP rises in the ischemic tissue [118], which should favor the opening probability of the calcium channels (see Factors Affecting the Calcium Current, above), thus theoretically increasing the calcium current during myocardial ischemia. Second, the free energy change of hydrolysis of ATP is reported to decrease during metabolic inhibition [119], which may decrease the calcium current. The dependence of calcium current on ATP is demonstrated by the injection of isolated myocytes by

ATP [120], or intracellular dialysis with ATP [121]. Furthermore, experiments with patch clamping also indicate that the opening of the calcium channel depends on a metabolic substance (perhaps ATP?) at its cytosolic face [51]. If the calcium current is in fact decreased by ischemia, the question arises of whether calcium channel blockers would be effective in preventing ischemic damage and arrhythmias. There is controversy in the literature regarding the efficacy of calcium channel blockers in the prevention of necrosis [122], and ischemic arrhythmias [107]. It is possible that the possible beneficial effects on ischemia by calcium channel blockers are not mediated by a direct effect on the ischemic myocardium, but rather by reducing the severity of ischemia mediated through an increased coronary flow and/or a decreased heart rate [107,123-126].

Conclusion

Various mechanisms exist in the cellular membrane to regulate the concentration of intracellular calcium ions, which in turn play an important role in normal and abnormal cellular function.

Of the various entry and exit pathways for calcium in the cell membrane, the influx of calcium ions through channels in the cell membrane is discussed. The influx of calcium ions will be associated with an electric current, called the calcium current, since there is a displacement of charge.

The calcium current plays an important role in the generation of the plateau of the cardiac action potential, allowing the entry of calcium ions into the cell for contraction to occur. The calcium current is also involved in conduction of impulses and in pacemaker activity of the nodal tissue.

The channel in the membrane that controls the flow of the calcium current 1) is highly selective for calcium ions: 2) has two gates, the so-called activation gate and the inactivation gate; and 3) will only allow calcium ions to pass provided that both gates are in the open position. For these reasons, on a perturbation of the membrane (a stepwise change to more positive potentials) the calcium current rapidly switches on (activation gates opening) before it decreases again as a function of time (because the inactivation gates close).

That the above sequence of events is not merely hypothetical, is illustrated by a recent advance in the field of electrophysiology. With the patch clamp technique, the flow of the calcium current through individual calcium channel can now be measured. There exist two types of calcium channels, a T-type (fast) which plays a role in pacemaker activity and the initiation of the action potential in nodal tissue, and a L-type (slow) which is probably responsible for calcium entry during the plateau of the action potential.

The calcium current is also modulated by neurotransmitters in normal physiologic conditions. Adrenaline, for example, increases the calcium current by increasing the probability of the calcium channel to be in the open state, while acetylcholine decreases the calcium current.

The function of the calcium current during pathologic states of the cardiovascular system, as in ischemic heart disease, remains undefined and is a subject for future work.

The calcium current is affected by other cations (some with a blocking effect, the so-called inorganic calcium channel blockers) and some that can pass through the calcium channel. The calcium current can also be blocked by a group of organic compounds referred to as "calcium channel blockers" or "calcium channel antagonists." These drugs are often used in the management of heart disease and hypertension.

References

1. Hodgkin AL, Huxley AF, Katz B. Measurement of current-voltage relations in the membrane of the giant axon of loligo. *J Physiol* 1952;116:424–448.
2. Fatt P, Ginsborg BL. The ionic requirements for the production of action potentials in crustacean muscle fibers. *J Physiol* 1958;142:516–543.
3. Hoffman BF, Suckling EE. Effect of several cations on transmembrane potentials of cardiac muscle. *Am J Physiol* 1956;186:317–324.
4. Noble D. A modification of the Hodgkin-Huxley equations applicable to Purkinje fiber action and pacemaker potentials. *J Physiol* 1962;160:317–352.
5. Coraboeuf E, Boistel J, Distel R. L'action de la quinidine sur l'activite electrique elementaire du tissu conducteur du coeur de chien. *C R Acad Sci (Paris)* 1956;242:1225–1228.
6. Niedergerke R. Movement of Ca in beating ventricles of the frog. *J Physiol* 1963;167:551–580.
7. Orkand RK, Niedergerke R. The dual effect of calcium on the action potential of the frog's heart. *J Physiol* 1966;184:291–311.
8. Deck KA, Kern R, Trautwein W. Voltage clamp technique in mammalian cardiac fibers. *Pflugers Arch* 1964;280:50–62.

9. Reuter H. The dependence of slow inward current in Purkinje fibers on the extracellular calcium-concentration. *J Physiol* 1967;192:479-492.

10. Brown HF, Clark A, Noble SJ: Identification of the pacemaker currents in frog atrial muscle. *J Physiol* 1976; 258:521-545.

11. Noma A, Irisawa H. A time- and voltage-dependent potassium current in the rabbit sinoatrial node cell. *Pflugers Arch* 1976;366:251-258.

12. DiFrancesco D. A study of the ionic nature of the pacemaker current in calf Purkinje fibers. *J Physiol* 1981; 314:377-393.

13. Noble D. *The Initiation of the Heartbeat.* Oxford University Press, Oxford, 1975.

14. Weidmann S: Effect of current flow on the membrane potential of cardiac muscle. *J Physiol* 1951;115:227-236.

15. McAllister RE, Noble D, Tsien RW. Reconstruction of electrical activity of cardiac Purkinje fibers. *J Physiol* 1975; 251:1-59.

16. Attwell D, Cohen I, Eisner D, et al. The steady-state TTX sensitive ("window") sodium current in cardiac Purkinje fibers. *Pflugers Arch* 1979;379:137-142.

17. Carmeliet E. Slow inactivation of the sodium current in rabbit cardiac Purkinje fibers. *Pflugers Arch* 1987;408:18-26.

18. Noble D. The surprising heart: A Review of recent progress in cardiac electrophysiology. *J Physiol* 1984;353:1-50.

19. Beeler GW, Reuter H: The relation between membrane potential, membrane currents and activation of contraction in ventricular myocardial fibers. *J Physiol* 1970;207:211-220.

20. Allen DG, Blinks JR: Calcium transients in aequorin-injected frog cardiac muscle. *Nature* 1978;273:509-513.

21. Wier WG, Isenberg G: Intracellular [Ca^{2+}] transients in voltage clamped cardiac Purkinje fibers. *Pflugers Arch* 1982,392:284-290.

22. Fabiato A. Calcium-induced release of calcium from the cardiac sarcoplasmic reticulum. *Am J Physiol* 1983;245:C1-C14.

23. Beeler GW, Reuter H, Membrane calcium current in ventricular myocardial fibers. *J Physiol* 1970;207:191-209.

24. New W, Trautwein W. The ionic nature of slow inward current and its relation to contraction. *Pflugers Arch* 1972;334:24-38.

25. Reuter H. Divalent cations as charge in excitable membranes. *Prog Biophys Mol Biol* 1973;26:1-43.

26. Reuter H. Time- and voltage-dependent contractile responses in mammalian cardiac muscle. *Eur J Cardiol* 1973;1/2:177-181.

27. Gettes LS, Reuter H. Slow recovery from inactivation of inward currents in mammalian myocardial fibers. *J Physiol* 1974;240:703-724.

28. Kohlhardt M, Krause H, Kuebler M, Herdey A. Kinetics of inactivation and recovery of the slow inward current in the mammalian ventricular myocardium. *Pflugers Arch* 1975; 355:1-17.

29. Trautwein W, McDonald TF, Tripathi O. Calcium conductance and tension in mammalian ventricular muscle. *Pflugers Arch* 1975;354:55-74.

30. McDonald TC, Trautwein W. Membrane currents in cat myocardium: Separation of inward and outward components. *J Physiol* 1978;274:193-216.

31. Isenberg G. Cardiac Purkinje fibers. The slow inward

current component under the influence of modified $[Ca^{2+}]_i$. *Pflugers Arch* 1977;371:61-69.

32. Reuter H, Scholtz H. A study of the ion selectivity and the kinetic properties of the calcium dependent slow inward current in mammalian cardiac muscle. *J Physiol* 1977; 264:17-47.

33. Isenberg G, Klockner U. Calcium currents of isolated bovine ventricular myocytes are fast and of large amplitude. *Pflugers Arch* 1982;395:30-41.

34. Lee KS, Tsien RW. Reversal of current through calcium channels in dialysed single heart cells. *Nature* 1982;297: 484-501.

35. Hume JR, Giles WR: Ionic currents in single isolated bullfrog atrial cells. *J Gen Physiol* 1983;81:153-194.

36. Mitchell MR, Powell T, Terrar DA, Twist VW. Characteristics of the second inward current in cells isolated from rat ventricular muscle. *Proc R Soc Lond B* 1983;219:447-469.

37. Baumgarten CM, Isenberg G. Depletion and accumulation of potassium in the extracellular clefts of cardiac Purkinje fibers during voltage clamp hyperpolarization and depolarization. *Pflugers Arch* 1977;368:19-31.

38. Ochi R. The slow inward current and the action of manganese ions in guinea pig's myocardium. *Arch Gen Physiol* 1970;316:81-94.

39. Bassingthwaighte JB, Reuter H. Calcium movements and excitation-contraction coupling in cardiac cells. In: *Electrical Phenomena in the Heart. In:* de Mello WC, ed. New York: Academic Press, 1972;353-395.

40. Kohlhardt M, Bauer B, Krause H, Fleckenstein A. Selective inhibition of the transmembrane Ca conductivity of mammalian fibers by Ni, Co and Mn ions. *Pflugers Arch* 1973;339:115-123.

41. Hess P, Tsien RW. Mechanism of ion permeation through calcium channels. *Nature* 1984;309:453-456.

42. Vereecke J, Carmeliet E. Sr action potentials in cardiac Purkinje fibers. I. Evidence for a regenerative increase in Sr conductance. *Pflugers Arch* 1971;322:60-72.

43. Kohlhardt M, Herdey A, Kubler M. Interchangeability of Ca ions and Sr ions as charge carriers of the slow inward current in mammalian myocardial fibers. *Pflugers Arch* 1973;344:149-158.

44. Rougier O, Vassort G, Garnier Y, et al. Existence and role of a slow inward current during the frog atrial action potential. *Pflugers Arch* 1969;308:91-110.

45. Ochi R. Manganese-dependent propagated action potentials and their depression by electrical stimulation in guinea pig myocardium perfused by sodium-free media. *J Physiol* 1976;263:139-156.

46. Kiltzner T, Morad M. The effects of Ni^{2+} on ionic currents and tension generation in frog ventricular muscle. *Pflugers Arch* 1983;398:267-273.

47. Carmeliet E. Influence of lithium ions on the transmembrane potential and cation content of cardiac cells. *J Gen Physiol* 1964;47:501-530.

48. Chesnais JM, Coraboeuf E, Sauviat MP, Vassas JM: Sensitivity to H, Li, and Mg ions of the slow inward current in frog atrial fibers. *J Mol Cell Cardiol* 1975;7:627-642.

49. Hamill OP, Marty A, Neher E, et al. Improved patch-clamp techniques for high-resolution current recording from cells and cell-free membrane patches. *Pflugers Arch* 1981;391:85-100.

50. Reuter H, Stevens CF, Tsien RW, Yellen G. Properties of

single calcium channels in cardiac cell culture. *Nature* 1982;297:501-504.

51. Cavalie A, Ochi R, Pelzer D, Trautwein W. Elementary currents through Ca^{2+} channels in guinea pig myocytes. *Pflugers Arch* 1983;398:284-297.

51a. Carbone E, Lux HD. A low voltage-activated, fully inactivating Ca channel in vertebrate sensory neurons. *Nature*, 1984;310:501-502.

52. Nilius B, Hess P, Lansman JB, Tsien RW. A novel type of cardiac calcium channel in ventricular cells. *Nature* 1985; 316:443-446.

53. Reuter H. Uber die Wirkung von adrenalin auf den cellulairen Ca-umsatz des meerschweinchenvorhofs. *Naunyn Schmiedeberg's Arch Exp Pathol Pharmakol* 1965;251: 401-412.

54. Meinertz T, Nawrath H, Scholtz H. Stimulatory effects of dB-cAMP and adrenaline on myocardial contraction and ^{45}Ca exchange. Experiments at reduced calcium concentration and low frequencies of stimulation. *Naunyn Schmiedeberg's Arch Exp Pathol Pharmakol* 1973;279: 327-338.

55. Otsuka M. Die wirkung van adrenalin auf Purkinje-fasern von Saugetierherzen. *Pflugers Arch* 1958;266:512-517.

56. Carmeliet E, Vereecke J. Adrenaline and the plateau phase of the cardiac action potential. *Pflugers Arch* 1969;313: 300-315.

57. Ingebretzen WR, Friedman WF, Mayer SE: Isoproterenol-induced restoration of contraction in K^+-depolarized hearts: relationship to cAMP. *Am J Physiol* 1981;24:H187-H193.

58. Vassort G, Rougier O, Garnier D, et al. Effects of adrenaline on membrane inward currents during the cardiac action potential. *Pflugers Arch* 1969;309:70-81.

59. Reuter H. Localization of beta adrenergic receptors, and effects of noradrenaline and cyclic nucleotides on action potentials, ionic currents and tension in mammalian cardiac muscle. *J Physiol* 1974;242:429-451.

60. Reuter H, Scholtz H. The regulation of the calcium conductance of cardiac muscle by adrenaline. *J Physiol* 1977; 264:49-62.

61. Brum G, Osterreider W, Trautwein W. β-Adrenergic increase in the calcium conductance of cardiac myocytes studied with the patch clamp. *Pflugers Arch* 1984;401:111-118.

62. Ingebretzen WR, Becker E, Friedman WF, Mayer SE. Contractile and biochemical responses of cardiac and skeletal muscle to isoproterenol covalently linked to glass beads. *Circ Res* 1977;40:474-484.

63. Giotti A, Ledda F, Mannaioni PF: Effects of noradrenaline and isoprenaline, in combination with α- and β-receptor blocking substances, on the action potential of cardiac Purkinje fibers. *J Physiol* 1973;229:99-113.

64. Watanabe AM, Besch HR: Cyclic adenosine monophosphate modulation of slow calcium influx channels in guinea pig hearts. *Circ Res* 1974;35:316-324.

65. Trautwein W, Tanigtuchi J, Noma A. The effect of intracellular cyclic nucleotides and calcium on the action potential and acetylcholine response of isolated cardiac cells. *Pflugers Arch* 1982;392:307-314.

66. Osterrieder W, Brum G, Hescheler J, Trautwein W. Injection of subunits of cyclic AMP-dependent protein kinase into cardiac myocytes modulates Ca^{2+} current. *Nature* 1982;298:576-578.

67. Sperelakis N, Schneider J: A metabolic control mechanism for calcium ion influx that may protect the ventricular myocardial cell. *Am J Cardiol* 1976;37:1079-1085.

68. Hutter OF: Mode of action of autonomic transmitters on the heart. *Br Med Bull* 1957;13:176-180.

69. Hoffman BF, Cranefield PF. *Electrophysiology of the heart.* New York: McGraw-Hill, 1960.

70. Giles W, Noble S. Changed in membrane currents in bullfrog atrium produced by acetylcholine. *J Physiol* 1976; 261:103-123.

71. Ten Eick R, Nawrath H, McDonald TF, Trautwein W. On the mechanism of the negative inotropic effect of acetylcholine. *Pflugers Arch* 1976;361:207-213.

72. Nargeot J, Garnier D. The action of muscarinic agents and antagonistic drugs on frog atrial fibers. *J Pharmacol* 1982; 13:431-445.

73. Hartzell HC, Simmons MA. Comparison of the effects of acetylcholine on calcium and potassium currents in frog atrium and ventricle. *J Physiol* 1987;389:411-422.

74. Carmeliet E, Ramon J. Electrophysiological effects of acetylcholine in sheep cardiac Purkinje fibers. *Pflugers Arch* 1980;387:197-205.

75. Carmeliet E, Ramon J: Effect of acetylcholine on time-dependent currents in sheep cardiac Purkinje fibers. *Pflugers Arch* 1980;387:217-223.

76. Carmeliet E, Mubagwa K. Changes by acetylcholine of membrane currents in rabbit cardiac Purkinje fibers. *J Physiol* 1986;371:201-217.

77. Fishmeister R, Hertzell HC. Mechanism of action of acetylcholine on calcium current in single cells from frog ventricle. *J Physiol* 1986;376:183-202.

78. Mubagwa K, Carmeliet E. Electrophysiological effects of acetylcholine on rabbit cardiac Purkinje fibers. *Arch Int Pharmacol Ther* 1981;249:326.

79. Ledda F, Mantelli L, Mugelli A. Blockade of burimaride of the restorative effect of histamine in tetrodotoxin-treated heart preparations. *Br J Pharmacacol* 1976;57:247-249.

80. Ouedraogo CO, Garnier D, Nargeot J, Pourrias B. Electrophysiological and pharmacological study of the inotropic effects of adrenaline, dopamine and tryptamine on frog atrial fibers. *J Mol Cell Cardiol* 1982;14:111-121.

81. Allen DG, Cohen NM, Dhallan RD, Rogers TB. Angiotensin II increases the calcium current in neonatal rat single cardiac myocytes. *Proc Physiol Soc* 1987;C49.

82. Opie LH. Calcium, calcium ions, and cardiovascular disease. In: *Calcium antagonists and cardiovasuclar* Disease. Opie LH, ed. New York: Raven Press, 1984:1-8.

83. Kass RS, Tsien RW. Multiple effects of calcium antagonists on plateau currents in cardiac Purkinje fibers. *J Gen Physiol* 1975;66:169-192.

84. Nawrath H, Ten Eick RE, McDonald TF, Trautwein W. On the mechanism underlying the action of D-600 on slow inward current and tension in mammalian myocardium. *Circ Res* 1977;40:408-414.

85. Fleckenstein A. Specific pharmacology of in myoardium, cardiac pacemakers, and vascular smooth muscle. *Ann Rev Pharmacol Toxicol* 1977;17:149-166.

86. Kass RS. Nisoldipine. A new, more selective calcium current blocker in cardiac Purkinje fibers. *J Pharmacol Exp Ther* 1982;223:446-456.

87. Kanaya S, Katzung BG. Effects of diltiazem on transmembrane potential and current of right ventricular papillary muscle of ferrets. *J Pharmacol Exp Ther* 1984;228:245-251.

88. Lee KS, Tsien RW. Mechanism of calcium channel blockade by verapamil, D600, diltiazem and nitrendipine in single dialysed heart cells. *Nature* 1983;302:790-794.

89. Bayer R, Kalusche D, Kaufmann R, Mannhold R. Inotropic and electrophysiological actions of verapamil and D-600 in mammalian myocardium. II. effects of optical isomers on transmembrane action potentials. *Naunyn-Schmiedeberg's Arch Pharmacol* 1975;290:81-97.

90. Tsien RW, Hess P, Lansman JB, Lee KS. Current views of calcium channels and their response to calcium antagonists and agonists. In: Zipes DP, Jalife J, eds. *Cardiac Electrophysiology and Arrhythmias.* New York: Grune & Stratton, 1985, 19-29.

91. Ehara T, Kaufmann R. The voltage- and time-dependent effects of (−)-verapamil on the slow inward current in isolated cat ventricular myocardium. *J Pharmacol Exp Ther* 1978;207:49-55.

92. McDonald TF, Pelzer D, Trautwein W. On the mechanism of slow calcium channel block in the heart. *Pflugers Arch* 1980;385:175-179.

93. Trautwein W, Pelzer D, McDonald TF, Osterrieder W. AQA 39, a new bradycardiac agent which blocks myocardial calcium (Ca) channels in a frequency- and voltage-dependent manner. *Naunyn Schmiedeberg's Arch Pharmacol* 1981;317:228-232.

94. Osterrieder W, Pelzer D, Yang Q-F, Trautwein W. The electrophysiologic basis of the bradycardic action of AQA 39 on the sinoatrial node. *Naunyn Schmiedeberg's Arch Pharmacol* 1981;317:233-237.

95. Vitek M, Trautwein W. Slow inward current and action potential in cardiac Purkinje fibers. *Pflugers Arch* 1971; 323:204-218.

96. Gibbons WR, Fozzard HA. Slow inward current and contraction of sheep cardiac Purkinje fibers. *J Gen Physiol* 1975;65:367-384.

97. Droogmans G, Callewaert G. Ca^{2+}-channel current and its modification by the dihydropyridine agonist BAY k 8644 in isolated smooth muscle cells. *Pflugers Arch* 1986;406:259-265.

98. Bean BP. Two kinds of calcium channels in canine atrial cells. Differences in kinetics, selectivity, and pharmacology. *J Gen Physiol* 1985. 86:1-30.

99. Lee E, Lee KS, Noble D, Spindler AJ. A new, very slow inward Ca current in single ventricular cells of adult guinea pig. *J Physiol* 1984;346:75P.

100. Lee E, Lee KS, Noble D, Spindler AJ. Further properties of the very slow inward currents in isolated single guinea pig ventricular cells. *J Physiol* 1984;349:48P.

101. Cavalie A, Pelzer D, Trautwein W. Fast and slow gating behavior of single calcium channels in cardiac cells. Relation to activation and inactivation of calcium-channel current. *Pflugers Arch* 1986;406:241-258.

102. Opie LH. Effects of regional ischemia on metabolism of glucose and fatty acids. Relative rates of aerobic and anaerobic energy production during myocaridal infarction and comparison with effects of anoxia. *Circ Res* 1976; 38:(Suppl 1):I52-74.

103. Hearse DJ, Garlick PB, Humphrey SM. Ischemic contracture by the myocardium: mechanisms and prevention. *Am J Cardiol* 1977.39:986-993.

104. Katz AM, Tada M. The "stone heart": A challenge to the biochemist. *Am J Cardiol* 1972;29:578-580.

105. Shen AC, Jennings RB. Kinetics of calcium accumulation

in acute myocardial ischemic injury. *Am J Pathol* 1972; 67:441-452.

106. Clusin WT, Bristow MR, Baim DS, et al. The effects of diltiazem and reduced serum ionized calcium on ischemic ventricular fibrillation in the dog. *Circ Res* 1982;50:518-526.

107. Coetzee WA, Dennis SC, Opie LH, Muller CA. Calcium channel blockers and early ischemic ventricular arrhythmias: Electrophysiological versus anti-ischemic effects. *J Mol Cell Cardiol* 1987;19(Suppl 2):77-97.

108. Carmeliet E. Cardiac transmembrane potentials and metabolism. *Circ Res* 1978;42:577-587.

109. Kleber AG. Resting membrane potential, extracellular potassium activity, and intracellular sodium activity during acute global ischemia in isolated perfused guinea-pig hearts. *Circ Res* 1983.52:442-450.

110. Isenberg G, Vereecke J, van der Heyden G, Carmeliet E. The shortening of the action potential by DNP in guinea-pig ventricular myocytes is mediated by an increase of a time-independent K conductance. *Pflugers Arch* 1983; 397:251-259.

111. Noma A, Shibasaki T. Membrane current through adenosine-triphosphate-regulated potassium channels in guinea-pig ventricular cells. *J Physiol* 1985;363:463-480.

112. Kakei M, Noma A, Shibasaki T. Properties of adenosine-triphosphate-regulated potassium channels in guinea-pig ventricular cells. *J Physiol* 1985;363:441-462.

113. McDonald TF, MacLeod DP. Metabolism and the electrical activity of anoxic ventricular muscle. *J Physiol* 1973; 229:559-582.

114. Schneider JA, Sperelakis N. The demonstration of energy dependence of the isoproterenol-induced transcellular Ca^{2+} current in isolated perfused guinea-pig hearts. An explanation for mechanical failure of ischemic myocardium. *J Surg Res* 1974;16:389-403.

115. Kohlhardt M, Haap K, Figulla HR. Influence of low extracellular pH upon the Ca inward current and isometric contractile force in mammalian ventricular myocardium. *Pflugers Arch* 1976;366:31-38.

116. Vogel S, Sperelakis N. Blockade of myocardial slow inward current at low pH. *Am J Physiol* 1977;233:C99-C103.

117. Kurachi Y. The effects of intracellular protons on electrical activity of single ventricular cells. *Pflugers Arch* 1982; 394:264-270.

118. Podzuweit T, Dalby AJ, Cherry GW, Opie LH. Cyclic AMP levels in ischemic and non-ischemic myocardium following coronary artery ligation: Relation to ventricular fibrillation. *J Mol Cell Cardiol* 1978;10:81-94.

119. Allen DG, Morris PG, Orchard CH, Pirolo JS. A nuclear magnetic resonance study of metabolism in the ferret heart during hypoxia and inhibition of glycolysis. *J Physiol* 1985;361:185-204.

120. Taniguchi J, Noma A, Irisawa H. Modification of the cardiac action potential by intracellular injection of adenosine triphosphate and related substances in guinea pig single ventricular cells. *Circ Res* 1983;53:131-139.

121. Irisawa H, Kokubun S. Modulation by intracellular ATP and cyclic AMP of the slow inward current in isolated single ventricular cells of the guinea pig. *J Physiol* 1983; 338:321-337.

122. De Leiris J, Richard V, Pestre S. Calcium antagonists and experimental myocardial ischemia and infarction. In: Opie LH, ed. *Calcium antagonists and Cardiovascular Disease.* New York: Raven Press, 1984, 105-115.

123. Tosaki A, Szekeres L, Hearse DJ. Diltiazem and the reduction of reperfusion-induced arrhythmias in the rat: Protection in secondary to modification of ischemic injury and heart rate. *J Mol Cell Cardiol* 1987;19:441-451.
124. Beeler GW, Reuter H. Voltage clamp experiments on ventricular myocardial fibers. *J Physiol* 1970;207:165-190.
125. Carbone E, Lux HD. A low voltage-activated, fully inactivating Ca channel in vertebrate sensory neurones. *Nature* 310:501-502.
126. Kleber AG, Janse MJ, Wilms-Schopmann FJG, et al. Changes in conduction velocity during acute ischemia in ventricular myocardium of the isolated porcine heart. *Circulation* 1986;73:189-198.

CALCIUM CHANNEL ANTAGONISTS: PART I: FUNDAMENTAL PROPERTIES: MECHANISMS, CLASSIFICATION, SITES OF ACTION

SUMMARY. Ca^{2+} channel antagonists are agents that interact with the voltage-dependent Ca^{2+} channel in a highly specific way. The prototype agents of cardiovascular importance are verapamil, nifedipine, and diltiazem, in historical order of appearance. These agents all have different molecular structures and bind separately with receptor sites located in or near the calcium channel, at molecular sites still to be fully identified. There are probably three distinct receptor sites (V, N, D) which stand in relation to the "gate" of the long-acting "L" calcium channel. There is probably overlap among the receptor sites, especially between the V and D sites to explain their common properties. All three agents inhibit the voltage-dependent calcium channel in vascular smooth muscle and also myocardial slow calcium channels. The ratio of the arterial to the myocardial effect is an index of the arterial selectivity, generally held to be a desirable property because the negative inotropic effect is usually a liability. The general clinical impression that nifedipine is the agent most active in vascular tissue in relation to the myocardial effect is supported by data on the relative potencies of these three agents on blood perfused dog preparations and by a comparison of the potency on rat vascular (portal vein) versus myocardial effects. Nonetheless all three agents are highly active in the inhibition of K^+-induced vascular contractions (nifedipine 10^{-9} M to 10^{-8} M; verapamil 10^{-7} M to 10^{-6} M; and diltiazem 5×10^{-7} M to 10^{-6} M; concentrations for 50% inhibition of K^+-induced vascular contractions in rat or rabbit aorta; comparative data for resistance vessels not available). The clinical impression that verapamil and diltiazem are more active on nodal tissue is also supported by a comparison of potencies on blood perfused dog nodal preparations in comparison with effects on coronary flow, with verapamil and diltiazem being approximately 10× more potent on the AV node than increasing coronary blood flow, so that the nodal effect is first detected. These basic pharmacological properties explain why all these three agents have clinical effects relevant to inhibition of vascular contraction (antihypertensive and antianginal effects) and only verapamil and diltiazem have clinically relevant inhibitory effects on the AV node (inhibition of supraventricular tachycardias).

Mechanisms of Action of Calcium Antagonists

Possible sites of calcium modulation

Calcium ions are concerned with a variety of important cardiovascular functions, including the regulation of the inotropic state of the myocardium, generation of impulses in the sinus and the AV nodes, and regulation of the tone of vascular smooth muscle including coronary arteries and peripheral resistance arterioles. The action of calcium antagonists in opposing the myocardial effects of calcium was emphasized by Fleckenstein [1,2]. *Calcium channel antagonists* specifically regulate the voltage-dependent entry of calcium ions into a variety of tissues of which the most important from the cardiovascular point of view are the myocardium, nodal tissues, and vascular smooth muscle. Alternate names (Table I-1) for calcium antagonists are calcium channel blockers, or slow channel blockers, or calcium entry inhibitors. To be a member of the calcium channel antagonist class of compounds, a drug must block the slow calcium channel by a direct action on the cell membrane channel itself (and not indirectly via metabolic depression or acidosis, for example), and this action must be relatively specific for the voltage-dependent calcium channel in contrast to other types of voltage-dependent ion channels (eg. fast Na^+ channel or delayed rectifier K^+ channel) [3].

Calcium modulation and intracellular calcium regulators. Strictly speaking, calcium antagonists are part of a larger group of agents, the *calcium modulators,* which include the intracellular calcium regulators (next section), and also the *calcium facilitators* such as the calcium channel agonists which enhance calcium entry through the calcium channel (for overall classification, see [4]).

Work on intracellular calcium regulators is still in its infancy. Ryanodine, an insecticide, is the prototype of such agents acting on the sarcoplasmic reticulum. Ryanodine inhibits calcium ion flux across the sarcoplasmic reticulum and is thought to have antiarrhythmic properties. Other agents acting on calcium ion flux in and out of the sarcoplasmic reticulum are caffeine and local anesthetics such as procaine. *Calmodulin regulators* are also at an early stage of description, so that there are few absolute specific compounds available at present. Interaction with calmodulin may be a nonspecific effect of certain dihydropyridines such as felodipine. Therefore from the practical point of view, calcium antagonists remain the only pharmacological agents capable of regulation of calcium ion movements acting on the calcium current.

Indirect regulation by beta-adrenergic receptor blockers. Beta-adrenergic antagonists are profound indirect regulators of intracellular calcium ion movements, and act to decrease the rate of contraction (less

Ca^{2+} entry because less phosphorylation of the calcium channel protein), the rate of relaxation (effects on uptake of calcium by sarcoplasmic reticulum and on troponin) and the peak force of contraction (lower peak intracellular Ca^{2+} concentration). The molecular differences between the sites of action of beta-blockers and calcium antagonists are considered in a later section.

Blood levels versus therapeutic effects. This review will frequently refer to the pharmacological effects of various concentrations of calcium antagonists. Therefore it is important to bear in mind the unbound circulating concentrations thought to occur in humans at therapeutic doses of these agents (Table I-1).

Sarcolemmal binding sites for calcium antagonists

It must first be stressed that each of the major calcium antagonists of cardiovascular interest, namely verapamil, nifedipine, and diltiazem, has an entirely different molecular structure. It is therefore logical that they should bind differently to the sarcolemma. One of the early models was that of Murphy et al. [5] the so-called "unitary model" in which the dihydropyridine site was allosterically acted upon by the secondary verapamil-diltiazem site. As more experience was gained, the concept of three separate sites took hold with, however, allowance for some degree of overlap between the sites (Figure I-1).

Now workers recognize at least three and probably four distinct molecular binding sites for the following types of agents: dihydropyridines such as nifedipine,

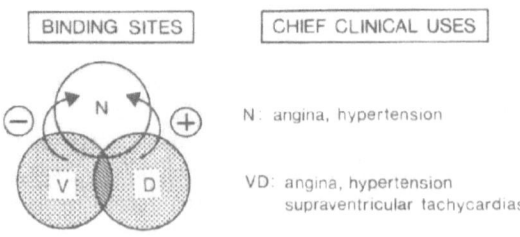

Fig. I-1. A cartoon model of the proposed interaction between the verapamil (V), nifedipine (N), and diltiazem (D) receptor sites. Diltiazem facilitates binding at the N site while verapamil inhibits such binding. From International Society and Federation of Cardiology Working Group [121].

verapamil, diltiazem, and diphenylalkylamines such as flunarizine [6-10]. Of these the sites for dihydropyridines, verapamil and diltiazem are of cardiovascular importance. Currently it seems that the three site model with more verapamil-diltiazem overlap than V-N or D-N overlap is closest to clinical reality. This issue will, however, be settled by physico-clinical studies currently under way.

The dihydropyridine site. Nifedipine and all other dihydropyridines (DHP) bind in a highly specific way to the DHP site, previously thought to be the unitary site of action of calcium antagonists because both verapamil and diltiazem also interact with it [5]. The DHP site should identify the binding of nifedipine, but for technical reasons other DHPs such as radiolabelled nitrendipine or nimodipine are usually used. The dihydropyridine site may be near the calcium channel or part of it; it must interact with the calcium channel because a new group of dihydropyridines have a positive, not negative, inotropic effect [11].

The verapamil site. Verapamil binds to another spatially separated ("allosteric") site, possibly nearer to the "inner mouth" of the calcium channel, less specifically to inhibit labelled-DHP binding in a complex biphasic way [6].

The diltiazem site. Diltiazem interacts with a third site, also allosterically linked to the DHP site, yet interacting in an opposite way to verapamil so that labelled-DHP binding is enhanced.

Table I-1. Alternate names for calcium antagonists*

Name Proposed	Point of Emphasis
Ca^{2+}-antagonist	Original observations by Fleckenstein: reversal by external Ca^{2+} of verapamil-induced cardiodepressant effect.
Ca^{2+}-channel antagonist (or inhibitor or blocker)	Selective inhibition by these agents of the Ca^{2+}-dependent component of the cardiac action potential
Ca^{2+}-entry antagonist (or blocker)	Allows for inhibition of calcium entry by channels not operated by depolarization
Slow channel antagonist (or inhibitor or blocker)	Slow inward calcium channel also carries Na^+ ions in some experimental conditions (although 100:1 preference for Ca^{2+})

*Modified from Opie [120].

Are verapamil and diltiazem really different? Recent studies emphasize differences between the verapamil and diltiazem binding sites [4,9,10]. Verapamil and diltiazem also have different effects on 5-HT$_2$ (5-HT = 5-hydroxytryptamine = serotonin) receptors with only verapamil interacting with these receptors [12]. Clinically, the overlap in indications and contraindications between verapamil and diltiazem is significant, and both agents are clearly separate from nifedipine and the other DHPs [13]. Only verapamil and diltiazem are of therapeutic use in supraventricular tachycardias, stressing their greater effect on the AV-node than in the case of nifedipine. Electrophysiologically, the explanation may be that verapamil and diltiazem are "use-dependent" (see next section: Voltage and frequency-dependent block).

Projected model for calcium channel

The concentration of calcium in the extracellular fluid is about 1,000× higher than in the cytosol. The properties of the lipid bilayer are such that there is a low rate of calcium ion penetration from without to within the cardiac cells. A higher rate of entry of calcium ions is partially or chiefly regulated by the properties of the calcium channel. In drawing up a provisional model of this channel, reliance has been placed on the more established modulated receptor hypothesis of Hondeghem and Katzung [14] for the sodium channel; the latter has both "activation" and "inactivation" gates [15]. A similar type of model for the calcium channel is now being proposed (Figure I-2). "The concept that dihydropyridines act by sterically plugging the channel is being modified in favor of a model in which binding of the dihydropyridine stabilizes the channel in a mode in which no openings occur" [16]. An important point is that calcium channel blockers preferentially block channels which have already been inactivated, for example, by ischemia [17], thereby changing the "state" of the channel [18]. Binding to inactivated channels is about 1,000× higher than to resting channels [19]. Some of the properties of calcium channels have been reviewed and are as follows [3,20].

Biochemical composition. Calcium channels are usually isolated from the T-tubules of skeletal muscle where calcium channels are abundant (and apparently have no known function). It is presumed on some experimental basis that these skeletal muscle calcium channels are the same as those of cardiac and vascular smooth muscles. The protein of each calcium channel has three polypeptide subunits, alpha,β and gamma with a total molecular weight of about 220,000 [18];

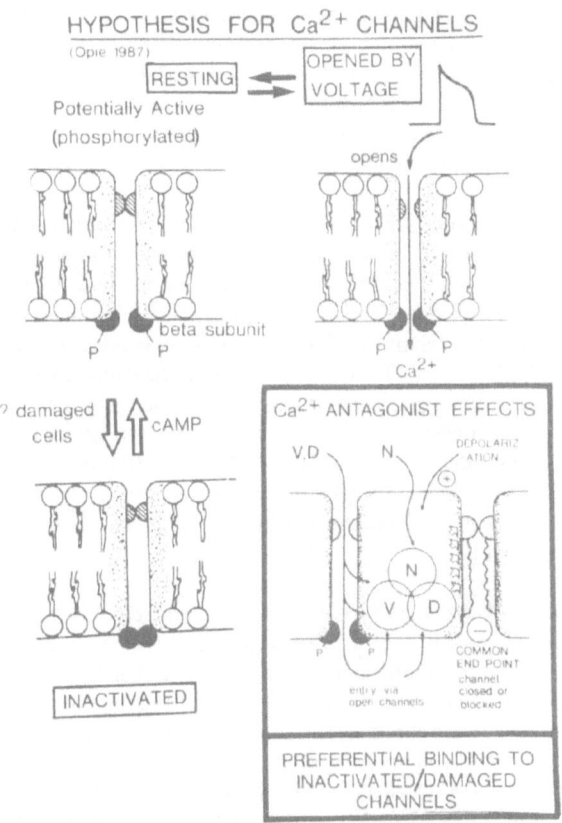

Fig. I-2. Cartoon model of calcium channel, based on concepts of International Society and Federation of Cardiology Working Group [121], Spedding [8], Glossmann et al. [7], Sperelakis [3], and Sanguinetti and Kass [19].

other estimates are of similar magnitude. The large alpha subunit (molecular weight about 150,000–160,000) is the site of DHP binding [21,22].

Calcium channel subdivision: L and T types. Recently a distinction has been made among the L, T, and N channels [23–25]. The L (long-lasting) channels have two modes of gating, mode 1 with short openings and mode 2 with long openings. Calcium antagonists change the opening mode of the L channels to a preponderance of short rather than long-acting channels, and also switch to long-lived closed states (mode 0; [24]). The T (transient) channels have short bursts of openings and do not interact with calcium antagonists. The T channels "open" at a lower voltage so that T channel activity presumably accounts for the earlier phases of spontaneous depolarization of the sinoatrial node, and L channel activity for later phases. The N (nervous) channels found in the neurotransmitter junctions of terminal neurons have properties in between those of the L and T channels [26], and are insensitive to calcium antagonists. The exact significance of these different types of calcium channels still needs clarification but is clearly going to be important.

Studies with the "voltage-patch" technique have shown that the calcium channel opens in bursts [27]. First the T and then the L channels open during progressive depolarization [23]; likewise T channels close before L channels. The probability of combined channel opening (T and L) increases as the transsarcolemmal voltage becomes more positive than -50 mV, and then decreases with further depolarization as the driving force decreases [27]. The inactivation of the voltage-dependent calcium inflow depends both on the voltage and on the internal calcium ion concentration [28].

Voltage and frequency-dependent block. Calcium channel antagonist drugs can reach the channel-associated receptor in one of two ways: either through the open channel or through the bilipid membrane to reach the channel [19]. In the case of verapamil, which is in the charged form at pH 7.4, lipid penetration is low so that entry is via the open state—this sequence explains why verapamil is "frequency-dependent" (or "use-dependent"). Similar arguments presumably hold for diltiazem. Once these agents have interacted with the channel-associated receptor, the channel becomes inactivated by the drug. Verapamil fails to interact markedly with the calcium channels even when they are depolarized to -45 mV, unless there is added positive passing to voltages above this level [19]. Dihydropyridines (nisoldipine, nitrendipine, nifedipine, etc.) interact with the calcium channel at similar voltages without added pulsing because they are lipophilic and capable of reaching the channel-associated receptor by penetration of the lipid bilayer [19]. The dihydropyridines interact preferentially with the inactivated state of the calcium channel. Nicardipine, being more water soluble than nifedipine, is more likely to have a use-dependent component with entry via the calcium channel in the open state [19].

Voltage and binding. Whether depolarization directly alters DHP binding is controversial. Green et al. [16] found an increased receptor density during K^+-induced depolarization without changes in the binding constant. Kokubun et al. [29] found an increased binding affinity of depolarized cultured neonatal rat heart cells during depolarization. More data are awaited.

Sodium and potassium ions. External sodium and calcium ions [30] are required for calcium channels to "open"; however, the calcium channels are highly selective for calcium ions [31]. External potassium only indirectly influences calcium channel opening. A high extracellular potassium concentration will depolarize the cell, thereby indirectly "closing" the calcium channel by closing the sodium channel. When the calcium channels close, voltage-dependent calcium influx ceases. Some data suggest that the channel-independent calcium influx may still occur via the sodium-calcium exchange mechanism [32] possibly contributing to the action potential plateau.

Beta-adrenergic stimulation. Beta-adrenergic stimulation [33,34] by an elevation of intracellular cyclic AMP levels and protein kinase activation, phosphorylates the α and β sub-units of the channel to change its molecular properties [3,18,35]. It is the L type channels which are activated by β-adrenergic agonists [23,24,36].

Receptor vs. depolarization operated channels. In the case of vascular smooth muscle, clear arguments have been made [37–40] for the differentiation between depolarization (= voltage) operated channels and receptor-operated channels. These claims still require objective study with new voltage and patch-clamp techniques. Receptor-operated channels may respond to alpha-adrenergic stimulation in vascular smooth muscle. However, α-stimulation is not thought to be an important mechanism of Ca^{2+} entry in the myocardium except in certain abnormal circumstances, such as congestive heart failure. Another possible source of receptor channel stimulation in the vascular smooth muscle is angiotensin-II, which also activates phosphoinositide (PI) hydrolysis [41]. In isolated rat cardiac myocytes, angiotensin-II increases Ca^{2+} current equally by voltage-dependent mechanism and an increase in calcium conductance [42], so that about half the angiotensin-II effect could be mediated by receptor-operated channels [41]. Thus both α-stimulation [43] and angiotensin-II may increase Ca^{2+} conductance through the phosphoinositide system, which could still presumably be voltage sensitive. Thus even in vascular smooth muscle the evidence for a receptor-operated voltage-independent calcium channel is not firm. In the myocardium, during beta-adrenergic agonist stimulation, additional voltage stimulation is required to open the calcium channel [30]. Thus for practical purposes in the myocardium there are only voltage-operated channels.

Calcium channel density. The density of the calcium channels has been estimated at about 0.1 calcium channels per μm^2 of the surface of cardiac cells in culture, compared with a sodium channel density of 16 per μm^2; this difference explains the much greater amplitude of the 'fast' sodium current (for references, see Table 4-2 in [44]. Nevertheless, the rate of calcium flux through the channel is extremely rapid and has been estimated at 3 million cations per second in the intact heart.

Calcium channels of skeletal muscle and brain. Calcium channels are found in tissues with a slow response type of action potential including the sinus and atrioventricular nodes of the heart, the myocardium, the vascular smooth muscle, and the T-tubules of skeletal muscle. L type calcium channels, found on neuronal bodies, appear to play a negligible role in central nervous system conduction, although N type channels, found on terminal neurons, may be concerned with the regulation of noradrenaline release into the neurotransmitter cleft. The function of calcium channels in two sites is still largely unknown. First, T-tubules of skeletal muscle are frequently used for isolation of DHP and other binding sites, yet calcium antagonists have no known clinical effects on skeletal muscle. Secondly, the role of the newly described N channels in nervous tissue are at an early stage of clinical dissection.

Different types of calcium channels in different tissues? To explain different effects of different calcium channel antagonists on various vascular beds and on nodal as opposed to myocardial contractile tissue, some investigators suggest that these drugs bind with different affinities to different populations of calcium channels. Because of the importance of depolarization in governing closure of the calcium channels by calcium antagonists [19], the existence of different resting membrane potentials in different blood vessels seems a plausible explanation for the arterial selectivity of DHP and regional arterial differences to various agents [45]. It must be emphasized that many "properties" of the calcium channel refer to that of the myocardial or skeletal sarcolemma, whereas the major clinical site of action is vascular smooth muscle or nodal tissue.

"Visual aid" model of calcium channel

In the absence of a clear relation between calcium antagonist binding to the receptor sites and a direct link to the effects on the calcium channel, all schemes must be hypothetical. Previously it has been thought that the nifedipine site must be superficial and the verapamil and diltiazem sites less superficial because of their marked use dependency. The latter agents therefore should enter when the calcium channel is open, accumulate within the cell [45A], and act deeply in the sarcolemma or on the inner layer [46]. The modern concept of the overlapping but interacting binding sites for V, D, and N and the proposal that lipid solubility governs the speed of onset of nifedipine [47] and the mode whereby it reaches the channel receptor [19] makes any simplified scheme unlikely. The accompanying cartoon (Figure I-2) is therefore a *highly schematic visual aid* of the cardiac calcium channel. Of particular note in comparison with previous models is 1) the close interaction of the DHP site with the inactivation gate; 2) the possibility of overlap between the N, V, and D sites, and 3) the possibility that the N site is "deeper" into the sarcolemma than previously thought (compare with Figure 2 in [20]).

Calcium antagonists vs. beta-adrenergic blockers: comparative molecular sites of action and differences

The above model for the calcium channel predicts that there could be close overlap between the properties of calcium agonists and beta-adrenergic agonists, and calcium antagonists and beta-adrenergic antagonists (beta-blockers). The properties of beta-receptor agonists are thought to be expressed by an elevation of intracellular cyclic AMP which activates protein kinases which in turn 1) phosphorylate the alpha and beta subunits of the calcium channel to change the inactivated state to a resting state, which can then be opened upon voltage-depolarization; 2) phosphorylate phospholamban to activate the calcium pump of the sarcoplasmic reticulum, thereby enhancing the rate of Ca^{2+} uptake, and 3) phosphorylate troponin-I to desensitize actin, which may enhance the rate of relaxation (Figure I-3).

Molecular differences between beta-adrenergic receptor inhibition and calcium antagonism. Beta-re-

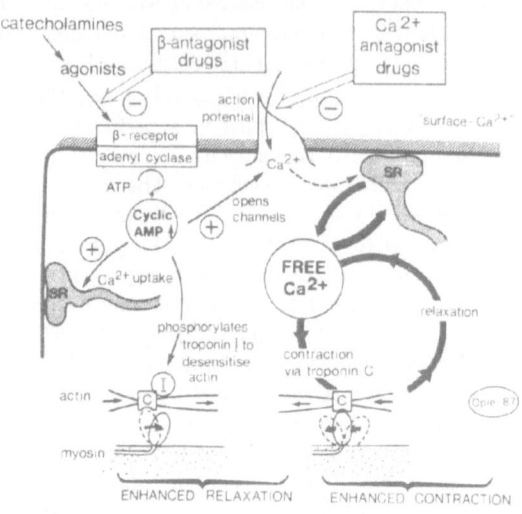

Fig. I-3. Schematic representation of different intracellular effects of calcium antagonists vs. β-antagonist drugs. Note that β-antagonist drugs inhibit formation of cyclic AMP with consequent effects on all aspects of intracellular calcium ion movements (calcium ion entry, calcium ion uptake into the SR, and contraction-relaxation cycle). Calcium antagonist drugs act on only one of these aspects, namely calcium ion entry. From Opie [120].

ceptor inhibition increases the number of inactivated channels, whereas calcium antagonists increase the number of blocked channels, so that both will decrease the probability of calcium channel opening [27]. However, the DHPs have a far higher affinity (perhaps $1,000\times$ more; [19,48] for the inactivated than for the resting channels, so that the combination of beta-antagonism and calcium antagonism should profoundly inhibit calcium channels. This is a subject for further work.

In the myocardium and nodal tissue, the indirect calcium blocking effects of beta-blockade and the direct effects of calcium antagonism mean that both types of agents would act similarly to decrease the effect of voltage-depolarization in opening calcium channels, so that both beta-blockers and calcium antagonists will have a common effect of being negatively inotropic and negatively chronotropic.

In vascular smooth muscle, beta-adrenergic blockers inhibit the formation of cyclic AMP as in other tissues. Yet there is an additional site of action of cyclic AMP, namely the myosin light chain kinase, which is inhibited by cyclic AMP. Removal of cyclic AMP therefore promotes vascular (and bronchial) smooth muscle contraction. This is the critical difference between beta-adrenergic blockers and calcium antagonists.

Reversal of verapamil effects by beta-adrenergic agonists. Fleckenstein's group found that beta-adrenoceptor agonists opposed the specific action of high-dose verapamil (10^{-5}M) in inhibiting myocardial contractility [2]. The effect of isoproterenol was very similar to an increased extracellular calcium. Thus calcium channel antagonists and beta-adrenergic agonists had opposing effects on transsarcolemmal calcium influx. However, calcium channel antagonist did not have beta-adrenergic blocking qualities, because verapamil was unable to inhibit an isoproterenol-induced tachycardia or inotropic response [49]. Verapamil could not prevent catecholamine-induced increases in the tissue level of cyclic AMP nor activation of adenylate cyclase; rather, verapamil blocked the transsarcolemmal calcium influx provoked by either catecholamines or by an increased external calcium [50].

The reversal of the effects of calcium channel antagonists by beta-adrenergic agonists is worth stressing for the practical therapy of patients suffering from overdose by calcium channel antagonists. However, the calcium channels closed by the calcium channel antagonists are probably different from those opened by the beta-adrenergic agonists, because the latter help to open channels in a state of physiological inactivity, whereas the calcium channel antagonists act preferentially on pathologically inactivated channels. Thus the beta-agonist-antagonist effect is descriptive rather than a true pharmacological agonist-antagonist interaction.

Classification of Calcium Antagonists

Recently there have been many proposals for classification of the calcium antagonists in an attempt to introduce some order into the properties of the different agents. These agents are those with a highly specific action on the voltage-dependent calcium channels. Historically the original descriptions of Fleckenstein need consideration. The term *calcium antagonist* was originally emphasized by Fleckenstein [1,2] who described suppression of the calcium current in ventricular muscle and the reversal of such suppression by an increased external calcium concentration. He stated [2] that verapamil and other calcium channel antagonists abolished "the contractile response of the guinea-pig papillary muscle in a low concentration without any significant change in the single fiber action potentials." Such agents did not "affect the simultaneous sodium movements which are connected with the action potential" [2]. The potency of the individual agents was as follows: each molecule of verapamil antagonized approximately 200 calcium ions whereas nifedipine 1 molecule antagonized up to several thousand calcium ions. Calcium antagonists also protected from isoproterenol-induced myocardial calcium overload even though those compounds did not have beta-adrenoceptor blocking effects. Meanwhile, however, a critical therapeutic property of calcium antagonists, namely the inhibition of the calcium-dependent tension development in vascular smooth muscle, was the focus of early independent studies by Godfraind and Kaba at about the same time [51]: "In polarized arterial smooth muscle, adrenaline probably increases both membrane permeability to extracellular calcium ions and intracellular mobilization of sequestered calcium. Cinnarizine antagonizes selectively the increase in membrane permeability to Ca^{++}ions."

Terminology

For historical reasons, the term "calcium antagonist" is preferred to calcium channel blocker or slow channel blocker, although to some extent both terms are electrophysiologically correct [52]. Nonetheless it must be emphasized that the calcium antagonists actually act by altering the gating characteristics of the calcium channel so that more channels are in the closed state. A major problem with the term calcium antagonist has been that the effect of verapamil on the atrioventricular node is not clinically antagonized by high concentrations of external calcium [53]; however, lower concentrations (up to double) are effective [54]. Although the term calcium antagonist is far less exact than "calcium channel antagonist" (Table I-1), for practical purposes the former is frequently used to describe the agents in question.

Classification of the International Society and Federation of Cardiology

In order to arrrive at a classification suitable for clinicians, a Working Committee of the International Society and Federation of Cardiology met in Washington, D.C. at the time of the World Congress of Cardiology in 1986 [20]. From the cardiovascular point of view, the Committee recommended a practical classification (Table I-2) in which the three *highly specific calcium antagonists* were regarded as 1) verapamil; 2) the dihydropyridines such as nifedipine; and 3) diltiazem. These three compounds appear to have different but probably overlapping binding sites on the myocardial and vascular smooth muscle sarcolemma (Figure I-1). These three highly specific compounds meet the original criteria of Fleckenstein for Group A agents.

Less specific agents (Fleckenstein's Group B) still have an interaction with the N binding site, as shown in the case of the combined sodium-calcium blockers such as bepridil, tiapamil, and lidoflazine which deserve special emphasis because of a greater probability of being effective against ventricular arrhythmias by virtue of sodium channel blockade. Cinnarizine and flunarizine, which also interact with the N site, have no cardiovascular therapeutic indications at present, and were not considered in detail by the Committee. (They are fully covered by Godfraind et al. [4].) Other less specific agents which do not interact with the N site include perhexiline, prenylamine, fendiline, and others.

In addition, a new category of *nonspecific agents* (Class C agents) was proposed to include those agents such as chlorpromazine which have nonspecific calcium antagonist properties. These correspond to the compounds in Group IIB of Godfraind et al. [4].

The table summarizing the recommendations of the Committee is reproduced (Table 1-1).

Other classifications

Among the other classifications recently proposed (see [8]), that of Godfraind et al. [4] is the most detailed and that of the World Health Organization the briefest (Table III of [55]). These are compared with the classification of the International Society and Federation of Cardiology in Table 1-2. In essence, the WHO classification recognizes agents specific to slow calcium channels including V, D, and N types of compounds, and the nonselective compounds including flunarizine, cinnarizine, and the combined Na^+/Ca^{2+} blockers.

Functional classification. From a clinical point of view, all calcium channel blockers thus far described have a vasodilating effect. However, the site of "preferred action" may vary — nifedipine-like compounds are "most" active on the peripheral resistance arterioles, some dihydropyridines are selectively active on the cerebral circulation (nimodipine), and compounds like flunarizine are still under study but might be more active on the vessels involved in peripheral vascular disease. Whether there are such fundamental

Table 1-2. Classification of calcium antagonists of ISFC (International Society and Federation of Cardiology [121], based on that of Fleckenstein, compared with that of Godfraind et al. [4] and chemical classification of World Health Organization (1987)

International Society and Federation of Cardiology (modified Fleckenstein)	Godfraind et al. (1986)	World Health Organization (1987)
Calcium antagonists	Calcium entry blockers	Calcium antagonists
A. Highly specific on voltage-dependent Ca^{2+} channels; three binding sites, all interact with DHP site Veramapil, nifedipine, diltiazem (V,N,D)	IA. Selective for myocardial slow Ca^{2+} channel: verapamil, nifedipine, diltiazem	1. Selective for slow Ca^{2+} channels: verapamil, nifedipine, diltiazem
B. i. Less specific Ca^{2+} antagonists also interacting with DHP site:	IB. Selective (vascular) but no myocardial effects: flunarizine, cinnarizine	2. Non-selective for slow Ca^{2+} channels: a. Diphenylpiperazines (cinnarizine, flunarizine)
(a) Sodium-calcium blockers bepridil, tiapamil, lidoflazine		b. Prenylamine derivatives
(b) Flunarizine, cinnarizine	IIA. Sodium-calcium blockers including prenylamine, perhexiline	c. Others (bepridil, perhexiline)
ii. Other less specific Ca^{2+} antagonists noninteractive with DHP site: prenylamine, perhexiline		
C. Primary site of action elsewhere with incidental Ca^{2+} antagonist activity	IIB. Primary site of action elsewhere	

DHP = dihydropyridine binding site.

differences remains to be seen by more detailed and careful studies.

From the practical point of view, *the calcium channels in nodal tissue, in myocardial tissue, and in vascular smooth muscle, all appear to have somewhat different characteristics although they share the property of being the site of action of calcium channel antagonists.* Whether there are truly different types of calcium channels in different sites, or whether the same channel responds differently in different tissues according to different patterns of regulation (such as different resting membrane potentials or different allosteric regulatory factors or different responses to the Ca^{2+} agonist factors), remains to be established. These aspects are discussed by Nayler et al. [56] and Godfraind [57].

Physiological Sites of Action of Calcium Antagonists

The critical question is which pharmacological effects can be achieved at therapeutic plasma concentrations (Table I-3). This may seem a long leap of faith from a consideration of binding sites. However, Godfraind [57] has shown a "pharmacotherapeutic cascade" (Table I-4) whereby concentrations of a calcium antagonist interacting with the binding sites are similar to those interacting at a cellular level (Ca^{2+} fluxes and action potentials) and also concentrations causing vasodilation in animal and human arterial tissue. All these values are similar to the three plasma levels circulating in man and having clinical effects such as those on angina. In contrast to this "relevant" progression is the situation in the smooth muscle of the gastrointestinal tract, where nifedipine and verapamil are experimentally both active in similar concentrations (nanomolar), yet only verapamil causes constipation. Some other unexplained factor must be at work to cause these differences.

Vascular smooth muscle and its calcium channel

In vascular smooth muscle, there are four mechanisms whereby calcium may enter: the receptor-operated channel, the potential-operated channel, a downhill calcium "leak," and calcium-sodium exchange. For simplicity the receptor-operated channel will be referred to as the ROC, and the potential-operated or depolarization-operated channel as POC or DOC. The inward calcium leak system may give rise to vascular contraction in the absence of a calcium uptake system [40]. In addition, calcium-sodium exchange probably

Table I-3. Comparative therapeutic levels of verapamil, nifedipine, and diltiazem in humans*

	Verapamil	Nifedipine	Diltiazem
Therapeutic level in man			
ng/ml	80 to 400	25 to 100	50 to 300
molecular weight	455	346	415
molar value	2 to 8×10^{-7} M	0.5 to 2×10^{-7} M	1 to 7×10^{-7} M
protein binding	about 90%	about 95%	about 85%
molar value, corrected for protein binding	2 to 8×10^{-8} M	0.3 to 1×10^{-8} M	1 to 5×10^{-8} M

*From Opie [20].

Table I-4. Comparison of basic and clinical properties of the calcium antagonist, nifedipine (based on Tables II and III, in Godfraind [57])

Level of Pharmacological Action	Qualitative Effects	Quantitative Parameter	Value (nM) in	
			Rat Aorta	Human Coronary Artery
Molecule	Binding to Ca^{2+} channel	K_i	4^a	—
Cell	Changes in Ca^{2+} fluxes and action potentials	I_{50}	2^b	—
Tissue in vitro	Smooth muscle relaxation	IC_{50}	2^b	$3,30^c$
Clinical effect	Antianginal	Therapeutic free drug levels	—	7-20 (3-10, Table I-3)

^{a}K_i, for displacement of nitrendipine by nifedipine.
^{b}Concentration of nifedipine producing 50% inhibition with $^{45}Ca^{2+}$ influx (I_{50}) or contraction (IC_{50}) evoked by K^+ depolarization.
^{c}Inhibition of contractions evoked by K^+ depolarization (3nM) or serotonin (30 nM).

but not certainly operates in vascular smooth muscle (for discussion see [58]) and may have importance in linking vasoconstriction with excess intracellular sodium found in some models and types of hypertension.

L and T components of depolarization-operated channels (DOCs). DOCs have now been investigated with voltage-clamp techniques on isolated vascular cells [24,36,59] showing two types of calcium currents similar to those found in canine atrial cells where they are classified as T (transient) and L (longlasting). As in the heart, the T type channel is insensitive to the calcium antagonists. Both T and L types are strongly voltage-dependent.

Are there really receptor-operated channels (ROCs)? ROCs were initially thought to be of considerable importance in vascular smooth muscle because calcium entry could be mediated by norepinephrine independently of voltage changes. At present a reasonable explanation for this phenomenon is that alpha-1 adrenergic stimulation can both enhance calcium ion entry by increasing Ca^{2+} conductance [43] (a process which could also be voltage-dependent) and intracellular messengers such as IP_3 may act to release calcium from the sarcoplasmic reticulum. A truly non-voltage-dependent receptor-operated channel has been shown in voltage-clamped segments of arterioles of guinea-pig small intestine [60]. Thus to show the operation of a ROC in the absence of depolarization requires voltage-clamp techniques. However, with this technique, norepinephrine can increase Ca^{2+} current flow in the rabbit ear artery independently of receptor stimulation [36] so that the real evidence for receptor-operated channels working independently of voltage is weak.

Contraction-relaxation cycle in vascular smooth muscle. This cycle is dependent on a rise and fall of internal calcium ion concentrations (Figure I-4). The sources for calcium contraction in vascular smooth muscle are several-fold, as previously discussed, and include downhill leaks, voltage-operated channels, receptor-operated channels, and exchange mechanisms. However, in addition a major source of calcium is from the sarcoplasmic reticulum, from whence it may be released in the absence of depolarization by an alpha-1-mediated intracellular messenger system involving inositol triphosphate (IP_3). For full expression of alpha-1-agonist stimulation, Ca^{2+} must be derived from two sources, both external, and the sarcoplasmic reticulum [61]. The activity of the alpha-1-stimulated messenger system is dependent on the hydrolysis of phosphotidyl inositol to IP_3 and is insensitive

VASCULAR CONTRACTION

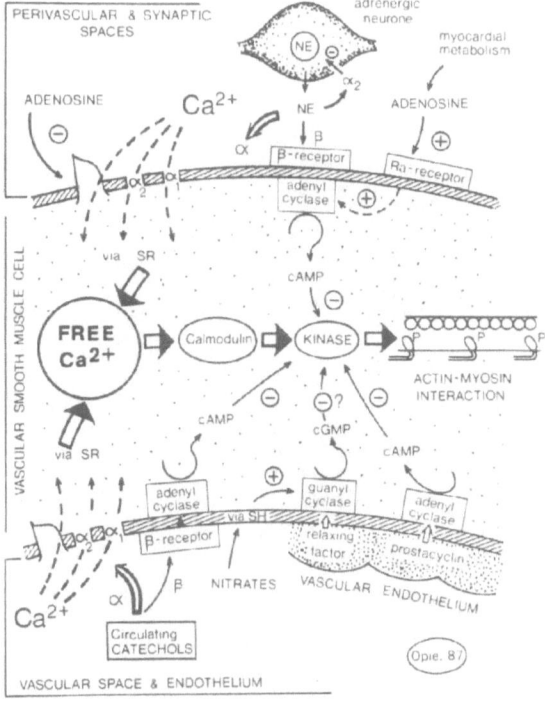

Fig. I-4. Mechanism of coronary artery spasm and role of calcium in causing vasoconstriction. For site of action of calcium antagonists, see Figure I-5. According to these concepts, calcium antagonists should relieve coronary artery spasm and β-adrenergic blockers exaggerate the phenomenon. From Opie and Maseri [131]. (Figure copyright: LH Opie).

to calcium antagonism [62], at least not in the aorta. Such internal calcium release system is theoretically unlikely to respond to calcium antagonism, as also supported by some (but not all) experimental evidence [63]. On the other hand, alpha-2-stimulation may evoke Ca^{2+} influx which may be inhibited by calcium antagonists (Figure I-5), depending on the type and site of blood vessel [57].

Functional differences between vascular smooth muscle (VSM) and myocardial cells. First, intracellular calcium elevations can be achieved by two different mechanisms in VSM, namely voltage-operated calcium channel depolarization and intracellular mobilization of calcium in response to receptor stimu-

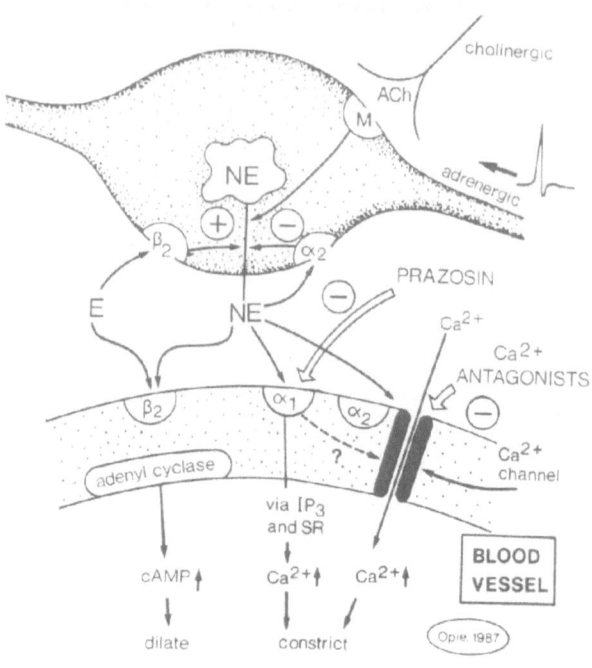

Fig. I-5. Proposed role of calcium antagonists on vascular smooth muscle adrenoceptors. There are thought to be two types of α-receptors on vascular smooth muscle: the α_1-receptors which are inhibited by prazosin, and the α_2-receptors, which are inhibited by calcium antagonists. β-adrenergic receptor blockers may inhibit the vasodilatory effects of cyclic AMP to allow unopposed α-adrenergic-mediated vasospasm. ACh = acetylcholine, E = epinephrine, M = muscarinic receptor, NE = norepinephrine.

lation. A second difference, stemming from the first, is in the contribution of external calcium. In the myocardium, external Ca^{2+} is essential for contraction. In VSM, external Ca^{2+} becomes more important with decreasing vessel diameter [64]. Hence logically the alpha-1-IP_3 sarcoplasmic reticulum system should become correspondingly less important as the vessel diameter decreases. Experimental proof of this supposition must be obtained. A third difference between VSM and myocardium lies in the control of the contractile mechanism. The enzyme myosin light chain kinase [65] is thought to phosphorylate the light chains of myosin to facilitate interaction of myosin ATPase with the thin actin filaments. The intracellular calcium regulator protein calmodulin is essential for the activation of the light chain in vascular smooth muscle. The effect of calmodulin is inhibited by cyclic AMP, explaining why beta-adrenergic receptor stimulation relaxes VSM. Relaxation may also be obtained by dephosphorylation of the myosin light chains in response to cyclic GMP which explains the vasodilation caused by nitrates and nitroprusside, which both increase smooth muscle cyclic GMP levels [66,67]. A fourth and important difference between VSM and myocardium lies in the non-ATP-requiring actin-myosin interaction, involving *dephosphorylated latch bridges* [68,69] which come into operation as the calcium ion concentration falls and have the capacity to sustain tone when the initial ATP-mediated contraction is over.

Sensitivity of vascular smooth muscle to calcium antagonists. Clinically the impression has been that the DHPs are most potent in their arteriolar vasodilating effects, followed by verapamil and diltiazem, although few truly comparative studies exist (Table I-5). The rat portal vein is claimed to be a suitable model for the hemodynamically important vessels of the periphery, and nifedipine is about 10× more potent in its inhibition of vascular contraction than verapamil, which again is somewhat more potent than diltiazem [70]. Some other approximate potencies on coronary artery smooth muscle are given by Chaffman and Brogden [71]; in general, nifedipine is an order of magnitude more powerful than diltiazem or verapamil which are roughly equipotent.

Calmodulin inhibition in vascular smooth muscle. Calmodulin is the tissue Ca^{2+}-receptor, whose level stays constant. It lacks tissue specificity and consists of a single polypeptide of molecular weight 16,700 with up to four Ca^{2+} binding sites. Activated calmodulin (Ca^{2+}-calmodulin) binds to target enzymes in a 1:1 ratio and regulates many critical enzymes of Ca^{2+}-metabolism, such as myosin light chain kinase, phosphorylase kinase, adenylate cyclase, guanylate cyclase, and calcium-dependent phosphodiesterases, and the Ca^{2+}-ATPase responsible for calcium extrusion. Calmodulin may seem to be an ideal target for drug action aimed at calcium modulation. As yet, however, no specific calmodulin antagonists have been discovered (see [72]). Even if a specific calmodulin inhibitor were to be discovered, the nature of the numerous enzyme interactions of calmodulin is so marked that a true inhibition could have unexpected results including inhibition of calcium extrusion, so that more than simple vasodilation could be possible. Some calcium antagonists have calmodulin inhibitory properties which may explain some of the properties of perhexiline, prenylamine, and fendiline [73]. Some

Table 1-5. Relative potencies of verapamil, nifedipine, and diltiazem on coronary arteries, aorta, and portal vein

	Verapamil	Nifedipine	Diltiazem	Reference
Isolated pig coronary artery K^+-contracted, IC_{50}	10^{-7} M	8×10^{-9} M	2×10^{-7} M	Fleckenstein [122]
Isolated dog coronary artery strips, ID_{50} for relaxation	2×10^{-7} M	10^{-7} M	3×10^{-6} M	Millard et al. [79]
Aorta, rabbit, K^+-contracted IC_{50}	10^{-7} M to 10^{-6} M	10^{-9} M to 3×10^{-8} M	5×10^{-7} M to 10^{-6} M	Godfraind et al. [4]
Aorta, rat (as above)	7×10^{-8} M to 10^{-7} M	10^{-9} M to 5×10^{-9} M	2×10^{-7} M	Godfraind et al. [4]
Resistance vessels, various origins, K^+-contracted	No data	10^{-9} M to 2×10^{-8} M	6×10^{-7} M	Godfraind et al. [4]
Resistance vessels, various origins, NE-induced contractions	No data	$2 \cdot 7 \times 10^{-8}$ M	10^{-8} M	Godfraind et al. [4]
Ratio of potencies in increasing coronary blood flow in conscious dog	1.3	20	1	Millard et al. [79]
Relative potentices on coronary blood flow in blood perfused dog papillary muscle	2	100	1	Taira [48]
Relative potencies on coronary blood flow in blood perfused dog papillary muscle	2	25	1	Himori et al. [123]
Portal vein, spontaneous contraction, IC_{50}	4×10^{-7} M	4×10^{-8} M	6×10^{-7} M	Ljung [70]

Table 1-6. Comparative direct negative inotropic effects of verapamil, nifedipine, and diltiazem

Preparation	Verapamil	Nifedipine	Diltiazem	Reference
Isolated guinea-pig atrium 40% reduction contractile force	5×10^{-6} M	5×10^{-7} M	5×10^{-4} M	Henry et al. [81]
Isolated dog trabecular muscles ID_{50} at 60 min	2×10^{-7} M	1×10^{-7} M	4×10^{-7} M	Millard et al. [79]
Langendorff guinea-pig heart, dP/dt approx 50% reduction	10^{-7} M	10^{-7} M	$>10^{-6}$ M	Millard et al. [79]
Isolated dog Purkinje fibers, IC_{50}	4.2×10^{-8} M	$(1.4 \times 10^{-8}$ M)*	3×10^{-7} M	Lathrop et al. [116]
Peak papillary muscle isolated and paced, peak force, IC_{50}	5×10^{-7} M	5×10^{-7} M	5×10^{-6} M	Ljung [70]
Ratio vascular (portal vein) inhibition versus negative inotropic effect	1.4	14	7	Ljung [70]

*Nisoldipine, not nifedipine.

dihydropyridines, such as felodipine, may have a relatively minor interaction with vascular smooth muscle calmodulin [74,75].

Myocardial effects of calcium antagonists: negative inotropism vs. vasodilatory potency

Of considerable importance is the ratio of the potency of these agents on vascular smooth muscle versus their potency in the myocardium, when nifedipine is 14 times more potent on VSM, diltiazem 7 times, and verapamil only 1.4 times (Table I-6). Thus the clinical impression that verapamil is the most negatively inotropic of the three agents seems valid. However, it must be emphasized that these figures are the result of the relative effects in afterload reduction in comparison with a direct negative inotropic effect; if only negative inotropism is considered, nifedipine is in fact most potent. Another important point is that the effects on the myocardium are highly stereospecific [76].

Besides the effect of simultaneous peripheral vasodilation to unload the heart (Figure I-6), several other factors influence the potential negative inotropic effect of calcium antagonists. First, vasodilation may call forth a reflex sympathetic response so that there is an indirect positive inotropic effect on the myocardium; this mechanism, although frequently emphasized, cannot be the sole explanation for the effects of nifedipine because left ventricular function in patients receiving nifedipine is not depressed when β-blockade is added [77]. Even in beta-blocked patients when there is a direct negative inotropic effect of added nifedipine, there is still an increased LV stroke output [78]. Secondly, there is a withdrawal of parasympathetic tone, most marked in the case of nifedipine [79], which will have the indirect effect of enhancing sympathetic tone independently of the presence or absence of beta-blockade. Thirdly, calcium antagonists may interact with phosphodiesterase. Iijima et al. [80] have shown that intracellular application of nifedipine and nicardipine actually increase the calcium current, probably these agents have as a side-effect inhibition of phosphodiesterase activity, thereby increasing cyclic AMP and therefore being less negatively inotropic than might be expected. However, in vascular smooth muscle, both the direct inhibition of calcium current and the indirect effects of phosphodiesterase inhibition will cause vasodilation.

Differential effects on vascular smooth muscle vs. myocardium. Although in systems diltiazem has almost no effective negative inotropic effect [81], so that this compound could be virtually free of any negative inotropic potential, other data [70] show that diltiazem has a negative inotropic potential lying between nifedipine and verapamil (Table 1-6). It is critical to consider that in clinical practice that the direct negative inotropic effect of all calcium antagonists must be taken into consideration with the vasodilating effects. Furthermore, the inotropic state of the myocardium may sensitize the failing heart to calcium antagonists [82]. Furthermore, unexpected severe hypotensive reactions may occur to calcium antagonists including diltiazem [83]. In the case of verapamil, there is a selective interaction with ischemic tissue [84,85]. There is also very substantial experimental work showing that calcium antagonists can protect against some aspects of ischemic [86] or hypoxic injury [87]. However, clinical data question this concept of "cardioprotection" from ischemic injury (see Part II of this review). Furthermore, it is impossible to extrapolate from the available experimental data to all clinical situations, so that prudence and caution will always be required when considering the clinically relevant properties of these drugs.

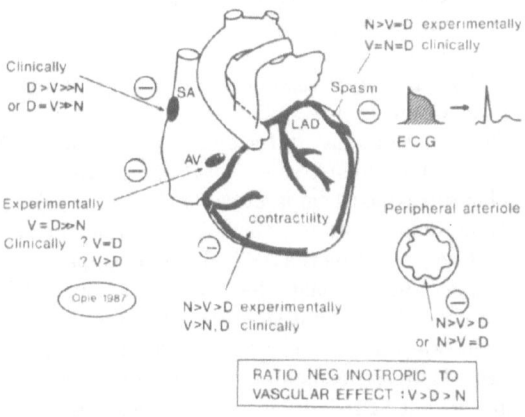

Fig. I-6. Proposed comparable potencies of three major calcium antagonist drugs: V = verapamil, D = diltiazem, N = nifedipine. These potencies are based on a consideration of literature reports and on isolated organ studies. However, the suggested potencies may not accurately reflect any particular experimental or clinical situation and must therefore be regarded as provisional. Clinical decisions must always be made after a careful consideration of all the pharmacological effects of the drug which can be expected in that particular patient.

Nodal tissue and calcium antagonists

Atrioventricular node. The slow calcium current (with L and T components) predominates in true AV nodal cells, although there may be other currents such as the slow sodium current [88], and an outward potassium current [89]. The reasons why nifedipine does not directly affect the AV (and sinus) nodes, except in high concentrations (Table I-7), could be structural or because nifedipine is not use-dependent (Figure I-2) or because of functional differences between the calcium channel of the nodal tissue and that of the myocardium. For example, in clinical practice, the inhibitory effect of verapamil on the atrioventricular node is not counteracted by an increased external calcium ion concentration [90], although calcium antagonism can be found pharmacologically at low calcium levels up to 2 times normal [54]. Thus the term calcium antagonist does not optimally describe the verapamil effect on the AV node. Alternatively, the calcium channel of atrioventricular-nodal tissue could be the same in structure as that of the myocardium and vascular smooth muscle, but merely exposed to different stimuli during supraventricular tachycardias, namely very rapid repetitive firing. Thus verapamil and diltiazem, being use-dependent, would "enter" rapidly through the increased opening of the AV nodal calcium channels to exert their inhibitory effects on the calcium channel, thereby stopping excess opening and ultimately causing the reentry circuit to be inhibited (for proposed molecular mechanisms, see [19]).

Clinical comparison of calcium antagonists on AV node. Clinically few studies show exact comparative effects of verapamil, diltiazem, and nifedipine on AV nodal (and sinus) tissues, although published data allow some rough comparative conclusions (Table I-7). Some workers estimate that diltiazem has less of an inhibitory effect on the AV node than verapamil [91], whereas others estimate that the effect is equal [48]. In one clinical comparative study [92], verapamil was about two-thirds more potent than diltiazem on a dose basis. However, comparative blood concentrations of the circulating free drugs were not measured.

Current in sinoatrial node. In addition to the slow inward calcium current, other depolarizing currents in the sinus node are a decaying outward potassium current and (at certain voltages) an inward current (I_f) which may all play a role in the pacemaker process. Furthermore, the calcium current can now be split into two components, the initial T (transient current), not sensitive to calcium antagonists, and the later onset L (long-lasting current), sensitive to calcium antagonists. Such multiple currents mean that verapamil and diltiazem, both acting on only one of the two types of Ca^{2+} currents, have only modest direct effects on the sinus node depolarization process. However, in the presence of sick sinus syndrome, the inhibitory effects of either agent can be serious. Again, there have been few comparable pharmacological studies of diltiazem and verapamil on the SA node, but diltiazem may have less direct depressant effect than verapamil [48].

Verapamil and diltiazem effects on the SA node. Both verapamil and diltiazem have inhibitory effects on the SA node (Table I-8). Clinically, bradycardia is more consistently found with diltiazem, but this may merely reflect the baroreceptor sensitivity whereby the peripheral vasodilatory effects are more readily translated into reflex sympathetic stimulation of the sinus node in the case of verapamil. This difference cannot be due to a direct effect on baroreceptor reflexes which are only slightly attenuated by diltiazem and more markedly attenuated by verapamil [79]; rather the reflex stimulation by verapamil probably indicates a more potent vasodilator effect (Table I-8).

Renal effects of calcium antagonists

Bauer and Reams [93] reviewed the renal effects of calcium antagonists. From the short-term point of view, verapamil, nifedipine, and diltiazem all increase urinary flow rate and urinary sodium excretion. From the long-term point of view, none of these three alters urinary kinetics. However, other second generation DHPs such as felodipine, nitrendipine, and nicardipine may all have a longer term effect. Amlodipine, a very recently introduced dihydropyridine, has a sustained diuretic effect over 6 weeks in rats [47]. In one study not reviewed by Bauer [94] nifedipine was thought to have a delayed diuretic effect coming on after some weeks.

Although part of the diuretic effect is explained by an increase in renal plasma flow, there appears to be a direct effect on renal tubular sodium excretion. In one small series of 8 patients [93] with low pretreatment GFRs, there was an increase of nearly 50% apparently sustained for several months. In the case of diltiazem, the mechanism may be an inhibition of the pressure-induced constriction of the afferent renal arteriole [95]. Furthermore, efferent arteriolar pressure may also fall with diltiazem, so that there is improved in-

Table 1-7. Effects of verapamil, nifedipine, and diltiazem on atrioventricular (AV) nodal preparations

	Verapamil	Nifedipine	Diltiazem	Reference
Excised superfused rabbit atrium with AV node				
Concentration required for 50 percent increase in effective refractory period	2.2×10^{-7} M	2.9×10^{-7} M	2.2×10^{-7} M	Kawai et al. [124]
Intact dog open chest				
Relative potencies on A-H conduction	1:1	[3:1]*	1:1	Lathrop et al. [116]
Relative potencies on coronary resistance	1:1	[30:1]*	1:1	Lathrop et al. [116]
A-H vs coronary effects	1:1	[0.1:1]*	1:1	Lathrop et al. [116]
Blood perfused preparations				
Isolated perfused dog AV node, relative potency of doses causing atrioventricular 2nd or 3rd degree block	1/2	1	1/2	Narimatsu and Taira [125]
Ratio of effects on AV node versus coronary flow	10:1	1:1	10:1	Table 1 and Figure 9, Narimatsu and Taira [125]
AV node versus contractile force	7:1	1:1	20:1	Ono and Hashimoto [126]

* = nisoldipine, not nifedipine.

Table 1-8. Comparative potencies of verapamil, nifedipine, and diltiazem on isolated sinoatrial nodal preparations

	Verapamil	Nifedipine	Diltiazem	Reference
Excised superfused rabbit atrium				
Concentration required for 50% sinus slowing	4.4×10^{-6} M	2.9×10^{-6} M	2.4×1^{-6} M	Kawai et al. [124]
Isolated superfused guinea-pig atrium				
Concentration required for 20% slowing of sinus rate	10^{-6} M	10^{-5} M	10^{-8} M	Henry et al. [81]
Blood perfused preparations				
Relative potency of negative chronotropic effects	1	1	1/3	Ono and Hashimoto [126]
Relative vasodilator potency in perfused papillary muscle	1/12	1	1/26	Ono and Hashimoto [126]
Ratio chronotropic to vasodilator potency	12:1	1:1	9:1	Ono and Hashimoto [126]

trarenal hemodynamics without glomerular hyperfiltration [96].

The significance of the diuretic effect of calcium antagonists is as follows: 1) although most vasodilators cause reactive sodium and water retention, these agents do not (see next section); 2) the diuretic effect may contribute to the antihypertensive effect; and 3) the pedal edema caused by calcium antagonists as a group is not due to overall water or sodium retention [97].

Renin, catecholamines, and aldosterone

In general, the *plasma renin activity* (PRA) is left unchanged or somewhat increased by calcium antagonists [93]. Acute and chronic effects may differ. Rapidly acting calcium antagonists such as nifedipine and nicardipine are more likely to increase the renin activity than slower onset agents such as nitrendipine, diltiazem, and verapamil [98]. However, in some studies diltiazem shows no acute increase in renin levels but during chronic administration levels may rise up to 2–3 times [71]. Felodipine increases renin activity and catecholamine levels, with both these effects being abolished by metoprolol [99].

Plasma catecholamines rise with nifedipine but not with verapamil during acute and chronic therapy of hypertension [98,100,101,102]. Presumably the powerful vasodilatory effect of nifedipine is the critical difference. However, Nayler and Sturrock [103] have reported that both verapamil and diltiazem are able to inhibit the release of noradrenaline from ischemic and reperfused hearts; recent extension of these data (as yet not fully published) suggests that chronic verapamil administration to rats results in catecholamine depletion.

Plasma aldosterone does not increase with nifedipine, even when PRA and angiotensin-II rise, suggesting that calcium is involved in aldosterone release [104,105]. In contrast, hydralazine evokes both a rise in PRA and in aldosterone, explaining the tendency to fluid retention and true edema [104]. In the case of nifedipine, pedal edema is a local phenomenon [97].

Metabolic effects of calcium antagonists

Glucose. Insulin release in response to hyperglycemia or insulin is calcium-mediated. The fear has been that the calcium antagonists may impair insulin release with a consequent tendency to hyperglycemia. However, proven hyperglycemia as a result of calcium antagonist therapy remains rare. Unexpectedly verapamil may have a mild hypoglycemic effect, perhaps by inhibition of hepatic glycogenolysis [105]. Nifedipine, although reported to cause deterioration of glucose tolerance or hyperglycemia in isolated reports, appears in reality to have no such effects upon careful testing [107,108]. However, long-term effects of calcium antagonists on glucose tolerance of patients remains to be reported.

Potassium. In general, the sodium diuresis of calcium antagonists is not accompanied by potassium loss [93]. However, hypokalemia has been reported in some patients given nifedipine as a third-line agent in the treatment of severe hypertension [109], while Landmark [94] showed a chronic K^+-losing effect of nifedipine.

Sodium. During prolonged nifedipine administration, serum sodium falls slightly [94], exchangeable sodium increases [105], and body weight is unchanged [94] or slightly increased [105].

Blood lipids. In general, calcium antagonists are thought to have little or no effect on blood lipids, thereby distinguishing this category of agents from the beta-blockers. However, no strict trials compare these two types of agents for potential effects on blood lipids.

Effects on nonvascular smooth muscle

Gastrointestinal muscle. Depolarization-operated channels in GI smooth muscle resemble those found in vascular smooth muscle [8]. Diltiazem and nifedipine can clinically relieve an increased lower esophageal pressure. Verapamil is well known for its capacity to induce constipation; why this side-effect should be so much more common with verapamil is not known. In vitro, the potencies of the various agents on gastrointestinal smooth muscle is nifedipine > verapamil = diltiazem [4]. Verapamil has apparently not been tested for possible beneficial effect in diarrhea. Although calcium antagonists have some potency on bronchial smooth muscle, they are less potent on this site than on other vascular smooth muscle [57].

Bronchial smooth muscle. In patients with exogenous asthma, diltiazem may decrease the dose of inhaled histamine required; however, diltiazem is not effective against exercise or cold-induced asthma [71]. (For further data on other calcium antagonists, see Part III of this review.) It is not known why the bronchial smooth muscle is relatively ineffective in its bronchodilator response to calcium antagonists.

Table 1-9. Comparative potencies of verapamil, nifedipine, and diltiazem on alpha-receptor binding

Receptor Subtype	Ligand	Tissue	Value Calculated	Verapamil	Nifedipine	Diltiazem	Reference
Alpha$_1$	3H-prazosin	Rat LV	K_D	10^{-5} M	No effect	No effect	Motulsky et al. [127]
Alpha$_1$	3H-prazosin	Rat LV	K_i	6×10^{-7} M	No data	No data	Karliner et al. [128]
Alpha$_1$	3H-prazosin	Rat heart	K_i	5×10^{-7} M	4×10^{-6} M	7×10^{-6} M	Corr and Sharma [129]
Alpha$_1$	3H-prazosin	Rat heart membranes	K_i	5×10^{-6} M	$>2 \times 10^{-4}$ M	1.7×10^{-4} M	Nayler et al. [130]
Alpha$_2$	3H-clonidine	Rat brain membranes	K_i	8×10^{-6} M	$>10^{-4}$ M	15×10^{-6} M	Nayler et al. [130]
Alpha$_2$	3H-yohimbine	Human platelets	K_D	10^{-6} M	$>10^{-4}$ M	$>10^{-4}$ M	Motulsky et al. [130]

Hemostasis and clotting

Nifedipine 10 mg given to normal volunteers prolonged clotting time and lessened thrombolysis time [110]. Nifedipine inhibits changes in platelet function induced by exercise [111]. Interactions of other calcium antagonists with platelets have also been reported [71,112].

Nonspecific interactions with alpha-adrenoceptors

The most important of these is the alpha-1-blocking capacity of verapamil (Table I-9). The failure of calcium antagonists to interact directly with the alpha-2 receptor does not exclude the possibility that alpha-2 receptor agonist mediated Ca^{2+} entry is inhibited by calcium antagonists as proposed by Van Meel et al. [113] and Van Zwieten et al. [114].

Nonspecific sodium channel effects

Verapamil and diltiazem may both inhibit the fast sodium current [115] as may nisoldipine [116]; however, the concentrations required (10^{-4} M in the case of verapamil and nifedipine) are those which also cause excitation-contraction uncoupling [116]. When dealing with the antiarrhythmic effects, a noncalcium antiarrhythmic effect of verapamil operates at levels of about 10^{-6} M [117], but there is no proof that this activity depends upon inhibition of the sodium channel. Thandroyen et al. [118] found that d-verapamil 10^{-7} M did not alter the maximal rate of depolarization of guinea-pig papillary muscle (dV/dt_{max}). Assuming that this index reflects sodium channel activity, between 10^{-4} M and 10^{-5} M dl-verapamil is required to inhibit the sodium channel [119]. In contrast, agents such as bepridil, tiapamil, and lidoflazine are combined sodium/calcium channel blockers [119], which interact with the DHP site, therefore being specific from the Ca^{2+} point of view although not specific from the point of view of having a major site of action other than on the calcium channel. Finally, agents such as perhexiline and prenylamine do not interact with the DHP site (Table I-2) yet are approximately equally effective on sodium and calcium channels [4]. All agents with added Na^+ blocking capacity may be less specific calcium antagonists yet being more likely to have ventricular antiarrhythmic qualities.

References

1. Fleckenstein A, Tritthard H, Fleckenstein B, Herbst A, Grun G. A new group of competitive Ca antagonists (iproveratril, D600, prenylamine) with highly potent inhibitory effects on excitation-contraction coupling in mammalian myocardium (abstr). *Pflug Arch Physiol* 1969;307:25.

2. Fleckenstein A. Specific inhibitors and promoters of calcium action in the excitation-contraction coupling of heart muscle and their role in the prevention or production of myocardial lesions. In: Harris P, Opie LH, eds. *Calcium and the heart.* London: Academic Press, 1971, 135.

3. Sperelakis N. Properties of calcium-dependent slow action potentials, and their possible role in arrhythmias. In: Opie LH, ed. *Calcium antagonists and cardiovascular disease.* New York: Raven Press, 1984, 277-291.

4. Godfraind T, Miller R, Wibo M. Calcium antagonism and calcium entry blockade. *Pharmacol Rev* 1986;38:321-416.

5. Murphy KMM, Gould RJ, Largent BL, et al. A unitary mechanism of calcium antagonist drug action. *Proc Natl Acad Sci* 1983;80:860-864.

6. Glossmann H, Ferry DR, Lubbecke F, et al. Calcium channels: direct identification with radioligand binding studies. *Trends Pharmacol Sci* 1982;3:431-437.

7. Glossmann H, Ferry DR, Goll A, et al. Calcium channels: basic properties as revealed by radioligand binding studies. *J Cardiovasc Pharmacol* 1985;7(Suppl 6):S20-S30.

8. Spedding M: Calcium antagonist subgroups. *Trends Pharm Sci* 1985;6:109-114.

9. Garcia ML, King VF, Siegl PKS, et al. Binding of Ca^{2+} entry blockers to cardiac sarcolemmal membrane vesicles. *J Biol Chem* 1986;261:8146-8157.

10. Balwierczak JL, Johnson CL, Schwartz A. The relationship between the binding site of [^{3}H]d-cis-diltiazem and that of other non-dihydropyridine calcium entry blockers in cardiac sarcolemma. *Molec Pharmacol* 1987;31:175-179.

11. Schramm M, Thomas G, Towart R, et al. Novel dihydropyridines with positive inotropic action through activation of Ca^{2+} channels. *Nature* 1983;303:535-537.

12. Defeudis FV. Calcium antagonist subgroups *Trends Pharm Sci* 1985;6:237-238.

13. Opie LH, Singh BN: Calcium channel antagonists. In: Opie LH, ed. *Drugs for the heart,* second expanded edition. Orlando: Grune and Stratton, 1987, 34-53.

14. Hondeghem L, Katzung BG. Time and voltage-dependent interactions of antiarrhythmic drugs with cardiac sodium channels. *Biochim Biophys Acta* 0978;472:373-398.

15. Weld FM, Coromilas J, Rottman JN, et al. Mechanisms of quinidine-induced depression of maximum upstroke velocity in ovine cardiac Purkinje fibers. *Circ Res* 1982;50:369-376.

16. Green FJ, Farmer BB, Wiseman GL, et al. Effect of membrane depolarization on binding of [^{3}H] nitrendipine to rat cardiac myocytes. *Circ Res* 1985;56:576-585.

17. Kanaya S, Arlock P, Katzung BG, et al. Diltiazem and verapamil preferentially block inactivated calcium channels. *J Mol Cell Cardiol* 1983;15:145-148.

18. Catterall WA, Curtis BM. Molecular properties of voltage-sensitive calcium channels. In: Lichtlen PR, ed. *6th International Adalat Symposium.* Amsterdam: Excerpta Medica, 1986, 375-382.

19. Sanguinetti MC, Kass RS. Voltage-dependent block of calcium channel current in the calf Purkinje fiber by dihydropyridine calcium channel antagonists. *Circ Res* 1984; 55:336-348.

20. Opie LH. Calcium ions, drug action and the heart - with special reference to calcium channel blockers (calcium antagonist drugs). In: Denborough MA, ed. *The role of calcium in drug action.* Oxford: Pergamon Press, 1987,103-138.

21. Glossmann H, Striessnig J, Hymel L, et al. Purification and reconstitution of calcium channel drug receptor sites. *Ann NY Acad Sci* 1987, in press.

22. Schwartz A. Mechanisms of action of calcium channel modulators: an update. *Ann NY Acad Sci* 1987, in press.

23. Bean BP. Two kinds of calcium channels in canine atrial cells. Differences in kinetics, selectivity and pharmacology. *J Gen Physiol* 1985;86:1-30.

24. Hess P, Lansman JB, Nilius B, et al. Calcium channel types in cardiac myocytes: Modulation by dihydropyridines and β-adrenergic stimulation. *J Cardiovasc Pharmacol* 1986; 8(Suppl 9): S11-S21.

25. Reuter H, Porzig H, Kokubun S, et al. Calcium channels in the heart: properties and modulation by dihydorpyridine enantiomers. *Ann NY Acad Sci* 1988;522:16-24.

26. Wagner JA, Guggino SE, Reynolds IJ, et al. Calcium antagonist receptors. *Ann NY Acad Sci* 1988;522:116-133.

27. Reuter H: Electrophysiology of calcium channels in the heart. In: Opie LH, ed. *Calcium antagonists and cardiovascular disease.* New York: Raven Press, 1984, 43-51.

28. Tsien RW, Hess P, Landsman JB. Current views of cardiac calcium channels and their response to calcium antagonists and agonists. In: Zipes DP, Jalife J, eds. *Cardiac electrophysiology and arrhythmias.* Orlando: Grune and Stratton, 1985, 19-29.

29. Kokubun S, Prod'hom B, Becker C, et al. Studies on Ca channels in intact cardiac cells: voltage-dependent effects and cooperative interactions of dihydropyridine enantiomers. *Mol Pharmacol* 1986;30:571-584.

30. Schneider JA, Sperelakis N. Slow Ca^{2+} and Na^+ responses induced by isoproterenol and methylxanthines in isolated perfused guinea-pig hearts exposed to elevated K^+. *J Mol Cell Cardiol* 1975;7:249-273.

31. Matsuda H, Noma A. Isolation of calcium current and its sensitivity to monovalent cations in dialysed ventricular cells of guinea-pig. *J Physiol* 1984;357:533-573.

32. Mullins LJ. The generation of electric currents in cardiac fibers by Na/Ca exchange. *Am J Physiol* 1979;236:C103-C110.

33. Reuter H. Localization of beta-adrenergic receptors, and effects of noradrenaline and cyclic nucleotides on action potentials, ionic currents and tension in mammalian cardiac muscle. *J Physiol* 1974;242:429-451.

34. Reuter H, Scholtz A. The regulation of the calcium conductance of cardiac muscle by adrenaline. *J Physiol* 1977;264: 49-62.

35. Catterall WA, Takahashi M, Curtis BM. Molecular properties of dihydropyridine-sensitive calcium channels. *Ann NY Acad Sci* 1988;522:162-175.

36. Benham CD, Tsien RW. Noradrenaline increases L-type calcium current in smooth muscle cells of rabbit ear artery independently of α- and β-adrenoceptors. *J Physiol* 1987; 384:98P.

37. Bolton TB. Mechanisms of action of transmitters and other substances on smooth muscle. *Physiol Rev* 1979;59:606-718.

38. Towart R. The selective inhibition of serotonin-induced contractions of rabbit cerebral vascular smooth muscle by calcium antagonistic dihydropyridines. An investigation of the mechanism of action of nimodipine. *Circ Res* 1981;48: 650-657.

39. Van Breemen C, Mangel A, Fahim M, et al. Selectivity of calcium antagonist action in vascular smooth muscle. *Am J Cardiol* 1982;49:507-510.

40. Johns A, Leijten P, Yamamoto H, et al. Calcium regulation in vascular smooth muscle contractility. *Am J Cardiol* 1987;59:18A-23A.

41. Allen IS, Cohen NM, Dhallan RD, et al. Angiotensin II increases the calcium current in neonatal rat single cardiac myocytes. *J Physiol* 1987;384:74P.

42. Allen IS, Cohen NM, Dhallan RD, et al. Phorbol esters increase the rate of spontaneous beating in cultured neonatal rat cardiac myocytes. *J Physiol* 1987;384:77P.

43. Alvarez JL, Mongo KG, Vassort G. Effects of α_1-adrenergic stimulation on the Ca current in single ventricular frog cells. *J Physiol* 1987;384:76P.

44. Opie LH. *The heart: Physiology, metabolism, pharmacology and therapy.* London and Orlando: Grune and Stratton, 1984.

45. Nelson MT, Laher I, Worley J. Membrane potential regulates dihydropyridine inhibition of single calcium channels and contraction of rabbit mesenteric artery. *Ann NY Acad Sci* 1988;522:47-50.

45A. Lullman H, Timmermans PBMWM, Ziegler A. Accumulation of drugs by resting or beating cardiac tissue. *Eur J Pharmacol* 1979;60:277-285.

46. Payet MD, Schanne OF, Ruiz-Ceretti E, et al. Inhibitory action of blockers of the slow inward current in rat myocardium, a study in steady state and rate of action. *J Mol Cell Cardiol* 1980;12:187-200.

47. Burges RA, Gardiner DG, Carter AJ, et al. Amlodipine: Long-term natriuretic and antihypertensive activity in spontaneously hypertensive rats with developing and established hypertension. *Ann NY Acad Sci* 1987, in press.

48. Taira N. Differences in cardiovascular profile among calcium antagonists. *Am J Cardiol* 1987;59:24B-29B.

49. Nayler WG, McInnes I, Swann JB, et al. Some effects of iproveratril (Isoptin) on the cardiovascular system. *J Pharmacol Exp Ther* 1968;161:247-261.

50. Watanabe AM, Besch HR. Subcellular myocardial effects of verapamil and D600: Comparison with propranolol. *J Pharmacol Exp Ther* 1974;191:241-251.

51. Godfraind T, Kaba A. Blockade or reversal of contraction induced by calcium and adrenaline in depolarized arterial smooth muscle. *Br J Pharmacol* 1969;36:549-560.

52. Lee KS, Tsien RW. Mechanism of calcium channel blockade by verapamil, D600, diltiazem and nitrendipine in single dialysed heart cells. *Nature* 1983;302:790-794.

53. Hariman RJ, Mangiardi LM, McAllister RG, et al. Reversal of the cardiovascular effects of verapamil by calcium and sodium: Differences between electrophysiologic and hemodynamic responses. *Circulation* 1979;59:797-804.

54. Lang J, Timour-Chah Q, El Chebly M, et al. Effect of gradual rise in plasma calcium concentration on the impairment of atrioventricular nodal conduction due to verapamil. *J Cardiovasc Pharmacol* 1986;8:6-13.

55. Vanhoutte PM. The Expert Committee of the World Health Organization on Classification of Calcium Antagonists: The viewpoint of the rapporteur. *Am J Cardiol* 1987;59:3A-8A.

56. Nayler WG, Dillon JS, Daly MJ. Cellular sites of action of calcium antagonists and β-adrenoceptor blockers. In: Opie LH, ed. *Calcium antagonists and cardiovascular disease*. New York: Raven Press, 1984, 181-191.

57. Godfraind T. Classification of calcium antagonists. *Am J Cardiol* 1987;59:11B-23B.

58. Opie LH, Davey DA. Biological membranes in hypertension: Is control of intracellular calcium and other ions mediated by a membrane defect. *Ann NY Acad Sci* 1987; 488:154-173.

59. Hermsmeyer RK, Sturek M, Rusch NJ. Calcium channel modulation by dihydropyridine calcium antagonists in vascular muscle. *Ann NY Acad Sci* 1988;522:25-31.

60. Finkel AS, Hirst GDS, van Helden DF. Some properties of excitatory junction currents recorded from submucosal arterioles of guinea-pig ileum. *J Physiol* 1984;351:87-98.

61. Chiu AT, McCall DE, Thoolen MJMC, et al. Ca^{++} utilization in the constriction of rat aorta to full and partial α_1-adrenoceptor agonists. *J Pharmacol Exp Ther* 1986;238: 224-231.

62. Beckeringh JJ, Michel MC, Brodde O-E. The hydrolysis of phosphatidylinositol as a measure of the efficacy of alpha-adrenoceptor agonists in rat aorta. Presentation to NY Acad Sci, Feb 1987.

63. Ruffolo RR Jr., Nichols AJ. The relationship of receptor reserve and agonist efficacy to the sensitivity of α-adrenoceptor-mediated vasopressor responses to inhibition by calcium channel antagonists. *Ann NY Acad Sci* 1988; 522:361–376.

64. Folkow B, Hallback M, Jones JV, et al. Dependence on external calcium for the noradrenaline contractility of the resistance vessels in spontaneously hypertensive and renal hypertensive rats, as compared with normotensive controls. *Acta Physiol Scand* 1977;1:84-97.

65. Adelstein RS, Eisenberg E. Regulation and kinetics of the actin-myosin-ATP interaction. *Ann Rev Biochem* 1980;49: 921-956.

66. Rapaport RM, Murad F. Endothelium-dependent and nitrovasodilator-induced relaxation of vascular smooth muscle: role of cyclic GMP. *J Cycl Nucl Prot Phosphoryl Res* 1983;9:281-296.

67. Rapaport RM, Draznin MB, Murad F. Endothelium-dependent relaxation in rat aorta may be mediated through cyclic GMP-dependent protein dephosphorylation. *Nature* 1983;306:174-176.

68. Murphy RA, Gerthoffer WT. Cell calcium and contractile system regulation in arterial smooth muscle. In: Opie LH, ed. *Calcium antagonists and cardiovascular disease*. New York: Raven Press, 1984, 75-84.

69. Mras S. Effects of calcium on stress and myosin phosphorylation in swine carotid media. *J Cardiovasc Pharmacol* 1986;8(Suppl 8): S80-S84.

70. Ljung B. Vascular selectivity of felodipine. *Drugs* 1985;29 (Suppl 2):46-58.

71. Chaffman M, Brogden RN. Diltiazem: A review of its pharmacological properties and therapeutic efficacy. *Drugs* 1985;29:387-454.

72. Winslow E, Martorana M, Jones DNC, et al. Do calmodulin antagonists exert significant electrophysiological effects? Presentation to NY Acad Sci, Feb 1987.

73. Mannhold R. Calmodulin antagonistic actions of Ca antagonists. Presentation to NY Acad Sci, Feb 1987.

74. Bostrom S-L, Ljung B, Mardh S, et al. Interaction of the

antihypertensive drug felodipine with calmodulin. *Nature* 1981;292:777-778.

75. Walsh MP. Effects of felodipine (a dihydropyridine calcium channel blocker) and analogues on calmodulin-dependent enzymes. Presentation to NY Acad Sci, Feb 1987.

76. Quinn P, Briscoe MG, Nuttall A, et al. Species variation in arterial-myocardial sensitivity to verapamil. *Cardiovasc Res* 1981;15:398-403.

77. Winniford MD, Fulton KL, Corbett JR, et al. Propranolol-verapamil versus propranolol-nifedipine in severe angina pectoris of effort: a randomized, double-blind crossover study. *Am J Cardiol* 1985;55:281-285.

78. Joshi PI, Dalal JJ, Ruttley MSJ, et al. Nifedipine and left ventricular function in beta-blocked patients. *Br Heart J* 1982;45:457-459.

79. Millard RW, Lathrop DA, Grupp G, et al. Differential cardiovascular effects of calcium channel blocking agents: potential mechanisms. *Am J Cardiol* 1982;49:499-506.

80. Iijima T, Yanagisawa T, Taira N. Increase in the slow inward current by intracellularly applied nifedipine and nicardipine in single ventricular cells of the guinea-pig heart. *J Mol Cell Cardiol* 1984;16:1175-1177.

81. Henry P, Borda L, Schuchleib R. Chronotropic and inotropic effects of vasodilators. In: Lichtlen PR, Kimaur E, Taira N, eds. *International Adalat panel discussion.* Amsterdam: Excerpta Medica, 1979, 14-21.

82. Porter CB, Walsh RA, Badke FR, et al. Differential effects of diltiazem and nitroprusside on left ventricular function in experimental chronic volume overload. *Circulation* 1983;68:685-692.

83. Krebs R. Adverse effects with calcium antagonists. *Hypertension* 1983;5(Suppl 2):125-129.

84. Smith HJ, Goldstein RA, Griffith JM. Regional contractility. Selective depression of ischemic myocardium by verapamil. *Circ Res* 1975;54:629-635.

85. Lumley P, Robertson MJ. Experimental conditions can differentially affect calcium channel blocker potency in guinea-pig cardiac muscle. Presentation to NY Acad Sci, Feb 1987.

86. Schwartz A, Grupp G, Millard RW, et al. Calcium channel blockers: possible mechanisms of protective effects on the ischemic myocardium. *Am Physiol Soc* 1981;191-210.

87. Nayler WG, Grau A, Slade A. A protective effect of verapamil on hypoxic heart muscle. *Cardiovasc Res* 1976;10: 650-662.

88. Ruiz-Ceretti E, Zumino AP, Schanne OF. Effects of TTX and verapamil on the upstroke components of the action potential from the atrioventricular node of the rabbit. *J Mol Cell Cardiol* 1978;10:95-107.

89. Iijima T, Taira N. Effects of manganese ions and diltiazem on the spontaneous action potential of the canine atrioventricular node cell. *J Mol Cell Cardiol* 1983;15:863-866.

90. Weiss AT, Lewis BS, Halon DA, et al. The use of calcium with verapamil in the management of supraventricular tachyarrhythmias. *Int J Cardiol* 1983;4:275-280.

91. Singh BN, Nademanee K. Use of calcium antagonists for cardiac arrhythmias. *Am J Cardiol* 1987;59:153B-162B.

92. Rowland E, McKenna WJ, Gulker H, et al. Comparative effects of diltiazem and verapamil on atrioventricular conduction and atrioventricular reentry tachycardia. *Circ Res* 1983;52(Suppl 1): 163-168.

93. Bauer JH, Reams G. Short- and long-term effects of calcium entry blockers on the kidney. *Am J Cardiol* 1987; 59:66A-71A.

94. Landmark K. Antihypertensive and metabolic effects of long-term therapy with nifedipine slow-release tablets. *J Cardiovasc Pharmacol* 1985;7:12-17.

95. Loutzenhier R, Epstein M, Horton C. Inhibition by diltiazem of pressure-induced afferent vasoconstriction in the isolated perfused rat kidney. *Am J Cardiol* 1987;59:72A-75A.

96. Isshiki T, Amodeo C, Messerli FH, et al. Diltiazem maintains renal vasodilation without hyperfiltration in hypertension: Studies in essential hypertensive man and the spontaneously hypertensive rat. *Cardiovasc Drugs Ther*, 1987;1:359-366.

97. Guazzi MD, De Cesare N, Galli C, et al. Calcium-channel blockade with nifedipine and angiotensin converting enzyme inhibition with captopril in the therapy of patients with severe primary hypertension. *Circulation* 1984;70:279-284.

98. Muiesan G, Agabiti-Rosei E, Castellano M, et al. Antihypertensive and humoral effects of verapamil and nifedipine in essential hypertension. *J Cardiovasc Pharmacol* 1982;4:S325-S329.

99. Lijnen P, Fagard R, Amery A. The acute hemodynamic and humoral responses to felodipine and metoprolol in mild hypertension. Presentation to NY Acad Sci, Feb 1987.

100. Agabiti-Rosei E, Muiesan ML, Romanelli G, et al. Similarities and differences in the antihypertensive effect of two calcium antagonist drugs, verapamil and nifedipine. *J Am Coll Cardiol* 1986;7:916-924.

101. Kiowski W, Erne P, Bertel O, et al. Acute and chronic sympathetic reflex activation and antihypertensive response to nifedipine. *J Am Coll Cardiol* 1986;7:344-348.

102. Muiesan G, Agabiti-Rosei E, Romanelli G. Adrenergic activity and left ventricular function during treatment of essential hypertension with calcium antagonists. *Am J Cardiol* 1986;57:44D-49D.

103. Nayler WG, Sturrock WJ. An inhibitory effect of verapamil and diltiazem on the release of noradrenaline from ischaemic and reperfused hearts. *J Mol Cell Cardiol* 1983;16:331-344.

104. Hiramatsu K, Yamagishi F, Kubota T, et al. Acute effects of the calcium antagonist, nifedipine, on blood pressure, pulse rate, and the renin-angiotensin-aldosterone system in patients with essential hypertension. *Am Heart J* 1982;104:1346-1350.

105. Marone C, Luisoli S, Bomio F, et al. Body sodium-blood volume state, aldosterone, and cardiovascular responsiveness after calcium entry blockade with nifedipine. *Kidney International* 1985;28:658-665.

106. Rojdmark S, Andersson DEH. Influence of verapamil on human glucose tolerance. *Am J Cardiol* 1986;57:39D-43D.

107. Ravens KG. Effect of nifedipine on glucose tolerance in man. In: Lichtlen PR, ed. *6th International Adalat Symposium*. Amsterdam: Excerpta Medica, 1986, 367-371.

108. Daniels AR, Opie LH. Effect of slow-release nifedipine on glucose tolerance. In: Lichtlen PR, ed. *6th International Adalat Symposium*. Amsterdam: Excerpta Medica, 1986, 495-496.

109. Murphy MB, Scriven AJI, Dollery CT. Role of nifedipine in treatment of hypertension. *Br Med J* 1983;287:257-259.

110. Rademaker M, Thomas RM, Kirby JD, et al. Effect of nifedipine on haemostasis, clotting and thrombolysis in vitro in healthy volunteers. *Ann NY Acad Sci* 1987, in press.

111. Hiroki T, Morishita Y, Inoue T, et al. Effect of nifedipine on platelet aggregation response to exercise in patients with ischaemic heart disease. In: Lichtlen PR, ed. *6th International Adalat Symposium.* Amsterdam: Excerpta Medica, 1986, 504-507.

112. Palermo A, Bertalero B, Costantini C, et al. The effect of verapamil on platelet function. In: Fleckenstein A, Laragh JH, eds. *Hypertension—the next decade: Verapamil in focus.* London: Churchill Livingstone, 1987, 292-297.

113. Van Meel JCA, de Jonge A, Kalleman HO, et al. Vascular smooth muscle contraction initiated by postsynaptic alpha$_2$-adrenoceptor activation is induced by an influx of extracellular calcium. *Eur J Pharmacol* 1981;69:205-208.

114. Van Zwieten PA, van Meel CA, Timmermans BMWM. Functional interaction between calcium antagonists and the vasoconstriction by the stimulation of postsynaptic α_2-adrenoceptors. *Circ Res* 1983;52 (Suppl I):77-80.

115. Nayler WG, Poole-Wilson P. Calcium antagonists: Definition and mode of action. *Basic Res Cardiol* 1981;76:1-15.

116. Lathrop DA, Valle-Aguilera JR, Millard RW, et al. Myocardial tissue. *Am J Cardiol* 1982;49:613-620.

117. Thandroyen FT. Protective action of calcium channel antagonist agents against ventricular fibrillation in isolated perfused rat heart. *J Mol Cell Cardiol* 1982;14:21-32.

118. Thandroyen FT, Higginson L, Opie LH, et al. The influence of verapamil and its isomers on vulnerability to ventricular fibrillation during acute myocardial ischemia and adrenergic stimulation in isolated rat heart. *J Mol Cell Cardiol* 1986;18:645-649.

119. Osterrieder W. Inhibition of the fast Na$^+$ inward current by the Ca^{2+} channel blocker tiapamil. *J Cardiovasc Pharmacol* 1986;8:1101-1106.

120. Opie LH. Calcium ions, drug action and the heart—with special reference to calcium antagonist drugs. *Pharmac Ther* 1984;25:271-295.

121. International Society and Federation of Cardiology Working Group. Classification of calcium antagonists for cardiovascular diseases. *Am J Cardiol* 1987;60:630-632.

122. Fleckenstein A. Specific pharmacology of calcium in myocardium, cardiac pacemakers, and vascular smooth muscle. *Ann Rev Pharmacol Toxicol* 1977;17:149-166.

123. Himori N, Ono H, Taira N. Simultaneous assessment of effects of coronary vasodilators on the coronary blood flow and the myocardial contractility by using the blood-perfused canine papillary muscle. *Japan J Pharmacol* 1976;26:427-435.

124. Kawai C, Konishi T, Matsuyama E, et al. Comparative effects of three calcium antagonists, diltiazem, verapamil and nifedipine, on the sinoatrial and atrioventricular nodes. *Circulation* 1981;63:1035-1042.

125. Narimatsu A, Taira N. Effects on atrioventricular conduction of calcium antagonistic coronary vasodilators, local anaesthetics and quinidine injected into the posterior and the anterior septal artery of the atrioventricular node preparation of the dog. *Naunyn-Schmiedeberg's Arch Pharmacol* 1976;294:169-177.

126. Ono H, Hashimoto K. Ca^{2+} antagonism in various parameters of cardiac function including coronary dilation with the use of nifedipine, perhexiline and verapamil. In: Winbury MM, Abiko Y, eds. *Ischemic myocardium and antiangial drugs.* New York: Raven Press, 1979, 77-88.

127. Motulsky HJ, Snavely MD, Hughes RJ, et al. Interaction of verapamil and other calcium channel blockers with α_1- and α_2-adrenergic receptors. *Circ Res* 1983;52:226-231.

128. Karliner JS, Motulsky HJ, Dunlap J, et al. Verapamil competitively inhibits α_1-adrenergic and muscarinic but not β-adrenergic receptors in rat myocardium. *J Cardiovasc Pharmacol* 1982;4:515-520.

129. Corr PB, Sharma AD. Alpha-adrenergic mediated effects on myocardial calcium. In: Opie LH, ed. *Calcium antagonists and cardiovascular disease.* New York: Raven Press, 1984, 193-204.

130. Nayler WG, Thompson JE, Jarrott B. The interaction of calcium antagonists (slow channel blockers) with myocardial alpha adrenoceptors. *J Mol Cell Cardiol* 1982;14:185-188.

131. Opie LH, Maseri A. Vasospastic angina. In: Krebs R, ed. *Treatment of cardiovascular disease by Adalat* (nifedipine). Stuttgart: Schattauer, 1986, 231-258.

CALCIUM CHANNEL ANTAGONISTS: PART II: USE AND COMPARATIVE PROPERTIES OF THE THREE PROTOTYPICAL CALCIUM ANTAGONISTS IN ISCHEMIC HEART DISEASE, INCLUDING RECOMMENDATIONS BASED ON AN ANALYSIS OF 41 TRIALS

SUMMARY. An analysis of 41 trials of angina of all varieties confirms that calcium antagonists are an important advance and are now established therapy for these syndromes. In effort angina, verapamil in a dose of 360–480 mg daily is better than propranolol in standard doses. Although nifedipine is highly effective against vasospastic angina, its use in threatened myocardial infarction or severe unstable angina is not supported by recent studies, unless combined with a beta-blocker. Diltiazem has recently been tested with apparent benefit in non-Q-wave myocardial infarction. Otherwise, these calcium antagonist agents all seem to have approximate equipotency in clinical ischemic syndromes including effort and vasospastic angina. Subjective side effects seem most troublesome in the case of nifedipine. All three calcium antagonists, especially nifedipine, have been successfully combined with beta-blocker therapy, yet occasional additive negative inotropic or chronotropic or dromotropic interactions may occur when verapamil or diltiazem is added to beta-blockade, and occasionally the direct negative inotropic potential of nifedipine may become evident. The choice between the calcium antagonists is determined not only by the clinical picture but also by the anticipated side effects in a given patient and by the overall cardiovascular status. In patients with supraventricular tachycardias or sinus tachycardia, verapamil or diltiazem is preferred, whereas in patients with a resting bradycardia or borderline heart failure nifedipine is likely to be chosen.

The *major clinical indications* for calcium antagonists remain angina pectoris and the related ischemic syndromes, hypertension, and (for the use-dependent agents) supraventricular tachycardias. The first of these indications will be considered in this article together with a brief consideration of the mechanism of action of the calcium antagonists in each ischemic syndrome. In Part III of this review, hypertension and arrhythmias will be discussed, as well as a number of *lesser indications,* including acute myocardial infarction (AMI), obstructive cardiomyopathy, congestive heart failure, pulmonary hypertension, Raynaud's phenomenon, cerebral insuf-

70

ficiency, subarachnoid hemorrhage, peripheral vascular disease, bronchospasm, and migraine. Part IV will focus on drug side-effects and interactions, and Part V on new calcium antagonists.

Mechanisms and Experimental Background (Table II-1, Figure II-1)

The chief mechanisms proposed for the antianginal effects of calcium antagonists vary among verapamil, nifedipine, and diltiazem and include: 1) coronary vasodilation; 2), decreased myocardial oxygen demand (decreased afterload, a decreased heart rate, and a negative inotropic effect); 3) a favorable redistribution of blood flow to the ischemic areas; and 4) a "direct" cellular anti-ischemic effect.

Coronary vasodilation and increased oxygen supply. Because the calcium antagonists are coronary vasodilators, they are especially effective when coronary spasm or vasoconstriction is the cause of myocardial ischemia. Likewise, when spasm is added to organic stenosis to create "dynamic stenosis," then calcium antagonists should also relieve the ischemia. Various degrees of coronary spasm may also be invoked by exercise, so that coronary dilation may relieve exercise-induced angina. Experimentally, when exercise-induced coronary vasoconstriction is relieved by calcium antagonists, blood flow increases to the subendocardial zones [1].

Decreased myocardial oxygen demand. Calcium antagonists influence three of the determinants of the myocardial oxygen uptake. First, the afterload is reduced as peripheral vasodilation brings down the blood pressure. Second, some agents (especially diltiazem and in some studies verapamil) reduce the heart rate, whereas nifedipine may increase the heart rate.

Table II-1. Hemodynamic mechanisms for antianginal effect of calcium antagonists

	Verapamil	Nifedipine	Diltiazem
Afterload reduction (BP $\downarrow$)	+	+ +	+
Heart rate fall	0,+	0	+
Rate-pressure fall	+,±	0,±	+ +
Negative inotropic effect	+,+ +	0	±
Coronary vasodilation	+	+,+ +	+
Altered diastolic properties	+	+	+

Abbreviations: BP, blood pressure; + +, major effect; +, effect; ±, borderline effect; 0, no effect.

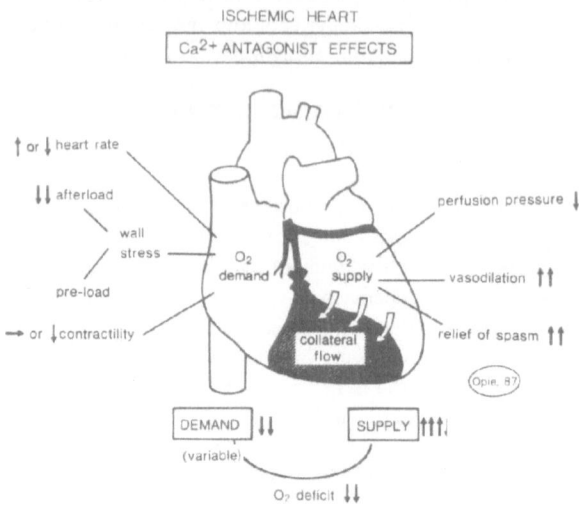

ISCHEMIC HEART

Ca²⁺ ANTAGONIST EFFECTS

Fig. Fig. II-1. Possible beneficial mechanisms of calcium antagonists on the ischemic heart. Note major role for coronary vasodilation and/or relief of spasm.

Third, there may be a direct negative inotropic effect to reduce the oxygen demand, evident especially in the case of verapamil.

Effect on models of myocardial infarction or regional ischemia. When considering the possible protection by calcium antagonists against regional ischemia, it is striking that the majority of studies showing myocardial protection relate to experiments in which calcium antagonists were given before coronary occlusion and not after [1,2]. There are, however, many exceptions to this rule[3] so that generalizations are not always possible. In all, it seems that these drugs have only a modest effect in limiting infarct size and may be most effective when the ischemic zone is small and the collateral flow adequate, as well as when there is early reperfusion [3]. In all these studies (Table II-2), the effects of calcium antagonists could be explained by the postulated favorable effects on the oxygen supply-demand equation.

Decreased reperfusion injury. During the reperfusion period after myocardial ischemia, there is a vigorous uptake of calcium by the myocardium which can become calcium overloaded. Part of this excessive uptake is susceptible to calcium antagonists [4], whereas part is not. The calcium antagonists act by basically limiting ischemic damage which in turn decreases the severity of reperfusion [5,6].

A "direct" cellular anti-ischemic effect. Whether, in addition to hemodynamic benefits, the calcium antagonists "directly" protect against ischemia is not clear. For example, work on hypoxic isolated guinea pig papillary muscle [7] shows that perfusion with verapamil has a direct protective effect. Isolated mitochondria from ischemic rabbit hearts are better functioning than those from ischemic hearts not pretreated by verapamil [4]. However, many such data can be explained by a negative inotropic effect of verapamil and, in the case of in vivo experiments, beneficial effects of pretreatment on the double-product. Table II-2 lists studies in which an additional protective effect was found which was not explicable by changes in the myocardial oxygen supply-demand ratio. In each case the "protective" dose was well above the therapeutic free blood levels in humans (compare with Table I-3, Part I).

However, where dose-response curves were undertaken in only a few studies so that the efficacy of the calcium antagonists at concentrations corresponding to the levels therapeutically effective in humans cannot be excluded unless specifically searched for. Watts et al. [8] varied verapamil from 7.5×10^{-8} to 2×10^{-6} M in experiments on the isolated ischemic rat heart and found improved function on reperfusion. Nifedipine 3×10^{-8} M started to have some protective effect in the rat heart with subtotal global ischemia followed by reperfusion [9], but a much better effect was found at 3×10^{-7} M nifedipine. In a coronary-ligated isolated working rat heart model of regional ischemia and developing infarction, 10^{-7} M nifedipine or diltiazem was required to reduce enzyme release. In such experiments with regional ischemia, it is impossible to exclude minor but critical redistribution of myocardial blood flow, unless specifically excluded.

In general, the concentrations of calcium antagonists with "direct" antihypoxic or anti-ischemic effects (see Table II-2) are well above the therapeutic levels in humans (around 10^{-8} M; see Table I-3 in Part I). Thus, the mechanisms for the antianginal effects of these agents, which will be discussed separately for each, should first be sought in favorable alterations in the myocardial oxygen supply-demand ratio, including calcium antagonist-induced coronary vasodilation and afterload reduction.

Chronic Stable Effort Angina

Angina is conventionally seen as an imbalance between the oxygen demand and supply. The benefit of beta-blockers is predominantly mediated by a reduc-

Table II-2. Protective concentrations of calcium antagonists in isolated heart preparations rendered ischemic ($\pm$ reperfusion) or hypoxic

Author	Drug	Effective Concentration	Preparation	Result
Yoon et al. [176]	Verapamil	10^{-6} M	Dog; cross-clamp Ischemia and cardioplegia	Improved mitochondrial respiration
Nayler et al. [7]	Verapamil	$1-2 \times 10^{-6}$ M	Perfused rabbit heart; hypoxic	Decreased hypoxic damage, no change in tissue Ca^{2+}
Bourdillon and Poole-Wilson [177]	Verapamil	2×10^{-6} M	Rabbit septum, 32°C, total ischemia and reperfusion	Verapamil decreased Ca^{2+} gain only if given preischemia. Acts by reduced cardiac work.
Bersohn and Shine [178]	Verapamil	5×10^{-7} M	Perfused rabbit heart. Maximum coronary dilation by dipyridamole.	Protection during ischemia and reperfusion only if given preischemia. Acts by reduced cardiac contractility.

Watts et al. [8]	Verapamil	7.5×10^{-8} M -2×10^{-6} M	Ischemic rat heart reperfused	ATP higher and function better
Henry et al. [179]	Nifedipine	10^{-7} M	Perfused rabbit heart	Prevention of ischemic contracture
Nayler [6]	Nifedipine	10^{-7} M	Perfused hypothermic rabbit heart	Improved postischemic recovery additive to hypothermia
De Jong et al. [9]	Nifedipine	3×10^{-8} M -3×10^{-7} M	Rat heart. Subtotal global ischemia with reperfusion.	Nifedipine reduces purine and lactate release in ischemia. Conserves ATP. Best effects at 3×10^{-7} M.
Cheung et al. [180]	Nifedipine Verapamil	10^{-6} M 10^{-6} M	Paced hypoxic cardiac myocytes	Protection achieved by inhibition of contractile activity
Weishaar and Bing [5]	Diltiazem	4×10^{-7} M	Working rat heart, global ischemia and reperfusion	D added 5 min before reperfusion reduced damage
Hamm and Opie [181]	Verapamil Nifedipine Diltiazem	3×10^{-7} M 1×10^{-7} M 1×10^{-7} M	Isolated perfused coronary-ligated working rat heart	Decreased enzyme release; D improved LV work. Lower concentrations of V/D/N ineffective.

Abbreviations: ATP, adenosine triphosphate; D, diltiazem; N, nifedipine; V, verapamil.

tion of the oxygen demand, whereas calcium antagonists chiefly increase the oxygen supply. However, calcium antagonists have additional modes of action, including peripheral vasodilation with afterload reduction (especially in the case of nifedipine) and a negative inotropic effect (especially in the case of verapamil).

Verapamil for Effort Angina

It is sometimes forgotten that the initial use of verapamil was in effort angina [10,11]. However, there were few double-blind control studies done until Sandler et al. [12] and Livesley et al. [13] compared verapamil with propranolol and found that 120 to 360 mg verapamil daily was the approximate equivalent of propranolol 300 mg daily. The same dose of verapamil (360 mg) is also the approximate equivalent of metoprolol 200 mg two times daily [14] or nifedipine 60 mg daily [15]. Several other studies attest to the benefits of verapamil in angina pectoris [16–21].

Verapamil compared with propranolol. (Table II-3). Six double-blind and one single-blind randomized studies on 117 patients are reviewed (see Table II-3). Taking into account dose variations, ten comparisons are possible. These comparisons are markedly dose-dependent. In four studies, high-dose verapamil (320 to 480 mg daily) was better than propranolol (240 to 320 mg). In four studies, verapamil (320 to 360 mg) was the equivalent of propranolol (255–320 mg). In two studies, low-dose verapamil (240 mg daily) was less effective than propranolol (160 to 300 mg). Indeed low-dose verapamil (240 mg) was either ineffective [22] or borderline benefit [13] when compared with placebo. The lowest dose of verapamil that might have antianginal efficacy on subjective symptoms but not electrocardiogram (EKG) parameters was 120 mg daily [12]. In all these studies, only propranolol caused withdrawal angina (2 of 22 patients) [23] and decreased vital capacity [22]. On the other hand, only high-dose verapamil caused symptomatic atrioventricular (AV) (1 of 14 patients) [24]. According to these analyses, verapamil might be given in a dose of at least 360 mg daily to achieve objective benefit in angina pectoris. At a higher dose of 480 mg/day, verapamil is more effective than propranolol at the possible risk of increased verapamil side effects, chiefly rhythm disturbances [24] and congestive heart failure [25]. It should be noted that the dose of 360 mg daily was also used by Khurmi and Raftery [26] in their open-label study extending over 4 months, whereas the studies with high-dose verapamil (480 mg daily) were only for 48 hours [24] or 1 week [23].

Verapamil plus propranolol. Hemodynamically this combination is quite acceptable provided that due care is taken for the possible added negative inotropic, chronotropic, and dromotropic effects [20,24]. Antianginal effects are more marked than with either agent acting singly [20,27–29]. In patients not responding optimally to propranolol alone (mean dose 255 mg), the addition of verapamil 360 or 480 mg has equal benefit. However, the combination of verapamil 360 mg daily and atenolol 100 mg daily, although improving antianginal control when compared with either agent singly, caused 4 of 15 patients to withdraw from a recent double-blind trial [29]. Therefore the combination verapamil–beta-blocker should be undertaken only with care and probably only in hospitalized patients. The possible hemodynamic dangers of the significant negative inotropic and chronotropic effects of verapamil when added to beta-blockers have been outlined in an acute study in which 40-, 80-, or 120-mg doses of verapamil were given orally to 15 patients with angina pectoris already receiving high doses of propranolol or metoprolol [30].

Mechanism of verapamil effect in effort angina. First, the rate-pressure product (which increases during exercise and is an index of the myocardial oxygen demand) usually falls. The hypotensive effect of verapamil reduces the afterload and double-product during exercise [31,32], especially when the heart rate also falls as in some studies [20]. However, the double-product can be unchanged even when verapamil has an antianginal effect [14]. Furthermore, when compared with propranolol, verapamil alters the double-product less [33], so that another mechanism must be sought to explain in full the antianginal effect of verapamil. Second, the prominent negative inotropic effect of verapamil should also decrease myocardial oxygen demand [24], yet in practice afterload reduction may balance this myocardial effect [33] unless intrinsic left ventricular (LV) function is severely reduced by disease. When the negative inotropic effect is elicited in experiments, it protects the ischemic myocardium [34]. The preferential action of verapamil on the ischemic as opposed to the nonischemic myocardium [35] enhances its negative inotropic effect relative to nifedipine [36]. Third, verapamil is a coronary vasodilator, although the increase in vascular diameter may be only modest and about half of that obtained by nitroglycerin [37]. During exercise a relative increase in coronary vascular tone may occur [38] so that coronary dilation during exercise could be of more importance than at rest. Fourth, Apstein and Grossman [39] have recently emphasized that an increased diastolic stiffness is an early change in angina pectoris.

Table II-3. Comparative effects of verapamil and β-blockade in one single-blind and six double-blind trials in chronic effort angina

Author	Trial Design	Patients (n)	Drug Test Period	Verapamil (V) Daily Dose	Propranolol (P) or Atenolol (A) Daily Dose	End-point	Result
Sandler et al. [12]	Pl, Seq, R, DB	16 No WOut	28 days	120 or 360 mg	P 300 mg	Clin, ex	V 360 = P 300
Livesley et al. [13]	Pl, Seq, R, DB	32 No WOut	28 days	240 or 360 mg	P 300 mg	Clin, ex	V 240 < P 300, V 360 = P 300
Leon et al. [24]	Pl, SB, R, CO	11 WOut	2 days	320 or 480 mg	P 100–320 mg (mean 225)	Clin, ex	V 320 = P 255, V 480 < P 255, V + P = best
Johnson et al. [22]	Pl, DB, R, CO, WOut	18	7 days	240 or 360 mg	P 160 or 240 mg	Clin, ex, Holter, radio	V 240 < P 160, V 360 > P 240
Sadick et al.	Pl, DB, Seq, R, L², no WOut	18	21 days	320 mg	P 320 mg	Ex, radio	V 320 = P 320

Frishman et al. [23]	Pl, DB, R, CO, WOut	20	7 days	240, 360, 480 mg	P 60, 160, 320 mg	Clin, ex	V 480 > P 320
Subramanian [20]	Pl, run-in, DB, CO, no WOut	22	28 days	360 mg	P 240 mg	Ex, Holter	V 360 > P 240
Findlay et al. [29]	Pl, R, DB, L^2, no WOut	11	21 days	360 mg	A 100 mg	Clin, ex, radio	V 360 = A 100 A + V best

Abbreviations: CO, crossover; DB, double-blinded; L^2, Latin square; Pl, placebo control; R, randomized; SB, single-blinded; Seq, sequential design; WOut, washout between active drug treatment phases.

V = P means that the clinical benefits are roughly comparable, for daily dose given in mg.

V > P means that V had more benefits than P.

Clin equals attacks of pain, nitroglycerin usage.

Ex equals formal exercise testing on treadmill or bicycle.

Holter equals Holter ambulatory monitoring for ST segment shifts.

Radio equals radionuclide left ventricular function by multigate pooled technique.

Verapamil can improve LV diastolic filling [40] and enhance early relaxation [41], thereby having another potential antianginal mechanism, while leaving LV systolic function unchanged.

Nifedipine for Effort Angina

The antianginal efficacy of nifedipine monotherapy has been shown both during acute and chronic administration. After one single oral dose of 10 or 20 mg nifedipine, the exercise time improves after 30 min [42] and the effect lasts for at least 3 and possibly 6 hours [43,44]. The effect of nifedipine in effort angina is considerably reduced in patients who smoke [45] which may have confounded some of the long-term studies. In contrast, nifedipine relieves coronary vasoconstriction induced by smoking [46].

During chronic studies, nifedipine 60 mg daily compared well with placebo, rendering 29% of patients angina-free and prolonging exercise time by 39% [20]. Nifedipine 10 mg three times daily reduced the anginal attacks and nitroglycerin usage; doubling the dose was not much more effective according to Sherman and Liang [47] nor according to Lynch et al. [48] who used complex ambulatory monitoring techniques. In another placebo-controlled crossover and parallel study [49], nifedipine 30 mg reduced anginal attacks and nitroglycerin use, but upward titration to a mean dose of 51 mg daily also prolonged exercise time. However, one-tailed p values were used, lessening the statistical force of the data.

Nifedipine compared with or combined with β-blockade. (Table II-4). Nifedipine has been compared with β-blockade in five studies on 128 patients, in three of which there was a crossover design and in two, randomization by the Latin square pattern. In three studies, the beta-blocker was propranolol and in one each atenolol or metoprolol. In three of the five trials, the beta-blocker was "better" than nifedipine, including the trial of Uusitalo et al. [50] on 54 patients. In one small trial [51], nifedipine seemed to be the equivalent of atenolol but a type II error may be evident because the mean results in every case favor atenolol. In only one trial (Higginbotham et al. [52] using the highest daily dose of nifedipine with a mean daily dose of 83 mg) was nifedipine equal to or better than propranolol; however, nifedipine side effects were common and found in 15 of 21 patients. In an acute study, Chaitman et al. [44] showed that a single dose of 20 mg nifedipine was better than low-dose propranolol (80 mg daily) or 0.6 mg sublingual nitroglycerin. However, in patients chronically dosed, nifedipine 60 mg/day was less effective than prop-

Table II-4. Comparative effects of nifedipine and β-blockers in chronic effort angina

Author	Trial Design	Patients (n)	Drug Test Period	Daily dose of Nifedipine (N)	Daily dose of Propranolol (P) or Metoprolol (M) or Atenolol (A)	End-point	Result
Lynch et al. [48]	Pl, R, DB, L^2	16	4 weeks	30–60 mg	P 240–480 mg	Clin	N 60 < P 480. N + P seemed best.
Kenmure and Scruton [182]	Pl, DB, CO, no WOut	21	2 weeks	30 mg	P 240 mg	Clin	N 30 < P 240. N + P best.
Higginbotham et al. [52]	Pl, R, SB, N titration, DB with CO, no WOut	21	5 weeks	30–90 mg (mean dose 83 mg)	P 240 mg	Clin, radio	N 90 = P 240.
Uusitalo et al. [50]	No Pl, R, DB, CO, no WOut	54	3 weeks	30 mg	M 200 mg	Clin, ex	N 30 < M 200. N + M best.
Findlay et al. [51]	Pl, DB, R, L^2, no WOut	16	12 weeks	60 mg	A 100 mg	Clin, ex, radio	N 60 = A 100, N + A = best
Acute study Chaitman et al. [44]	Pl, R, DB, WOut	15	Acute	20 mg single dose	P 80 mg single dose	Ex	N > P (time to angina, work)

Abbreviations: As in Table II-3; EKG, electrocardiogram.

ranolol 240 or 480 mg/day [48]. Likewise, nifedipine 20 mg three times daily was also somewhat less effective than atenolol 100 mg daily [51]. Finally, nifedipine 30 mg daily was less effective than metoprolol 200 mg daily [50]. In every case, however, the combination of nifedipine with beta-blocker appeared to be more effective in prevention of angina.

Provocation of angina by nifedipine. Nifedipine may provoke ischemia [53]. In the large open-label study of Stone et al. [54], between 10 and 20% of patients with refractory exertional angina had an increase in attack frequency and this increase was especially found in patients without features of coronary spasm. In the double-blind study of Subramanian et al. [19], 4 of 32 patients complained of chest pain and palpitations after 20 mg nifedipine. To avoid ischemic chest pain requires careful dose-titration [20,55]. In a retrospective review of over 3,000 patients with angina (mostly stable effort angina), Terry [56] found exaggeration of angina by nifedipine in only about 1% of the population: however, there is no information on the number of patients dropping out after an adverse effect such as chest pain experienced after the first dose.

Mechanisms for antianginal effect of nifedipine. The effects of nifedipine on effort angina are very complex and governed in part by 1) the extent of afterload reduction, variable from patient to patient; 2) the extent of reflex tachycardia, more marked during the acute than chronic phases of nifedipine administration [57]; 3) the contribution of coronary artery spasm and "dynamic stenosis" to the symptom of angina; 4) the risk of "coronary steal" with production of ischemic chest pain; and 5) the coronary artery anatomy.

The independence of the antianginal effect of nifedipine from the *rate-pressure product* during exercise, an index of myocardial oxygen demand, is shown in the study of Chaitman et al. [44] in which nifedipine 20 mg increased the rate-pressure product but also increased the work that could be undertaken. The increase in the rate-pressure product was due to a modest increase in the heart rate. In other studies too [43,52], nifedipine gave pain relief without a change in the rate-pressure product.

The *reflex tachycardia* can cause either an absolute [58] or a relative increase in the myocardial oxygen consumption which can be prevented either by giving the nifedipine by the intracoronary route [59] or by concomitant β-blockade [60]. Yet sometimes the effect of nifedipine in reducing the blood pressure outweighs that in increasing the heart rate so that the rate-pressure product falls [47]. Why nifedipine frequently but not always increases the heart rate (see Table II-3; [61]) is not known, but may depend in part on the age of the patient and the status of the baroreceptor control mechanisms. Furthermore, during chronic dosing, nifedipine may cause little or no reflex tachycardia, especially when given for the therapy of hypertension [57] but also angina [19]. When the *heart rate* was controlled in pacing-induced angina [62], the striking result of nifedipine administration was a reduction of the blood pressure and thereby a reduction of the double-product. Taking together all the evidence, the variable effect on the double-product shows that not only the oxygen demand is decreased, but that other antianginal mechanisms must be at work, as in the case of verapamil (see Verapamil for Effort Angina, above). In the study of Sherman and Liang [47], there was evidence for nifedipine causing both an increased oxygen supply and a decreased oxygen demand. During submaximal exercise, there was less ST depression for a given double-product, suggesting an improved oxygen supply. On the other hand, there was a fall of systolic pressure at submaximal exercise, showing a decreased oxygen demand because the rate-pressure product for any given workload was less with nifedipine [47].

The myocardial oxygen supply may be improved by nifedipine. In patients with exercise-induced angina and with left anterior descending coronary artery disease [63], half the patients failed to respond to 20 mg nifedipine and in that group there was no change in the great coronary vein flow nor in the calculated anterior regional coronary resistance. In contrast, in patients who responded to nifedipine coronary venous flow increased, coronary resistance decreased and the duration of exercise lengthened. Normally exercise induces an increase in coronary tone; nifedipine may reduce this effect by coronary vasodilation [43]. Animal studies also support the concept that nifedipine relieves an exercise-induced increase in coronary tone [38]. Thus an improved myocardial oxygen supply is the most likely mechanism by which nifedipine may improve exercise capacity in patients with stable exertional angina. If nifedipine reduces the exercise-induced increase in coronary tone, presumably mediated by catecholamine release during exercise, that would explain why there is no consistent benefit in pacing-induced angina [64] or why there may in fact be an adverse effect [65].

The coronary artery anatomy may also influence the effects of nifedipine. When there is a single stenotic coronary artery, exercise testing 16 minutes after nifedipine shows an improvement (judged by ST segment depression), but if there is an occluded coronary artery with collaterals, there is no improvement after nifedipine [66]. These data suggest that nifedipine may be most effective either in relieving "dynamic stenosis" [67] or in improving myocardial collateral blood flow, or in reducing the increase of coronary tone induced by exercise [38,43]. *Improved myocardial diastolic stiffness,* as induced by angina, may be a further antianginal mechanism [41].

Diltiazem for Effort Angina

In three studies, 120 mg diltiazem given acutely improved parameters of angina. Wagniart et al. [68] showed that the time to peak exercise was increased by 29% 3 hours after the acute dose; during the submaximal period of exercise, the rate-pressure product fell showing a decreased oxygen demand. In a similar study, Chaitman et al. [44] showed that the exercise time increased by 31% and improved work capacity was still present 8 hours after 120 mg diltiazem. In a third study, 120 mg diltiazem given acutely improved the ejection fraction in patients with mild impairment of myocardial performance [69]. These acute benefits can be translated into sustained antianginal effects. In a double-blind randomized trial on 57 patients, Hossack et al. [70] found benefit with doses up to 240 mg/day. In other smaller studies, doses up to 360 mg/ day have been used with benefit [29,71-74]. In the study of Lindenberg et al. [72], anginal frequency was reduced more by high dose (360 mg/day) than by 240 mg/day; however even 120 mg/day was effective. A sustained antianginal effect was shown in an open-label study over 4 months (diltiazem 360 mg daily) by Khurmi and Raftery [26]. The antianginal benefit of this dose of diltiazem was prolonged for up to 52 weeks [75] with few side effects.

Diltiazem compared with or combined with propranolol. When compared with propranolol (Table II-5) in five studies on 108 patients, diltiazem 240 to 360 mg daily was the approximate equivalent of propranolol 240 to 360 mg daily, or in some studies was better. Two studies [44,69] were acute so that chronic benefit cannot be predicted. One study compared the addition of diltiazem to propranolol [27], leaving only four truly comparable studies. In all these studies, diltiazem was the equivalent of propranolol (mean dose 120 to 360 mg in these four studies), or possibly diltiazem was better in one study [71]. The combination diltiazem 360 mg with propranolol 240 mg daily appeared to produce excess bradycardia and hypotension, with little added benefit beyond that of high-dose diltiazem itself [71]. A lower dose of each agent in combination (diltiazem 240 mg daily, propranolol 160 mg daily) gave a good response with little excess bradycardia and few symptomatic side effects [27]. Johnston et al. [27] suggest propranolol-diltiazem for combined therapy rather than propranolol-nifedipine or propranolol-verapamil because of the "low incidence of adverse clinical effects."

Mechanism of angina relief by diltiazem. As in the case of verapamil and nifedipine, the exact mode of antianginal effect is not known. The mechanism may include enhanced performance of the ischemic myocardium and reduction of the heart rate and blood pressure with a reduced double product [69,71,76,77]. Improved oxygen delivery may play a role yet the major factor seems to be a reduction in the rate-pressure product [77]. In this way the antianginal mechanism would appear to differ from that of nifedipine.

Withdrawal of Calcium Antagonists in Effort Angina

Verapamil. In patients with stable effort angina, abrupt withdrawal of verapamil 480 mg daily can safely be undertaken without causing symptoms of angina, whereas propranolol 320 mg daily may not be so withdrawn (2 of 20 patients had severe aggravation of angina [23]). Likewise, in the Danish study, verapamil was safely stopped in postinfarct patients. However, none of these studies used ambulatory monitoring. Lahiri et al. [78] showed that verapamil withdrawal led to an increased heart rate with an increased number of asymptomatic episodes of ST deviations; symptomatic episodes only marginally increased (although at $p < 0.05$) and nitroglycerin usage was unchanged. These studies show: 1) that calcium antagonist withdrawal syndrome can be subtle and not readily clinically manifest and 2) that verapamil withdrawal is less dangerous than that of propranolol, yet should still be undertaken with care and the drug properly tapered off.

Nifedipine. Whether or not there is a true withdrawal syndrome with nifedipine is controversial. Leisten et al. [79] distinguished between 1) aggravation of the underlying disease on removal of the marked coronary and peripheral vasodilator effects of nifedipine, which means that caution should be observed and the withdrawal probably should be gradual; and 2) a true withdrawal syndrome with enhanced clinical features so that the disease process itself seems worse, as in the case of β-blockade withdrawal. Gott-

Table II-5. Comparative effects of diltiazem and β-blockade in chronic effort angina

Author	Trial Design	Patients (n)	Drug Test Period	Daily Dose of Diltiazem	Daily Dose of Propranolol	End-point	Result
Hung et al. [71]	PI, R, DB, L^2, no WOut	12	2 weeks	360 mg	P 240 mg	Ex, radio	D = P or D > P D + P = D
Strauss and Parisi [74]	PI(SB), R, DB, CO, WOut	24	2 weeks	360 mg	P 80-320 mg (mean 276)	Clin, ex	D = P; D + P best in about half
Johnson et al. [27]	PI(SB), R, DB, CO, no WOut	19	4 weeks	240 mg (with P)	P 160 mg	Clin, ex	P + D > P
Subramanian [20]	PI(SB), R, DB, CO, no WOut	29	2 weeks	180-360 mg	P 240 mg	Ex, Holter	D 360 = P 240 D 180 < P 240
Humen et al. [183]	No PI, DB, L^2	24	2 weeks	240 mg (360 + P)	P 170 mg (mean)	Ex, radio	D 240 = P 170 D 360 + P 360 > D or P
Acute studies							
Anderson et al. [69]	R, DB, CO	12	Acute	120 mg	P 100 mg	Ex, radio	D > P. D improved ejection fraction
Chaitman et al. [44]	PI, R, DB, WOut	15	Acute	120 mg	P 80 mg	Ex	D > P

Abbreviations: As in Tables II-3 and II-4. D = diltiazem; P = propranolol lieb et al. [80] withdrew nifedipine or placebo abruptly from patients who were also receiving therapy with both nitrates and propranolol, and found no withdrawal effects; however continued therapy with propranolol and/or nitrates might have protected from withdrawal so that the whole subject needs much more careful investigation, along the lines of the verapamil study by Lahiri et al. [78].

Diltiazem. No reports of a withdrawal syndrome could be found, nor have any studies specifically been designed with this end in mind. Again, the subject warrants study.

Comparison of Calcium Antagonists in Effort Angina

Verapamil versus nifedipine. Proper comparisons are few (Table II-6). Dawson et al. [15] compared verapamil 360 mg daily (120 mg three times) with nifedipine capsules 60 mg daily (20 mg three times) over 4 weeks, including a comparison of 16-point precordial maps. Both agents increased workload in addition to lessening the severity of EKG ischemic changes. Both decreased the number of anginal attacks and the use of nitroglycerin; verapamil seemed better without reaching statistical significance in this small number of patients (n = 16). Ankle edema and palpitations were most common with nifedipine and constipation with verapamil. Using the same doses, Subramanian et al. [19] found that 11 of 28 patients became angina-free on verapamil and 8 of 28 with nifedipine. Exercise time and EKG parameters were all better with verapamil, using computer-assisted exercise testing and 24-hour ambulatory Holter monitoring for ST shifts. With a higher dose of nifedipine (80 mg daily, 20 mg four times), the effect on exercise time and subjective parameters (pain, nitroglycerin usage) was similar to the effects of verapamil 360 mg daily (120 mg three times) in a single-blind crossover study [81]. Both agents improved LV function during exercise.

Diltiazem versus nifedipine. Once again strict comparisons are few. Schurtz et al. [82], quoted by Chaffman and Brogden [83], compared two low doses of the two compounds, diltiazem 180 mg daily and nifedipine 30 mg daily. They found equipotency against angina in 20 patients. Single doses of nifedipine (20 mg) were equipotent to diltiazem (120 mg) and better than propranolol (60 mg) in prolonging exercise time for 3 hours [44]. Subramanian [20] only indirectly compared these two agents by using similarly selected patients and similar end-points (exercise time

Table II-6. Comparative effects of calcium antagonists in chronic effort angina

Author	Trial Design	Patients (n)	Drug Test Period	Daily Doses of Calcium Antagonists			End-point	Result
				Verapamil	Nifedipine	Diltiazem		
Dawson et al. [15]	Pl, R, DB, Seq, WOut	16	4 weeks	360 mg	60 mg	—	Clin	V = N
Subramanian et al. [19]	Pl, R, DB, CO, no WOut	28	4 weeks	360 mg	60 mg	—	Clin	V > N testing, Holter
Weiner et al. [84]	DB, CO, then parallel	46	6 weeks 9 months	480 mg	—	360 mg	Clin	D = V
Schurtz et al. [82]	Pl, R, DB, CO, no WOut	20	15 days	—	30 mg	180 mg	Ex	D = N (ex) D > N (EKG)
Khurmi and Raftery [26]	Initial Pl, then open-label parallel	45	16 weeks	360 mg	—	360 mg	Ex	D = V
Khurmi and Raftery [184]	Separate trials each vs. placebo	146	2–4 weeks	360 mg	60 mg	360 mg	Clin, ex testing	D, V > N (ex) V > N, D (pain)

Abbreviations: D, diltiazem; EKG, electrocardiogram; N, nifedipine; V, verapamil.

and freedom from pain). Diltiazem 360 mg was compared with placebo in a double-blind protocol, nifedipine 30 mg in a single-blind study versus placebo, and nifedipine 60 mg in a double-blind study versus verapamil (the latter study has already been referred to). Fifty percent of the diltiazem-treated subjects became pain-free while 5% of low-dose nifedipine, and 29% of high-dose nifedipine patients became pain-free. Such indirect comparisons leave much to be desired and more studies are required to compare nifedipine with diltiazem.

Verapamil versus diltiazem. Again, only limited data are available. In a double-blind randomized crossover study in 46 patients over 7 weeks (diltiazem 2 weeks, verapamil 2 weeks, placebo 3 weeks) after an initial 5-week single-blind dose-titration period, diltiazem 360 mg daily was the approximate equivalent of verapamil 480 mg daily [84]. Then followed an open-label follow-up study over 9 months (total study duration 1 year) which supported the marginal superiority of diltiazem because the treadmill time to development of symptoms improved more with diltiazem; also the time to onset of ST depression was longer and peak ST depression was less. However, none of these possible "differences" between diltiazem and verapamil were statistically significant. In the same study, side effects seemed low during the chronic phase (6 of 26 patients had constipation with verapamil; 4 of 20 patients had edema or flushing with diltiazem). However, patients had been carefully screened to exclude congestive heart failure and sinoatrial and AV conduction disease. In the Subramanian study [20] (see diltiazem versus nifedipine, above), indirect comparisons on different patients subject to a similar protocol suggest that diltiazem 360 mg (50% of patients angina-free) was less effective than verapamil 360 mg daily (71% of patients angina-free) or else of similar potency (equal prolongation of exercise time). In an open-label study over 4 months, Khurmi and Raftery [26] showed that diltiazem 360 mg daily improved exercise duration by 95%, verapamil 360 mg daily by 79%, and nicardipine 120 mg daily by 45%. (Nifedipine was not studied; nicardipine is closely related to nifedipine in its properties, requiring, however, roughly twice the dose of nifedipine. For further details on nicardipine, see Part V of this review series.) The rate-pressure product at peak exercise actually increased with nicardipine and decreased with diltiazem and verapamil, suggesting different modes of antianginal action. These studies suggest that verapamil is approximately as effective as diltiazem. However, the differences are not decisive.

*Calcium Antagonists Compared with or
Added to β-Adrenergic Blockade*

Diltiazem (240 mg daily), verapamil (360 mg daily), or
nifedipine (60 mg daily) all equally reduced the number of anginal attacks and the ST segment depression
(propranolol-nifedipine [P-N] being statistically the
best) when added to propranolol 160 mg daily [27].
Heart size increased and PR interval lengthened with
propranol-diltiazem (P-D) and propranolol-verapamil
(P-V) compared with P-N. Subjectively, most side effects occurred with P-V (chiefly constipation), then
with P-N (chiefly dizziness, leg swelling) and then
with P-D (incidence of side effects close to placebo).
Thus hemodynamically P-N was superior, and subjectively P-D was better. Propranolol-diltiazem or P-V
should not be used in the presence of heart failure. In
another double-blind crossover study aimed at a population of patients with angina not fully responsive to
propranolol (mean daily dose 229 mg), either verapamil 360 mg daily or nifedipine 60 mg daily was
added [28]. Verapamil was more effective than nifedipine in reducing anginal frequency, nitroglycerin
use, and the magnitude of ST depression with exercise. However, exercise times were similar with P-V
and P-N. Left ventricular ejection fraction was somewhat higher with P-N and the PR interval was shorter.
Symptomatic bradycardia occurred in two of ten
patients on P-V and was relieved by reducing the dose
of verapamil to 240 mg without sacrificing antianginal
efficacy. Thus P-V, although probably a better antianginal combination than P-N, was potentially the
more risky from the hemodynamic point of view unless
the verapamil dose was limited to 240 mg daily [28] or
the propranolol dose to 160 mg daily [27]. Verapamil
360 mg daily combined with atenolol 100 mg daily led
to 4 of 15 patients withdrawing from the trial [29].

*Efficacy of Calcium Antagonists in Effort
Angina: Summary*

Comparative data delineate different mechanisms for
the antianginal effects of verapamil, diltiazem, and
nifedipine. Hence different patients may respond differently to each agent. *Although the antianginal effects of these three agents are similar in most studies,
imperfect evidence suggests that nifedipine may be
marginally less effective on its own than verapamil or
diltiazem; further controlled trials are required. In
comparison with beta-blockade, nifedipine (worse
than beta-blockade in three of five studies) compared
less well than did verapamil (better than beta-block-*

ade in four of six studies) or diltiazem (equal to beta-blockade in four studies), possibly because of its tendency to cause a tachycardia. In contrast, nifedipine is easier and safer to combine with beta-blockade than the other two agents. The approximate daily dose equivalents of these agents are verapamil 360 to 480 mg, nifedipine 60 to 80 mg, diltiazem 360 mg, and propranolol 240 to 480 mg daily. In the case of nifedipine, it should be realized that to achieve the optimal dose requires titration, generally not done in these trials, and that the highest dose required may be more than usually used and may be up to 120 mg daily (see use in vasospastic angina, below). Furthermore, with prolonged nifedipine use the reflex sympathetic stimulation seems blunted; at least during the chronic therapy of hypertension there is no tachycardia induced by nifedipine [57,85]. Thus, possibly prolonged antianginal therapy with nifedipine might have given different results from those in the acute trials.

Angina Caused by Coronary Spasm: "Vasospastic Angina"

Mechanisms and Clinical Presentation

It is chiefly spasm of the large coronary arteries that is responsible for vasospastic angina. The regulation of such arteries differs from that of the coronary vascular resistance vessels, which are physiologically controlled by the metabolic demand of the myocardium and only secondarily by neurogenic mechanisms [86,87]. As recently reviewed [88], the large coronary arteries are regulated by a complex interaction between passive flow factors, neurogenic factors, and endothelial-platelet related factors. If the metabolic demand in the coronary vascular resistance vessels acts to increase myocardial blood flow, then the increased flow passing through the large coronary arteries will cause dilation which in turn may help to avoid ischemia in certain zones. Among the other vasodilating influences are the beta-adrenoceptors on the large coronary arteries, which are chiefly $beta_1$ in nature, purinergic stimuli including release of adenosine triphosphate (ATP) and to some extent adenosine, and vasodilatory prostaglandins such as prostacyclin. On the other hand, vasoconstrictory stimuli include cholinergic stimulation, release of thromboxane A_2 (probable but not yet definitely proven), and alpha-adrenergic stimulation (both $alpha_1$ and $alpha_2$-receptors are involved). Thus neurogenic mechanisms are of more importance than in the regulation of the coronary resistance vessels. In the genesis of coronary spasm, a critical interaction is that between the endothelium, platelets, and vasoconstrictors released from the platelets such as serotonin and thromboxane A_2. When the endothelium is damaged, certain vasodilator stimuli are blunted [89] and vasoconstrictor stimuli predominate. The endothelial relaxing factor [90] is of crucial importance. Certain agents which are vasoconstrictors in vascular tissue denuded of endothelium can, in the presence of endothelium, cause vasodilation. Such factors include histamine, serotonin, and some prostaglandins [91]. For example, serotonin, released from damaged platelets, becomes a vasoconstrictor when the endothelium is removed. Vasodilators may accordingly be divided into those which require the endothelium for their activity and those which do not, such as the nitrates [92]. In conditions where there is endothelial damage, as in atheroma, stimuli that are normally vasodilatory may become vasoconstrictive. Maintenance of endothelial integrity may be critical in avoiding coronary artery spasm. At present no therapeutic agents are available to restore endothelial integrity.

Diurnal variation of vasospastic angina. A marked diurnal variation in the incidence of attacks of coronary spasm underlies the high incidence of attacks from midnight to early morning, while the patient is asleep or at rest [93]. The explanation is complex and includes: 1) less production of hydrogen ions at night with a rise of blood pH and ionized extracellular calcium, 2) increased relative activity of the parasympathetic nervous system, and 3) rapid eye movement sleep with a sudden rise in sympathetic tone, acting via the alpha-receptors.

Clinical presentation of vasospastic angina. The diagnosis in a typical case of Prinzmetal's angina with electrocardiographic ST segment elevation is usually not in doubt; in such cases calcium antagonists rather than beta-blockers are usually the basic therapy. Although coronary spasm is a proven hypothesis to explain Prinzmetal's angina [87], it should not be forgotten that Prinzmetal described the combination of coronary spasm and organic coronary artery disease [94] and that two of Prinzmetal's original three patients went on to develop a classical myocardial infarction. Thus it is difficult to exclude underlying coronary artery disease which may cause associated ischemic syndromes, responding well to β-blockade, even if the spasm itself were to respond poorly. Another problem is that the more subtle features of lesser degrees of spasm [95] merge into "silent" ischemia and "mixed" angina (see below) in which calcium antagonists and beta-blockers may both be effective. Furthermore, the role of coronary spasm in silent ischemia and mixed angina is still unproved. Therefore the "edges" of the clinial picture of coronary spasms are now increasingly blurred.

The lack of clear definition of vasospastic angina may account for the apparent variability of the natural history. Pepine et al. [96] followed-up patients with ST elevation during angina or angiographic documentation of coronary spasm and observed that besides calcium antagonists, additional therapy including nitrates and beta-blockers was often required because the anginal attacks persisted. On the other hand, Previtali et al. [97] followed-up patients who also had ST elevation during pain but without specific angiographic proof of spasm. These patients responded well in hospital to calcium antagonist therapy and there was a complete remission of angina in 50% of them at 12 months. Presumably, underlying differences in the severity of associated coronary artery disease account for these apparent differences in the natural history of Prinzmetal's angina.

Comparisons of Calcium Antagonists in Open-Label Studies in Vasospastic Angina

All three major calcium antagonists are very effective in relieving coronary artery spasm causing Prinzmetal's variant angina. In an open-label study, nifedipine (40 to 160 mg/day) was strikingly effective, eliminating painful episodes in nearly two-thirds of patients while side-effects required withdrawal in only 5% of patients [98]. However, an important positive aspect of the Antman study was that coronary artery spasm was diagnosed by rigorous angiographic criteria. Another convincing unblinded study is that of Kimura and Kishida [99]. In 286 Japanese patients with typical Prinzmetal's angina, nifedipine 40 mg daily, diltiazem 160 mg daily, and verapamil around 240 mg daily were effective in 94, 91, and 86% of patients, respectively, irrespective of the presence or absence of organic coronary artery disease. Today these doses could be regarded as "low." Apparently the most effective therapy was the combination of nifedipine (mean daily dose 32 mg) and diltiazem (mean daily dose 100 mg tested in a small number of patients). However, there was neither crossover nor blinded evaluation nor strict dose-titration, nor do these Japanese patients necessarily have the same incidence of associated coronary artery disease as in America or Europe. In yet another open study, Waters et al. [100] showed long-term survival over 15 months of over 90% in patients receiving calcium antagonist therapy; nifedipine 80 mg daily was nearly similar to diltiazem 360 mg daily or verapamil 480 mg daily.

Direct proof of relief of angiographic spasm by calcium antagonists has been obtained in a small number of studies [101,102].

Calcium Antagonists for Vasospastic Angina: Placebo-Controlled and Comparative Studies

In a small but placebo-controlled study [103], nifedipine (10 to 20 mg every 4 hours) decreased the incidence of electrocardiographic ST segment deviations. In a second study, Schick et al. [104] showed that in patients responding to open-label nifedipine which was then withdrawn, 84% responded to reinstitution of nifedipine in a double-blind comparison with placebo. However, it should be noted that the study population was defined in advance by having a response to nifedipine during the course of their ordinary clinical care. In a third and complex study [105], verapamil and placebo were first compared in a long-term double-blind randomized trial lasting 9 months, and then open-label nifedipine was followed for 2 months. Although this trial design precludes strict comparison of verapamil and nifedipine, it should be noted that a mean nifedipine dose of 71 mg daily was the approximate equivalent of verapamil 450 mg daily, both being given in three to four daily doses, as judged by the reduction of chest pain, usage of nitroglycerin, and decreased ST segment deviation. The patients were treated throughout with isosorbide dinitrate (average daily dose 104 mg/day). Side effects of verapamil and nifedipine were similar, but subjectively worse for nifedipine in that seven of the patients had dose-limiting adverse effects and in one patient therapy was stopped because of orthostatic hypotension.

Diltiazem versus nifedipine. In 15 patients with angiographically proven spasm (spontaneous or ergonovine-induced), the effects of nifedipine (30 to 120 mg, mean 82 mg daily) were compared with diltiazem (90 to 360 mg, mean 257 mg daily); endpoints were the clinical attack rate and nitroglycerin usage [106]. Of the 15 patients, 9 had typical Prinzmetal's angina. These agents were approximately equipotent; however, 5 of 15 of the diltiazem and 12 of 15 of the nifedipine-treated patients ($p < 0.05$) had adverse reactions. In nine patients not responding well to monotherapy, combination nifedipine and diltiazem was attempted; all experienced side effects and only six tolerated the combined regime. Anginal attacks decreased from a mean of 1.75 during the placebo period; because of the open nature of this stage of the trial design, no statistical analysis could be undertaken. From these studies it may be concluded that in angiographically proven coronary spasm, diltiazem (mean dose 257 mg daily) and nifedipine (mean dose 82 mg daily) were about equipotent, with diltiazem having the edge as far as absence of side-effects was concerned.

Ergonovine-induced angina. Ergonovine is a coronary vasoconstrictor agent which may precipitate attacks of vasospastic angina, and has been used under careful control to evoke such attacks in patients for diagnostic purposes (Table II-7). In a study on 27 hospitalized patients with typical clinical Prinzmetal's angina [107], provocative testing with ergonovine was used to assess the efficacy of nifedipine (80 mg daily), diltiazem (360 mg daily), and verapamil (480 mg daily), given in randomized order. In one patient the dose of verapamil was decreased to 240 mg daily to avoid a sinus bradycardia. Of the patients, 18 of 27 responded to verapamil, 22 of 27 to nifedipine, and 22 of 27 to diltiazem. Some of the patients responded better to one drug than to the other two. During a 7-month (mean duration) follow-up period, 15 patients took the calcium antagonist drug that had converted the ergonovine result from positive to negative and 14 remained pain-free. Of the 12 patients who took a calcium antagonist that had failed to convert the ergonovine test, only 4 were pain-free. The message of this study is that different patients, all with vasospastic angina, may respond differently to the three calcium antagonists; it appeared difficult to select the best agent in advance.

Calcium Antagonists Compared or
Combined with Long-acting Nitrates
in Vasospastic Angina

Nifedipine versus dinitrate. Only two double-blind studies appear to have been undertaken. There were similar benefits of nifedipine (82 mg mean daily dose) and isosorbide dinitrate (66 mg mean daily dose) in 12 outpatients [108]. The major side effect of isosorbide was headache while pedal edema occurred during nifedipine therapy. Generally nifedipine was preferred to isosorbide because of the increased subjective benefit and fewer uncomfortable side effects [108]. Hill et al. [109] compared nifedipine with isosorbide dinitrate in a dose-titration procedure. With the number of anginal attacks and the use of nitroglycerin as end-points, nifedipine in a mean dose of 65 mg daily was approximately equivalent to isosorbide dinitrate in a mean dose of 75 mg daily. Some hypotension occurred during dose-titration with nifedipine.

Verapamil or nifedipine plus long-acting nitrates in vasospastic angina. In an open-label study, isosorbide dinitrate (mean daily dose 117 mg) was combined with verapamil (mean daily dose 453 mg) or nifedipine (mean daily dose 71 mg) [110]. During combination therapy by calcium antagonist-nitrate the frequency of angina and ST segment deviation was dramatically reduced. Verapamil-nitrate and nifedipine-nitrate were very similar in their potencies [109].

Calcium Antagonists Compared or Combined with beta-Blockade in Vasospastic Angina

Although beta blockers are widely regarded as inappropriate therapy for vasospastic angina, strict studies are few. If it can be assumed that transient EKG changes in patients with angina at rest are caused by spasm (an unproven but attractive hypothesis), then verapamil 400 mg daily was considerably better than propranolol 200 mg daily in reducing ST segment shifts from a control value of 11.9 to 2.6 per 24 hours (verapamil) whereas patients treated with propranolol showed no change [111].

Rebound After Cessation of Calcium Antagonist Therapy

In vasospastic angina, nifedipine therapy should not be abruptly halted because the frequency and duration of attacks may increase [114]. Nifedipine (40 to 80 mg/day), verapamil (80 to 120 mg four times per day), or isosorbide dinitrate (30 mg four times per day) all reduced the rebound phenomenon. In a placebo-controlled double-blind study, abrupt withdrawal of nifedipine increased the anginal attack rate although not to levels found before nifedipine had been started [104]. In unstable angina at rest, a condition not directly related to coronary spasm, nifedipine cessation caused worsening [80,115]. Apparently no information is available on possible rebound after cessation of verapamil therapy in patients with vasospastic angina. However, because nifedipine tends to increase circulating catecholamines [57] more than verapamil [116], there may be a greater chance of rebound with nifedipine than with verapamil. In the case of diltiazem, abrupt withdrawal of daily doses of 120 to 240 mg did not precipitate attacks in patients with Prinzmetal's angina [117].

Exertional Vasospasm

Sometimes vasospasm can be provoked by exertion, especially in the early morning [118]. This topic appears to be poorly studied with no double-blind studies. In four patients with exercise-induced coronary spasm [119], anginal attacks were not inhibited by propranolol but by diltiazem (90 mg) or nifedipine (20 mg). In a single patient, atenolol 100 mg daily was ineffective for exertional angina with ST segment elevation, but the addition of nifedipine 10 mg twice daily prevented the angina (Figure II-2; Opie et al. [120]).

Vasospastic Angina: Summary

Therapy with all the major three calcium antagonists is highly effective in vasospastic angina manifesting as Prinzmetal's variant angina. The various agents appear to be approximately equally effective. However, strict double-blind comparisons are not available. Nifedipine 60 to 80 mg daily is the rough equiva-

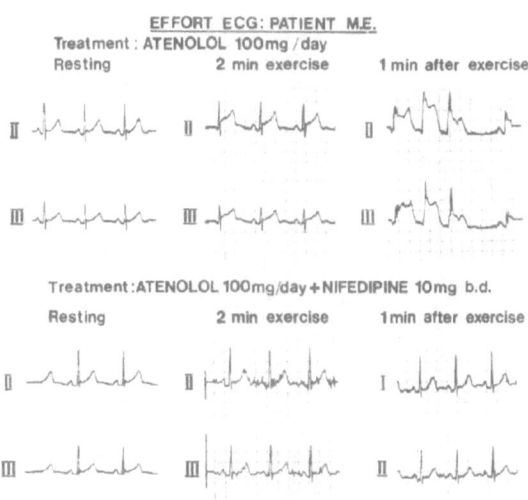

Fig. II-2. Exercise-induced ST elevation in patient with hypertension and angina pectoris (top panel). Note development of multiple ventricular premature systoles. After addition of nifedipine to atenolol (bottom panel), the EKG abnormalities reverted to normal. From [120] by courtesy of American Heart Journal.

Table II-7. Comparative effects of calcium antagonists in vasospastic angina

Author	Trial Design	Patients (n)	Drug Test Period	Evidence for Spasm	Daily Doses of Calcium Antagonists			End-point	Result
					Verapamil (V)	Nifedipine (N)	Diltiazem (D)		
Waters et al. [107]	R seq, no WOut. open-label	27	3 days	Repeated ergonovine	480 mg	80 mg	360 mg	Angina or EKG changes	N = D (81% benefit) V = 66% benefit
Prida et al. [106]	DB, CO; open-label for N+D phase	15	16 weeks	Angiospasm spontaneous or ergonovine	—	30–120 mg (mean 82)	90–360 mg (mean 257)	Clinical; ambulatory EKG	N = D; D fewer side effects; D (206 mg mean) + N (61 mg mean) best*
Pepine et al. [96]	Open-label	45	1 year	ST elevation with pain or angio spasm	(Mean 419 mg, n = 16)	(Mean 68 mg, n = 16)	(Mean 240 mg, n = 13)	Pain	D = N = 69% benefit V = 56% benefit

Abbreviations: As in Table II-3.

*D+N caused frequent side-effects while helping those patients who could tolerate the combination.

lent of isosorbide dinitrate 60 to 80 mg daily. Nifedipine or verapamil may be combined with isosorbide dinitrate (diltiazem has apparently not been tested). Whereas β-blockade on its own may exaggerate the condition or fail to benefit, the combination diltiazem-propranolol is as effective as diltiazem alone, so that diltiazem annulled the harmful effects of β-blockade. Efficacy of calcium antagonist agents in the case of vasospastic angina must not be extrapolated to angina at rest and unstable angina (see below).

"Silent" Ischemic Episodes

The Concept of "Silent" Ischemia

Increasingly, transient "silent" ischemia is detected in angina pectoris by continuous ST monitoring techniques. Such ST changes are yet another expression of the anginal syndrome, just as is pain. In simplified terms, it is "angina without anginal pain." There may be a spectrum of ischemia in which mild or moderately severe episodes may be "silent" and only more severe or prolonged episodes may reach the threshold for pain [121]. In addition, the threshold for angina varies among patients, so that a generalized defective perception of all painful stimuli may determine whether the ischemia is painful or not, rather than the severity or not the ischemia is painful or not, rather than the severity of the actual underlying ischemia being the operative factor [122]. Data starting to come through suggest that these "silent" ischemic episodes in patients with effort angina respond both to β-blockers and calcium antagonists [121].

ST Deviations in Normal Volunteers

In apparently normal patients without symptoms of coronary artery disease, ST segment shifts are not proof of ischemia. Indeed, such ST segment changes observed in 10 to 28 percent of asymptomatic healthy volunteers under the age of 40 [123] are not at all well understood and most unlikely to represent ischemia (many of the patients were women). Furthermore, the detection of such episodes does not warrant anti-ischemic therapy.

ST deviations in Patient with Stable Effort Angina

In patients with stable effort angina, "silent" episodes detected by ambulatory Holter techniques respond to the same therapy as does the underlying condition (Table II-8). Thus in the study of Lynch et al. [48], propranolol was more effective than nifedipine both in

Table II-8. Comparative effects of calcium antagonist therapy with β-adrenergic blockade in patients with chronic effort angina and spontaneous ST segment deviation on ambulatory EKG ("silent ischemia")

Author	Trial Design	Patients (n)	Drug Test Period	Episodes of ST deviations Per Day	Calcium Antagonist Daily Dose	β-Blocker Daily Dose	Effect on Incidence of ST Deviations
Oakley et al. [185]	Not B, No R	6	1 week	47/24 hr	N 60 mg	P 480 mg	N 48% fall, P 43% fall, N + P 83%
Cocco et al. [124]	SB, R, parallel	12	45 days	Not stated	N 20–30 mg	Pin 20–30 mg	N; rest ischemic episodes reduced in 6 or 7 Pin: rest episodes reduced in 1 of 5
Lynch et al. [48]	Pl, R, DB, L^2	16	4 weeks	About 5	N 30–60 mg	P 240–480 mg	N 30 mg: 35% fall, N 60 mg: 54% fall P 240 mg: 66% fall, P 480 mg: 70% fall N + P: low dose 85% fall, high dose 90% fall
Subramanian [20]	P(SB), DB, CO, no WOut	22	4 weeks	18 ± 1 on placebo	V 360 mg	P 240 mg	V = P = 75% fall in ischemic episodes

Abbreviations: N, nifedipine; P, propranolol; Pin, pindolol; V, verapamil; other abbreviations as in Table II-3.

relieving symptoms of angina and in decreasing the incidence of ST deviations (some of which were "silent"). Heart rate seems to be an important determinant of the development of EKG changes [124,125] in patients with effort angina, in that atenolol which decreased the heart rate had a better effect on electrocardiographic ischemia than did pindolol. Logically, therefore, diltiazem, which usually decreases heart rate, may be anticipated to be "better" for the control of episodes of EKG-monitored ischemia than nifedipine (such a study would be of great interest). This benefit of a reduced heart rate is also supported by the double-blind cross-over study of Subramanian et al. [19] in which verapamil 360 mg daily decreased the heart rate, whereas nifedipine 60 mg did not; verapamil was better than nifedipine in preventing ischemia as monitored by ST segment shifts.

ST Deviations in Patients with Angina at Rest and Transient Chest Pain

In patients with angina at rest and short-lived attacks of chest pain, several studies attest to the benefit of calcium antagonists [111,126,127]. For example, Rizzon et al. [127] found that transient ST deviations (60% "silent," 83% ST depression) were better controlled by nifedipine (120 mg daily) or verapamil (480 mg daily) than by isosorbide dinitrate (120 mg daily). In the study of Parodi et al. [111], over 1,600 ischemic episodes of ST segment shift were studied and 43% were "silent." The mean duration of pain was 6 minutes, whereas the mean duration of the "silent" episodes was about 3 minutes. In a careful study interspersed with three placebo periods, verapamil 400 mg daily was considerably better than propranolol 300 mg daily.

When intravenous nitrates are given in low doses, nitrates can reverse the consequences of "silent" ischemia [128]; in this study nitrate tolerance had probably not developed, whereas the high dinitrate dose in the study of Rizzon et al. [127] suggested that tolerance had developed. There is no proof that either calcium antagonists, nitrates, or beta-blockers by reversing "silent" ischemia can alter symptoms or prognosis in patients with ischemic heart disease.

ST Deviations in Unstable (Preinfarct) Angina

In patients with genuine unstable angina, added "silent" ischemic episodes indicate a poor prognosis [129] and may warrant specific aggressive therapy.

"Mixed" Angina

Although the term "mixed" angina has been widely used, the concept is now becoming controversial and the present ideal is to incorporate this category into other better established descriptions such as unstable angina or vasospastic angina, depending on the prominent clinical presentation. "Mixed" angina was defined by Maseri et al. [130] as angina in which two quite different basic pathophysiologic mechanisms were at work, namely, both an excessive increase in myocardial oxygen demand (secondary angina) and a transient impairment of coronary blood flow supply (primary angina). Stone et al. [54] used the term "mixed angina" to describe patients who had both classic exertional angina as well as clinically suspected coronary vasospasm, defined as occasional episodes of rest angina or by a variable effort threshold for the angina; however, patients with ST segment elevation during pain were excluded and vasospasm was not proven. Nifedipine therapy was thought to be most effective in patients with "pure" vasospasm and least effective in patients with classical exertional angina. For Andre-Fouet et al. [131], "mixed" angina meant the onset of spontaneous angina at rest in patients previously known to have effort angina; such patients responded equally well to diltiazem or propranolol therapy. However, these studies were not undertaken on an intention-to-treat basis but rather patients with "mixed" angina were retrospectively defined as a subgroup. Therefore the conclusions are subject to statistical reserve. *Formal therapeutic trials in patients with documented and proven "mixed" angina have not yet been reported. To prove that a component of "mixed" angina is caused by coronary vasospasm is no easy task because strictly speaking angiographic evidence is required [95,98].*

The occurrence of transient ST segment changes ("silent" ischemia) is not proof of a partially vasospastic etiology for the angina (see ST Deviations in Patients with Stable Effort Angina, above). New knowledge that these ST segment deviations respond to beta-adrenergic blockade in patients with effort angina makes only a vasospastic etiology seem unlikely. Thus the concept of preferential calcium antagonist therapy for "mixed" angina is at present purely conjectural and not supported by the data of Andre-Fouet et al. [131]. It is only when true coronary spasm is thought to be the cause of spontaneous angina in a patient who also has effort angina, that it is logical to prefer calcium antagonists to beta-blockade as first-line therapy. In other patients with effort angina and ST deviations, either calcium antagonists or beta-blockade may be selected according to other criteria such as side effects and expected tolerance [131].

Angina at Rest

Definition. Definitions are critical without being standard. Thus frequently "angina at rest" is confused with "unstable angina" which merges into preinfarction angina and threatened myocardial infarction. Both "angina at rest" and "unstable angina" are marked by spontaneous anginal pain at rest, not evoked by any known external factor. Yet it is particularly important to distinguish "angina at rest" with short-lived episodes of chest pain, usually less than 15 minutes [111], from the longer-lasting and much more serious attacks of true preinfarction unstable angina (see Unstable Angina with Threatened Infarction, below). For example, it seems as if the patients studied by Parodi et al. [111,126] and Rizzon et al. [127] had repetitive stable short-lived attacks of chest pain or electrocardiographic episodes with stable angina at rest, placing them in a different clinical category from patients with unstable angina or the "intermediate coronary syndrome" (Table II-9). Thus there are important differences between "stable angina at rest" [111] and "unstable angina at rest." Stone [121] likewise distinguishes between 1) "simply the presence of angina at rest with reversible ST-segment deviation," which is possibly due to coronary vasospasm; and 2) "unstable angina with its heterogeneous pathophysiology." Nonetheless it must be realized that in any given patient such distinctions may be arbitrary and that there is in fact a spectrum of conditions extending all the way from Prinzmetal's angina through angina at rest to unstable angina and myocardial infarction [95].

Verapamil. In several elegant studies, Parodi et al. [111,126,132] have shown the efficacy of verapamil 400 to 480 mg daily in controlling short-lived attacks of pain and ST segment deviations. In patients with (probably) more severe episodes of ischemia (because they were symptomatic and the number and length of attacks was increasing), both verapamil and propranolol were effective, although verapamil was more so [133]. However, these patients appear to belong to the category of those with true unstable angina pectoris.

Diltiazem. This agent has been used for angina at rest, although in the study of Andre-Fouet et al. [131] it is not clear how many of the attacks were really short-lived and how many were those of unstable

Table II-9. Effects of calcium antagonists alone or compared with β-adrenergic blockers in Prinzmetal's angina or angina at rest or unstable angina or threatened myocardial infarction

Clinical Condition Author Trial design	Patients (n)	Drug Test Period	Type of Angina and Coronary Angiography (CA) Findings	Calcium Antagonist or β-Blocker Doses and Effects	Conclusion
Prinzmetal's angina					
Previtali et al. [103] Pl, non-R, non-B, Seq, with WOut	14	2 days	Short-lived attacks of rest pain or of silent ischemia promptly relieved by NG. Thirteen of 14 patients: ST elevation with pain (Prinzmetal's angina) CA: 14 of 14 patients CAD	N 60–120 mg daily. 4-hourly doses. Episodes of ischemia fell from 21 to 1 per 48 hr.	N $\gg$ placebo in Prinzmetal's
Kimura and Kishida [99] Non-R, observational	286	25 days mean	Prinzmetal's angina (rest pain with ST elevation)	V 240 mg (around), N 40 mg, D 160 mg all reduce chest pain	N = D = V. Response rate 94, 91, and 86%.
Feldman et al. Pl, R, DB, followed by open label D for 16 months	12	70 days	Prinzmetal's angina (rest pain with ST elevation). Decreasing incidence with time.	D 120 or 240 mg/day, both effective. 6 patients pain-free. Two no change.	D > placebo in Prinzmetal's

Rest angina

Parodi et al. [111, 126] Pl, R, DB, multiple CO, WOut	10	2 days	Up to 180 episodes of EKG ischemia per 24 hr, mostly silent. Attacks of chest pain < 15 min. CA: 9 of 10 patients CAD. 2 of 10 patients spontaneous spasm.	V 400 mg daily reduced painful and silent episodes by about 80%; P 300 mg daily no effect. Note highly selected population (10 of 167 patients with unstable angina at rest).	V 400 ≫ P 300 in rest angina
Andre-Fouet et al. [131] No Pl, R, non-B, parallel	24	2 days	Patients with recent onset of rest pain. Some with unstable angina as here defined. CA: 24 of 36 patients CAD in total series	D (titrated to 540 mg daily, mean 280 mg) much better than P (titrated to 360 mg, mean 160) in patients with rest but no effort angina: D: 9 of 13 patients pain-free, P: 0 of 11 patients pain-free.	D 280 ≫ P 360 in rest angina

Mixed angina

Andre-Fouet et al. [131] No Pl, R, non-B, parallel	46	2 days	Effort and rest angina. Part of above series.	D (titrated as above) vs. P (titrated): D: 14 of 22 patients pain-free; P: 18 of 25 patients pain-free	D = P in mixed angina

(continued)

Table II-9 (continued)

Clinical Condition Author Trial design	Patients (n)	Drug Test Period	Type of Angina and Coronary Angiography (CA) Findings	Calcium Antagonist or β-Blocker Doses and Effects	Conclusion
Unstable angina Capucci et al (1983) Pl, R, DB (P:SB), CO, WOut	20	3 days	Variety from short-lived pain to pre-infarction state. CA: 12 of 14 patients severe CAD. 7 of 20 patients Prinzmetal's.	V (480 mg/day) reduced anginal attacks from 3 to 0.2/day (p<0.01). P (240 mg/day) reduced attacks to 1.6/day (p<0.01). NG usage fell from 2.9 to 0.1/day with V, 1.2 with P (p<0.05 for D vs P).	V 480 ≫ P 240 in recurrent rest angina mostly with severe CAD.
Theroux et al (1985) R, SB, parallel groups	100	28 days or longer	Unstable angina at rest. Prinzmetal's excluded. Crescendo angina or prolonged chest pain or early post-infarction angina, with poor long-term prognosis.	D (360 mg/day titrated) equal to P (240 mg/day titrated). 80% pain-free on leaving CCU. However 5 months later (mean time) only 20% pain-free and 40% need CABG.	D 360 = P 240 in unstable angina with threatened infarction.

Muller et al (1984a) R, DB, parallel groups followed by combined therapy	126	14 days	Angina <45 min; EKG changes or documented CAD. About three anginal attacks per day. Note trial designed to assess choice of therapy to be introduced or frequently added to background β-blockade.	N (80-120 mg daily). P 80-240 mg daily (added to background P in 67 patients, mean dose 115 mg). Isosorbide dinitrate 40-80 mg daily.	If prior β-blockade, N addition better than increased dose of β-blockade and/or nitrates. If no prior β-blockade, N less effective than conventional treatment (p<0.001).
HINT Study (1986) Pl, R, DB but code could be broken, parallel	338	2 days	Unstable, defined as angina at rest with variable ST segment changes or pain >15 min with ST segment changes or with previously documented CAD (post-infarction, CA).	N 60 mg daily seemed harmful: trial stopped. M 200 seemed beneficial. N + M seemed beneficial. In patients already on β-blockade, N beneficial.	N alone probably C/I in unstable angina; β-blockade or N + β-blockade better. In patients not already on a β-blocker, β-blocker treatment of first choice. In patients already on β-blocker, N improves.
Mauritson et al (1983) Pl, R, initial SB then DB then open label	10*	3 days	Recurrent angina up to 5 attacks per day with added silent St-deviations. Two patients worsen during trial. CA: 7 of 9 patients CAD: 5 of 9 patients ergonovine spasm	V 320-480 mg/day. V 320 mg in 5 patients on first day reduced anginal episodes from 5.4 to 2.2 per day (p<0.01), ST changes from 12.6 to 6.2 (p<0.005), and NG use from 2.9 to	V 320 initially highly effective. By third day only 6 of 10 patients pain-free despite V 480 dose.

(continued) |

Table II-9. (Continued)

Clinical Condition Author Trial design	Patients (n)	Drug Test Period	Type of Angina and Coronary Angiography (CA) Findings	Calcium Antagonist or β-Blocker Doses and Effects	Conclusion
				1.6 tablets daily (NS). On third day only 3 of 10 patients controlled on V 320. Of patients on V 480, only 2 of 7 were pain-free.	
Threatened myocardial infarction					
Muller et al. [144] Pl, R, DB, parallel	105	14 days	Threatened myocardial infarction chest pain > 45 min (66 other patients, AMI)	N (120 mg daily) similar to placebo, 75% develop AMI in both groups. Possible increase in early 2 week mortality with N taking threatened MI and AMI together.	N ineffective in threatened infarction. N also ineffective in limiting infarct size (enzyme release).

Abbreviations: AMI, acute myocardial infarction; CA, coronary angiography; CABG, coronary artery bypass graft; CAD, coronary artery disease; CCU, care unit; C/I, contraindicated; D, diltiazem; N, nifedipine; NG, nitroglycerin; Prinzmetal's, variant anginal pain with ST segment elevation; V, Verapamil; other abbreviations as in Table II-2.

[a]One additional patient with mild disease treated by placebo for 2 days, V 320 mg last day. Few symptoms throughout.

angina. In patients with exclusively spontaneous angina at rest, there was a mean of 4.7 episodes of chest pain per 48 hours, reduced to 0.8 by diltiazem (mean dose 260 mg daily) with no effect of propranolol (mean dose 160 mg daily).

Nifedipine. Previtali et al. [103] showed benefit also for nifedipine in the therapy of patients with angina at rest, in regard to whom it is specifically stated that all ischemic episodes were of brief duration and were promptly relieved by sublingual nitroglycerin. The data by Moll et al. [134], published only in abstract form, suggest that patients with angina at rest, in whom Prinzmetal's angina and severe anginal attacks are excluded, respond well to nifedipine (80 to 120 mg daily) with about 45% of the episodes improving (with a similar percentage for propranolol, 160 to 240 mg daily). The combination of the two drugs controlled 86% of the episodes.

In summary, in angina at rest several different patient populations may be involved (see Table II-9). These vary from 1) those with short-lived attacks of repetitive chest pain, hypothetically caused by coronary spasm or another cause of intermittent coronary obstruction, and accompanied by frequent ST segment deviations; to 2) the situation in unstable angina with threatened infarction where the pain is longer in duration and the situation is unstable, so that infarction is truly a risk. When considering the patients in the first category, the evidence for the benefit of verapamil is strongest, but all calcium antagonists are likely to work. When considering the patients in the second category (see Unstable Angina, below), nifedipine is less effective and is contraindicated unless accompanied by beta-adrenergic blockade. In patients with stable angina at rest, characterized by very short-lived episodes of chest pain and numerous transient ST segment deviations on the EKG, calcium antagonists are better than propranolol which may be ineffective.

Unstable Angina With Threatened Infarction

Definition. In true unstable angina, one of the following is required [135]: 1) crescendo angina, being the presence of anginal pain with a recent increase in frequency, intensity, and duration; or 2) acute coronary insufficiency ("intermediate coronary syndrome") with prolonged anginal pain poorly relieved by nitrates yet without electrocardiographic or enzyme evidence of AMI; or 3) spontaneous angina 3 to 30 days after the onset of AMI. This definition includes those patients with longer episodes of chest pain lasting 15 to 20 minutes or more and which may go onto myocardial infarction as end-point [136,137]. Two other definitions of unstable angina need to be considered. First, Conti et al. [138] regard patients with recent onset effort angina as also being in the category of "unstable" angina. However, in practice, their definition coincides well with that used here because 51 of their 57 patients presented with multiple daily episodes of ischemic cardiac pain, all but 1 had angina at rest, 40 were treated surgically, and of the 15 given medical therapy, 10 were potential candidates for surgery. Second, the Dutch Holland Interuniversity Nifedipine/Metoprolol Trial (HINT) Study [139] regarded "unstable" angina as chest pain at rest with variable ST-T changes or anginal pain lasting more than 15 minutes in patients with a documented history of infarction or unstable angina (note the circular definition) or with coronary artery disease or angiography. In this study, it was essential that pain relief be achieved by nitrates or by a single dose of fentanyl (a narcotic analgesic). This somewhat loose definition means that the patients studied in the Dutch trial might not have corresponded to those of Theroux et al. [140]; nonetheless early infarction was a frequent end-point so that, as a group, these patients indeed had preinfarction unstable angina.

Pathophysiology. The heterogeneous nature of the pathophysiology of unstable angina is now becoming apparent. Stone [121] and Forrester et al. [140] propose that unstable angina may be due to a dynamic interaction among several major mechanisms. Forrester et al. [141] stress that a ruptured or fissured or ulcerated atherosclerotic plaque may lead to a nidus for platelet aggregation and partial thrombosis, usually reversible in unstable angina. Stone [121] proposes that the plaque can act as a trigger for spasm-induced "dynamic stenosis," possibly by an interaction between platelets and the damaged endothelium, leading to release of vasoconstrictive substances including thromboxane A_2. *Thus, the four critical factors in the mechanism of unstable angina are the atherosclerotic plaque, the platelets, a partial thrombus, and coronary vasospasm. These heterogeneous factors demand a more complex approach to therapy,* especially when it is considered that prolonged pain and LV failure, as found in some patients with the "intermediate coronary syndrome," may lead to catecholamine release with consequences such as tachycardia and a metabolically based increased myocardial oxygen demand [142]. In view of such complexities, Hugenholtz [143] states that: "There will never be one therapy for every case of unstable angina pectoris, nor will there ever be the best therapy for unstable angina. There will only be an optimal therapy for that particular stage of the syndrome at that particular moment in time for that patient."

Nifedipine for True Unstable Angina at Rest

Nifedipine compared to nifedipine plus propranolol or nifidipine plus metoprolol in unstable angina. Although nifedipine is excellent therapy for short-lived episodes of chest pain and for Prinzmetal's angina, recent evidence shows that when used as sole therapy in true unstable angina, it is not as good as propranolol [144] and is probably detrimental [139]. In patients with ischemic pain exceeding 45 minutes, classified as having threatened myocardial infarction [145], nifedipine monotherapy actually increased mortality, with $p < 0.02$. These reservations about the use of nifedipine are supported by isolated case reports of adverse responses to this drug in unstable angina [146, 147]. In the HINT Study [139] (see Table II-9), nifedipine was clearly beneficial for patients with true unstable angina already on beta-blockade, yet the combination nifedipine-metoprolol was no better than metoprolol alone for patients not already receiving beta-blockade. Thus, in the latter category, β-blockade rather than nifedipine was recommended as first-line therapy. Nifedipine by itself seemed to increase the event rate by about 15% ("events" equal recurrent angina or AMI within 48 hours). Yet it should be noted that some of the patients allocated to primary nifedipine therapy had characteristics that put them into a somewhat worse risk group than patients randomized to β-blockade. The critical importance of separating off patients with Prinzmetal's angina from true unstable angina at rest is shown by Gerstenblith et al. [148]. Patients on propranolol were in addition given nifedipine or placebo; the difference favoring nifedipine was found specifically in those with ST segment elevation (indicating Prinzmetal's angina).

Diltiazem for Unstable Angina

Diltiazem compared with propranolol in unstable angina. (See Table II-9). In "true" unstable angina in which Prinzmetal's variant angina was excluded and in which the chest pain was prolonged so that admission to a coronary care unit was required, both the calcium antagonist diltiazem (360 mg daily) and propranolol (240 mg daily) were equally effective [140]. In a variable population of patients some with unstable angina at rest [131], diltiazem (mean dose around 280 mg/day) was regarded as more effective than propranolol (mean dose around 160 mg/day). It must be stressed that a number of these patients did not appear to have true unstable preinfarction angina as here defined, but rather angina at rest (see Angina at rest, below). In patients with both rest and exertional angina, propranolol was as effective as diltiazem in controlling attacks of pain [131]. In patients with unstable angina [140] with careful exclusion of Prinzmetal's vasospastic angina (defined as rest pain with ST elevation), diltiazem titrated up to a dose of 360 mg daily was no better than propranolol 240 mg daily. Of 50 patients, 14 of the patients treated with diltiazem were symptom-free after 1 month compared with 13 patients treated with propranolol. The number of chest pain episodes, 0.75 per day in the control condition, was decreased to 0.26 by diltiazem and 0.29 by propranolol (both $p < 0.05$).

Verapamil for Unstable Angina

Verapamil versus propranolol (see Table II-9). In the study by Capucci et al. [133], patients had only short-lived attacks of pain and others were seemingly on the way to infarction. Verapamil 480 mg/day was compared with propranolol 240 mg/day; both agents were effective, although verapamil seemed better. Propranolol, for example, reduced the incidence of attacks per day from 3.0 in the placebo period to 1.6 per day ($p < 0.01$), whereas verapamil reduced the incidence to 0.2 per day ($p < 0.01$). Nitroglycerin consumption appeared less with verapamil than propranolol and here the differences between the two drugs were significant ($p < 0.05$). This study lends support to the early use of calcium antagonists of the verapamil-diltiazem group in true unstable angina. In the follow-up study of patients treated for unstable at rest, verapamil continued to produce benefit without altering the natural history so that there was still a high incidence of death from myocardial infarction [149].

Unstable Angina: Summary

In true unstable angina, where infarction is threatened, there are arguments against the use of nifedipine so that it is usually contraindicated unless used together with beta-blockade [139,145]. Thus it seems preferable to use diltiazem or verapamil if calcium antagonist monotherapy is desired; however, no strict comparisons between these agents and nifedipine exist. In choosing between beta-blockade and diltiazem therapy, there appears to be no real difference in the one study [140], whereas the other study with a greater number of patients corresponding more to angina at rest than to true unstable angina showed greater benefit for diltiazem [131]. Verapamil was better than propranolol when a number of patients were also included who did not appear to have true preinfarction angina [133]. *Therefore the closer the patient is to threatened infarction, the stronger is the case for beta-blockade. On the other hand, the closer the patient is to Prinzmetal's vasospastic angina, the stronger is the case for calcium antagonists. These potential differences appear to be particularly important in the case of nifedipine.*

Acute Myocardial Infarction

Nifedipine for AMI

Nifedipine is among the best studied of the calcium antagonist agents in patients with acute myocardial infarction (AMI). Although nifedipine (10 mg sublingually) may improve a low cardiac output and reduce a high wedge pressure, as well as bringing down the blood pressure [150,151], on formal testing nifedipine has shown no benefit in two large multicenter trials [145,152]. In one of these trials, patients randomized to nifedipine showed some excess mortality [143]. In the giant nifedipine TRENT Study, in which nearly 3,000 patients were studied, nifedipine given 10 mg four times daily for 28 days showed neither benefit nor harm [153]. The TRENT Study also showed that patients on prior beta-blockade therapy had a reduced mortality, thereby reconfirming the benefits of beta-blockade as opposed to those of nifedipine. In another recent study [154], 98 patients were randomized on a double-blind basis to nifedipine or placebo with an average delay time of only 3–4 hours after onset of chest pain, and treatment was continued for 3 days. No significant differences were found in clinical or enzyme parameters and the mortality at 1 month was similar in both groups. All these studies show that there is no indication for routine use of nifedipine in AMI or threatened myocardial infarction [151]. The possible adverse effects of nifedipine in true unstable angina (see Unstable Angina, below) also suggest that nifedipine in the absence of β-blockade is not the therapy of choice in threatened myocardial infarction or actual AMI, unless the specific hemodynamic changes induced by nifedipine are desired.

Verapamil for AMI

In two studies [155,156], verapamil has apparently reduced parameters of myocardial infarction size when given intravenously and acutely. However, in a double-blind study on 217 patients [157], verapamil 0.1 mg/kg intravenously (mean 4 hours after onset of chest pain) followed by 120 mg three times daily did not reduce cumulative enzyme release. In a large double-blind study on 1,436 patients with AMI [158], half were treated with verapamil starting with an intravenous dose followed by 120 mg three times daily; there was neither any difference in the acute or chronic mortality. More patients were withdrawn from the verapamil group than from the placebo group due to the development of second- and third-degree heart block. In addition, heart failure was more frequent in the verapamil-treated group. The single benefit of verapamil treatment was a reduction in intermittent atrial fibrillation. These two Danish studies did not support the concept that verapamil might be beneficial in AMI. However, further retrospective and subgroup analysis [158], which is a procedure open to possible criticism, suggests decreased reinfarction and mortality in the verapamil group when the late results are considered (22–180 days). This concept would suggest that early adverse effects of verapamil balance the later beneficial effects. However, a formal trial would be required to prove this point. Verapamil is also not effective in preventing early postinfarction angina and reinfarction [159], although this small trial only studied 17 patients over 10 days, it was stopped because of the failure of verapamil to benefit.

Diltiazem for AMI

Diltiazem appears not to have been studied in the acute phase of the usual type of myocardial infarction with Q-wave development. In patients with non-Q-wave myocardial infarction (formerly called non-transmural or subendocardial infarction), diltiazem given as 90 mg every 6 hours and initiated 24–72 hours after the onset of infarction and continued for up to 14 days reduced the incidence of reinfarction and the frequency of refractory postinfarction angina without changing the low mortality of only 3 to 4% [160]. These studies suffer from three defects. First the statistical significance fades when the customary two-tailed p-test is used instead of the one-tailed test the authors preferred. Second, nearly two-thirds of the patients received beta-blockade so that the real comparison was between diltiazem plus beta-blockade versus placebo plus beta-blockade. Third, the study was limited to very early reinfarction, within 14 days, so that there can be no comparison with the beta-blocker studies in which mortality was reduced over a period of months and years. Nonetheless, the studies can be regarded as promising and worthy of further extension.

Calcium Antagonists in Postinfarction Follow-up

Recently Yusuf and Furberg [161] have summarized in abstract form their meta-analysis of data on acute short-term and long-term studies in patients treated with calcium antagonists following myocardial infarction. They used a method of analysis similar to that already used in their meta-analysis of beta-blockade post-infarction [162]. Overall, the data, which included one study on verapamil, four on nifedipine, one on diltiazem, and one on lidoflazine, all indicated about a 6% excess in mortality by treatment. Some benefit, unlikely to be more than about 6%, could not be excluded. Therefore, at present, calcium antagonists as a group cannot be recommended, especially in view of the recent negative diltiazem postinfarction trial [187].

Reperfusion Injury

Reperfusion damage is at least in part calcium mediated (and in part mediated by free radicals) and experimental reperfusion injury may respond in part to calcium antagonist treatment [163]. Reperfusion arrhythmias are also in part ameliorated by calcium antagonists as a group cannot be recommended, especially in view of the recent negative diltiazem postinfarction trial [187].

Ischemic Ventricular Tachycardia and Fibrillation

In patients with previous myocardial infarction, sudden death is reduced by beta-adrenergic receptor antagonism, presumably as a result of a decreased incidence of ventricular fibrillation. *Calcium ions may be involved in the genesis of ventricular fibrillation* [165–167]. An elevation of tissue cyclic adenosine monophosphate (AMP) in ischemic tissue could be linked to the onset of ventricular fibrillation [168–170] with calcium as the active "messenger" of cyclic AMP so that a calcium-dependent transient inward current may underlie the development of ventricular automaticity [167]. In the isolated rat heart model with ligation [165], the three first-generation calcium antagonists, verapamil, nifedipine and diltiazem, could all inhibit the fall in ventricular fibrillation threshold, especially in conditions of adrenaline stimulation, when l-verapamil inhibited the fall in the fibrillation threshold more than d-verapamil [171]. The inhibition by l-verapamil rather than by d-verapamil favors the view that the calcium channel antagonist effects of verapamil prevent the effect of external catecholamines on the ventricular fibrillation threshold. However, it should be noted that in the absence of external stimulation, both d- and l-verapamil isomers were equally effective, suggesting that another property besides calcium antagonism was also in operation, such as sodium antagonism.

Why Are Calcium Antagonist Agents Not More Effective in AMI and in Postinfarction Protection?

With some impressive experimental effects of calcium antagonists against myocardial ischemia (for review, see Nayler [1]) and infarct size (for review, see Kloner and Braunwald [3]) and reperfusion injury [172], as well as the reduction of ischemic ventricular arrhythmias in some experimental models (for review, see Coetzee et al [167]) and a possible antiatherogenic effect [173], it is highly disappointing that no specific benefit of calcium antagonist therapy has been shown either during or after AMI [161]. Some possible explanations are as follows.

First, the antiarrhythmic concentrations required usually exceed the ordinary therapeutic blood levels; Clusin et al. [166] delayed the onset but did not prevent ventricular fibrillation in dogs with therapeutic blood diltiazem concentrations. Second, in the case of nifedipine (not verapamil and diltiazem), reflex tachycardia and excess hypotension may limit some of the anti-ischemic benefit. Third, all the studies are not yet in, and diltiazem has shown promising results in non-Q-wave infarction [160]. Thus not enough careful studies have been done with calcium antagonists to exclude fully antiarrhythmic and anti-ischemic protection during the very early phase of AMI when the effect might be most evident [174].

Mortality in ischemic heart disease is complex and ill-understood, probably a combination of sudden death due to ventricular fibrillation and myocardial failure secondary to ischemic failure. Presumably ventricular fibrillation is due at least in part to excess β-adrenergic activity acting through a complex variety of mechanisms, including a lowered arterial plasma potassium, a general enhancement of the intracellular calcium ion movements through an elevation of myocardial cyclic AMP levels, and increased ischemic injury resulting from an increased oxygen demand. Calcium antagonists cannot be expected to counter all these effects. Put differently, enhanced calcium ion entry is only one of several possible arrhythmogenic mechanisms of beta-stimulation. Thus in acute infarct management it would seem more logical to decrease

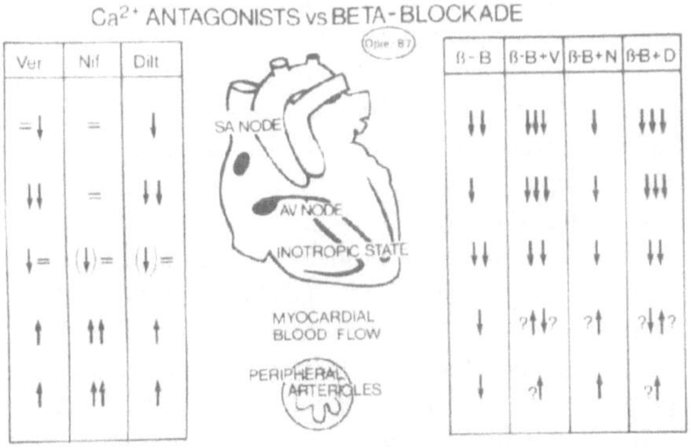

Fig. II-3. Proposed hemodynamic effects of calcium antagonists, singly or in combination with beta-blockade. Note that some of these effects are based on animal data and extrapolation to humans needs to be made with caution. Abbreviations: BB, beta-blockade; Dilt, diltiazem; Nif, nifedipine; Ver, verapamil. Copyright LH Opie.

potentially harmful excessive beta-stimulation by beta-adrenergic blockade than to use calcium antagonists. To settle this proposal, strict comparisons of beta-blockade versus calcium antagonists in the acute infarct state would have to be undertaken. Likewise these arguments can be applied to explain why post-infarct trials of calcium antagonists have thus far been so disappointing.

Percutaneous transluminal coronary angioplasty (PTCA). During this procedure there is a period of deliberate transient total ischemia at the site of coronary stenosis while balloon dilation takes place, followed by reperfusion. Both transient ischemia and reperfusion may respond to prophylactic therapy with calcium antagonists, which may be given locally at high concentrations. Therefore calcium antagonists are potentially promising in this situation [174] and need careful controlled evaluation.

Summary: Calcium Antagonists in Anginal and Ischemic Syndromes

Calcium antagonists are effective antianginal agents, acting in a complex fashion. As a group they offer an important and significant new advance in the therapy of these conditions and they are likely to be increasingly used. Nifedipine relieves chiefly arterial spasm and afterload; a compensatory tachycardia may offset some of the antianginal benefit in angina of effort. Verapamil, besides reducing afterload, has a negative inotropic effect which may also be offset by the afterload reduction; however, verapamil seems specifically to act on the ischemic zone. Diltiazem reduces afterload and usually has a mild negative chronotropic effect. The proposed mechanisms of all these agents in *effort angina* are still not well understood and it seems prudent to consider that they may improve myocardial oxygen supply by reduction of an exercise-induced increase in coronary tone. Furthermore, the effect on ventricular relaxation, impaired early in effort angina, needs consideration [175]. In *vasospastic angina,* coronary dilation is crucial in the relief of pain and ischemic episodes by calcium antagonists. In *unstable angina with threatened infarction,* coronary spasm by itself seems not an important mechanism, so that additional consequences of calcium antagonist therapy must be brought in to explain benefit, as bradycardia in the case of diltiazem and a negative inotropic effect in the case of verapamil. The emerging complexity of the etiology of unstable angina with an increasing emphasis on microthrombi and coronary obstruction rather than on spasm, may explain the failure of nifedipine to benefit unstable angina (threatened myocardial infarction) and its possible harm when given as monotherapy, whereas its combination with β-blockade is helpful. It is difficult to explain the absence of long-term postinfarction protection by calcium antagonists, with the possible exception of diltiazem for non-Q-wave infarction.

Comparisons of the efficacy of calcium antagonists with each other are difficult. Verapamil, the calcium antagonist in longest use and licensed for more indications than the others and hence the "drug for all seasons," does however have some disadvantages: 1) it frequently causes constipation, an adverse effect in patients with cardiovascular disease in whom straining at defecation can be especially harmful; and 2) it combines relatively poorly with beta-blockade (added negative inotropic, chronotropic, and dromotropic effects), even though with care this combination has been safely used. *Nifedipine* is excellent for vasospastic angina and short-lived attacks of rest angina, while in effort angina careful dose-titration avoids the occasional precipitation of ischemia. In unstable preinfarction angina, nifedipine may be contraindicated in the absence of beta-blockade, possibly because of nifedipine-induced tachycardia. Nifedipine usually combines well with beta-blockers. Even the latter combination may have added negative inotropic effects in patients with poor myocardial function. However, side effects of nifedipine are frequent. *Diltiazem* is well tested in effort angina, vasospastic angina, and unstable angina; there is also suggestive evidence for benefit in non-Q-wave myocardial infarction. Diltiazem traditionally has few side effects yet with the higher dose of 360 mg/day, now frequently used, side-effects including pedal edema are more common. The combination of diltiazem with β-blockade is theoretically easier than in the case of verapamil because of the lesser negative inotropic effect of diltiazem. Yet in practice adverse interactions have occurred, so that again more care is needed than with the nifedipine-beta-blocker combination.

In any given patient, the overall hemodynamic status and likely side effects of the various calcium antagonists might be important. For example, in a patient with a resting bradycardia or with borderline heart failure, nifedipine is likely to be chosen. In a patient with supraventricular or sinus tachycardia, diltiazem or verapamil is likely to be chosen above verapamil. In a patient with severe effort angina, combined beta-blockade-calcium antagonist therapy will probably be chosen, working up the doses to the limit of subjective and hemodynamic tolerance.

Compared with the β-adrenergic blocking agents, calcium antagonists have fewer contraindications for use in angina and, probably, fewer side effects (depending on the agent chosen). In particular, calcium antagonists do not interfere with exercise hemodynamics. Beta-blockers are known to give postinfarction protection and beta-blockade pretreatment lessens the mortality of myocardial infarction. Long-acting beta-blockers are readily available, allowing once-daily dosing, whereas even slow-release calcium antagonist preparations are not of proven value as once-daily therapy in angina pectoris. Beta-blockers are still chosen by many physicians as first-line antianginal agents unless 1) beta-blockers are contraindicated or 2) beta-blockers cause unwarranted side effects such as fatigue. Nevertheless, initial therapy with calcium antagonists is increasingly used because of the possibility of coexisting coronary spasm and the fact that there are fewer contraindications to calcium antagonists than to beta-blockers. *The different potential side effect profiles between calcium antagonists and beta-blockers and among the three prototypical calcium antagonists means that ultimately the choice between these agents will be tailored to the needs of the individual patient.*

References

1. Thaulow E, Guth BD, Ross J Jr: Role of calcium channel blockers in experimental exercise-induced ischemia. *Car-*

diovasc Drugs Ther 1987;1:503–512.

2. Nayler WG. Review. Calcium antagonists and the ischemic myocardium. *Int J Cardiol* 1987;15:267–285.

3. Kloner RA, Braunwald E. Effects of calcium antagonists on infarcting myocardium. *Am J Cardiol* 1987;59:84B–94B.

4. Nayler WG, Ferrari R, Williams A. Protective effect of pretreatment with verapamil, nifedipine and propranolol on mitochondrial function in the ischemic and reperfused myocardium. *Am J Cardiol* 1980;46:242–248.

5. Weishaar RE, Bing RJ. The beneficial effect of a calcium channel blocker, diltiazem, on the ischemic-reperfused heart. *J Mol Cell Cardiol* 1980;12:993–1009.

6. Nayler WG: Protection of the myocardium against post-ischemic reperfusion damage. The combined effect of hypothermia and nifedipine. *J Thorac Cardiovasc Surg* 1982; 84:897–905.

7. Nayler WG, Grau A, Slade A: A protective effect of verapamil on hypoxic heart muscle. *Cardiovasc Res* 1976; 10:650–662.

8. Watts JA, Maiorano LJ, Maiorano PC. Protection by verapamil of globally ischemic rat hearts: Energy preservation, a partial explanation. *J Mol Cell Cardiol* 1985;17:797–804.

9. De Jong JW, Harmsen E, De Tombe P, et al. Nifedipine reduces adenine nucleotide breakdown in ischemic rat heart. *Eur J Pharmacol* 1982;81:89–96.

10. Knoch G, Schlepper M, Witzleb E: Isoptin—a clinical study using normal subjects and patients with coronary disease. *Med Klin* 1963;58:1485–1491.

11. Tschirdewahn B, Klepzig H. Clinical studies on the effect of Isoptin and Isoptin S in patients with coronary insufficiency (in German). *Deutsche Med Wochensch* 1963; 88:1702–1710.

12. Sandler G, Clayton GA, Thornicroft SG. Clinical evaluation of verapamil in angina pectoris. *Br Med J* 1968;3:224–227.

13. Livesley B, Catley PF, Campbell RC: Double-blind evaluation of verapamil, propranolol and isosorbide dinitrate against a placebo in the treatment of angina pectoris. *Br Med J* 1973;1:375–378.

14. Arnman K, Ryden L. Comparison of metoprolol and verapamil in the treatment of angina pectoris (abstr). *Am J Cardiol* 1982;49:821.

15. Dawson JR, Whitaker NHG, Sutton GC. Calcium antagonists in chronic stable angina. Comparison of verapamil and nifedipine. *Br Heart J* 1981;46:508–512.

16. Andreassen F, Boye E, Christoffersen E, et al. Assessment of verapamil in the treatment of angina pectoris. *Eur J Cardiol* 1975;2/4:443–452.

17. Subramanian VB, Lahiri A, Paramasivan R, et al. Verapamil in chronic stable angina. *Lancet* 1980;i:841–840.

18. Hecht HS, Clew CYC, Burnam MH, et al. Verapamil in chronic stable angina: Amelioration of pacing-induced abnormalities of left ventricular ejection fraction, regional wall motion, lactate metabolism and hemodynamics. *Am J Cardiol* 1981;48:536–544.

19. Subramanian VB, Bowles MJ, Khurmi NS, et al. Rationale for the choice of calcium antagonists in chronic stable angina. An objective double-blind placebo-controlled comparison of nifedipine and verapamil. *Am J Cardiol* 1982; 50:1173–1179.

20. Subramanian VB. *Calcium Antagonists in Chronic Stable Angina Pectoris.* Amsterdam: Excerpta Medica, 1983;97–116, 217–229.

21. Weiner DA, Klein MD, Cutler SS. Efficacy of sustained-

release verapamil in chronic stable angina pectoris. *Am J Cardiol* 1987;59:215–218.

22. Johnson SM, Mauritson DR, Corbett JR, et al. Double-blind, randomized, placebo-controlled comparison of propranolol and verapamil in the treatment of patients with stable angina pectoris. *Am J Med* 1981;71:443–451.

22A. Sadick N, Tan ATH, Fletcher PJ, et al: A double-blind randomized trial of propranolol and verapamil in the treatment of effort angina. *Circulation* 1982;66:574–579.

23. Frishman WH, Klein NA, Strom JA, et al. Superiority of verapamil to propranolol in stable angina pectoris: A double-blind randomized crossover trial. *Circulation* 1982; 65(Suppl I):51–59.

24. Leon MB, Rosing DR, Bonow RO, et al. Clinical efficacy of verapamil alone and combined with propranolol in treating patients with chronic stable angina pectoris. *Am J Cardiol* 1981;48:131–139.

25. Pine MB, Citron D, Bailly DJ, et al. Verapamil versus placebo in relieving stable angina pectoris. *Circulation* 1982;65:17–22.

26. Khurmi NS, Raftery EB. Comparative effects of prolonged therapy with four calcium ion antagonists (diltiazem, nicardipine tiapamil and verapamil) in patients with chronic stable angina pectoris. *Cardiovasc Drugs Ther* 1987;1:81–87.

27. Johnston DL, Lesoway R, Humen DP, et al. Clinical and hemodynamic evaluation of propranolol in combination with verapamil, nifedipine and diltiazem in exertional angina pectoris: A placebo-controlled, double-blind, randomized, crossover study. *Am J Cardiol* 1985;55:680–687.

28. Winniford MD, Fulton KL, Corbett JR, et al. Propranolol-verapamil versus propranolol-nifedipine in severe angina pectoris of effort: A randomized, double-blind crossover study. *Am J Cardiol* 1985;55:281–285.

29. Findlay IN, MacLeod K, Gillen G, et al. A double-blind placebo-controlled comparison of verapamil, atenolol, and their combination in patients with chronic stable angina pectoris. *Br Heart J* 1987;57:336–343.

30. Packer M, Meller J, Medina N, et al. Hemodynamic consequences of combined beta-adrenergic and slow calcium channel blockade in man. *Circulation* 1982;65:660–668.

31. Patton JN, Vlietstra RE, Frye RL. Randomized, placebo-controlled study of the effect of verapamil on exercise hemodynamics in coronary artery disease. *Am J Cardiol* 1984;53:674–678.

32. Rouleau J-L, Chatterjee K, Ports TA, et al. Mechanism of relief of pacing-induced angina with oral verapamil: Reduced oxygen demand. *Circulation* 1983;67:94–100.

33. Singh BN, Chew CC, Josephson MA, et al. Pharmacologic and hemodynamic mechanisms underlying the anti-anginal actions of verapamil. *Am J Cardiol* 1982;50:886–893.

34. Urquhart J, Epstein SE, Patterson RE. Comparative effects of calcium-channel blocking agents on left ventricular function during acute ischemia in dogs with and without congestive heart failure. *Am J Cardiol* 1985;55:10B–16B.

35. Smith HJ, Goldstein RA, Griffith JM. Regional contractility. Selective depression of ischemic myocardium by verapamil. *Circulation* 1976;54:629–635.

36. Lumley P, Robertson MJ. Experimental conditions can differentially affect calcium channel blocker potency in guinea-pig cardiac muscle. Presentation to NY Acad Sci, Feb 1987.

37. Chew CYC, Brown G, Singh BN, et al. Effects of verapamil on coronary hemodynamic function and vasomobility rela-

tive to its mechanism of antianginal action. *Am J Cardiol* 1983;51:699-705.

38. Heusch G, Guth BD, Seitelberger R, et al. Attenuation of exercise-induced myocardial ischemia in dogs with recruitment of coronary vasodilator reserve by nifedipine. *Circulation* 1987;75:482-490.

39. Apstein CS, Grossman W. Opposite initial effects of supply and demand ischemia on left ventricular diastolic compliance: The ischemia-diastolic paradox. *J Mol Cell Cardiol* 1987;19:119-128.

40. Bonow RO, Leon MB, Rosing DR, et al. Effects of verapamil and propranolol on left ventricular systolic function and diastolic filling in patients with coronary artery disease: Radionuclide angiographic studies at rest and during exercise. *Circulation* 1981;65:1337-1350.

41. Bolognesi R, Cucchini F, Manca C, et al. Effects of verapamil and nifedipine on rate of left ventricular relaxation in coronary artery disease patients with normal systolic function. Presentation to NY Acad Sci, Feb 1987.

42. Atterhog JH, Ekelund LG, Melin AL: Effect of nifedipine on exercise tolerance in patients with angina pectoris. *Eur J Clin Pharmacol* 1975;8:125-130.

43. Ardissino D, de Servi S, Salerno JA, et al. Efficacy, duration and mechanism of action of nifedipine in stable exercise-induced angina pectoris. *Eur Heart J* 1983;4:873-881.

44. Chaitman BR, Wagniart P, Pasternac A, et al. Improved exercise tolerance after propranolol, diltiazem or nifedipine in angina pectoris: Comparison at 1, 3 and 8 hours and correlation with plasma drug concentration. *Am J Cardiol* 1984;53:1-9.

45. Deanfield J, Wright C, Krikler S, et al. Cigarette smoking and the treatment of angina with propranolol, atenolol and nifedipine. *N Engl J Med* 1984;310:951-954.

46. Winniford MD, Jansen DE, Reynolds GA, et al. Cigarette smoking-induced coronary vasoconstriction in atherosclerotic coronary artery disease and prevention by calcium antagonists and nitroglycerin. *Am J Cardiol* 1987;59:203-207.

47. Sherman LG, Liang C-S. Nifedipine in chronic stable angina: A double-blind placebo-controlled crossover trial. *Am J Cardiol* 1983;51:706-711.

48. Lynch P, Dargie H, Krikler S, et al. Objective assessment of antianginal treatment: A double-blind comparison of propranolol, nifedipine and their combination *Br Med J* 1980;281:184-187.

49. Mueller HS, Chahine RA. Interim report of multicenter double-blind, placebo-controlled studies of nifedipine in chronic stable angina. *Am J Med* 1981;71:645-657.

50. Uusitalo A, Arstila M, Bae EA, et al. Metoprolol, nifedipine and the combination in stable effort angina pectoris. *Am J Cardiol* 1986;57:733-737.

51. Findlay IN, MacLeod K, Ford M, et al. Treatment of angina pectoris with nifedipine and atenolol: Efficacy and effect on cardiac function. *Br Heart J* 1986;55:240-245.

52. Higginbotham MB, Morris KG, Coleman RE, et al. Comparison of nifedipine alone with propranolol alone for stable angina pectoris including hemodynamics at rest and during exercise. *Am J Cardiol* 1986;57:1022-1028.

53. Jariwalla AG, Anderson EG. Side effects of drugs. Production of ischaemic cardiac pain by nifedipine. *Br Med J* 1978;1:1181-1182.

54. Stone PH, Muller JE, Turi ZG, et al. Efficacy of nifedipine therapy in patients with refractory angina pectoris: Sig-

nificance of the presence of coronary vasospasm. *Am Heart J* 1983;106:644-652.

55. Deanfield J, Wright C, Fox K. Treatment of angina pectoris with nifedipine: Importance of dose titration. *Br Med J* 1983;286:1467-1470.

56. Terry RW. Nifedipine therapy in angina pectoris: Evaluation of safety and side-effects. *Am Heart J* 1982;104:681-689.

57. Kiowski W, Erne P, Bertel O, et al. Acute and chronic sympathetic reflex activation and antihypertensive response to nifedipine. *J Am Coll Cardiol* 1986;7:344-348.

58. Van Wezel HB, Bovill JG, Koolen JJ, et al. Myocardial metabolism and coronary sinus blood flow during coronary artery surgery: Effects of nitroprusside and nifedipine. *Am Heart J* 1987;113:266-273.

59. Schanzenbacher P, Liebau G, Deeg P, et al. Effect of intravenous and intracoronary nifedipine on coronary blood flow and myocardial oxygen consumption. *Am J Cardiol* 1983;51:712-717.

60. Schanzenbacher P, Gottfert G, Liebau G, et al. Coronary hemodynamic and metabolic effects of nifedipine in patients with coronary artery disease treated with betablocking drugs. *Am J Cardiol* 1985;55:33-36.

61. Sorkin EM, Clissold SP Brogden RN. Nifedipine. A review of its pharmacodynamic and pharmacokinetic properties and therapeutic efficacy in ischaemic heart disease, hypertension and related cardiovascular disorders. *Drugs* 1985; 30:182-274.

62. Emanuelsson H, Holmberg S. Mechanisms of angina relief after nifedipine: A hemodynamic and myocardial metabolic study. *Circulation* 1983;68:124-130.

63. Specchia G, de Servi S, Falcone C, et al. Effects of nifedipine on coronary hemodynamic findings during exercise in patients with stable exertional angina. *Circulation* 1983; 68:1035-1043.

64. Feldman RL, Hill JA, Conti R, et al. Effect of nifedipine on coronary hemodynamics in patients with left anterior descending coronary occlusion. *J Am Coll Cardiol* 1985;5: 318-325.

65. Kramer PH, Chatterjee K, Schwartz A, et al. Alterations in angina threshold with nifedipine during pacing induced angina. *Br Heart J* 1984;52:308-313.

66. Schulz W, Jost S, Kober G, et al. Relation of antianginal efficacy of nifedipine to degree of coronary arterial narrowing and to presence of coronary collateral vessels. *Am J Cardiol* 1985;55:26-32.

67. Lichtlen PR, Engel H-J, Rafflenbeul W. Calcium entry blockers, especially nifedipine, in angina of effort: possible mechanisms and clinical implications. In: Opie LH, ed. *Calcium Antagonists and Cardiovascular Disease.* New York: Raven Press, 1984;221-236.

68. Wagniart P, Ferguson RJ, Chaitman BR, et al. Increased exercise tolerance and reduced electrocardiographic ischemia with diltiazem in patients with stable angina pectoris. *Circulation* 1982;66:23-28.

69. Anderson JL, Wagner JM, Datz FL, et al. Comparative effects of diltiazem, propranolol, and placebo on exercise performance using radionuclide ventriculography in patients with symptomatic coronary artery disease: Results of a double-blind, randomized, crossover study. *Am Heart J* 1984;107:698-706.

70. Hossack KF, Pool PE, Steele P et al: Efficacy of diltiazem in angina of effort: A multicenter trial. *Am J Cardiol* 1982;49:567-572.

71. Hung J, Lamb IH, Connolly SJ, et al. The effect of diltiazem and propranolol, alone and in combination, on exercise performance and left ventricular function in patients with stable effort angina: a double-blind, randomized, and placebo controlled study. *Circulation* 1983; 68:560-567.

72. Lindenberg BS, Weiner DA, McCabe CH, et al. Efficacy and safety of incremental doses of diltiazem for the treatment of stable angina pectoris. *J Am Coll Cardiol* 1983; 2:1129-1133.

73. Go M, Hollenberg M. Improved efficacy of high-dose versus medium- and low-dose diltiazem therapy for chronic stable angina pectoris. *Am J Cardiol* 1984;53:669-673.

74. Strauss WE, Parisi AF. Superiority of combined diltiazem and propranolol therapy for angina pectoris. *Circulation* 1985;71:951-957.

75. Khurmi NS, Bowles MJ, O'Hara MJ, et al. Long-term efficacy of diltiazem assessed with multistage graded exercise tests in patients with chronic stable angina pectoris. *Am J Cardiol* 1984;54:738-743.

76. Weiner DA, Cutler SS, Klein MD. Efficacy and safety of sustained-release diltiazem in stable angina pectoris. *Am J Cardiol* 1986;57:6-9.

77. Joyal M, Cremer K, Pieper J, et al. Effects of diltiazem during tachycardia-induced angina pectoris. *Am J Cardiol* 1986;57:10-14.

78. Lahiri A, Dasgupta P, Rodrigues EA, et al. Acute drug withdrawal in patients with stable angina on long term treatment with verapamil. In: Raftery EB, ed. *Verapamil SR.* Langhorne: ADIS Press International, 1987;18-29.

79. Leisten L, Kuhlmann J, Ebner F. Side effects and pharmacodynamic interactions. In: Krebs R, ed. *Treatment of Cardiovascular Diseases by Adalat^R (nifedipine).* Stuttgart: Schattauer, 1986;279-314.

80. Gottlieb SO, Ouyang P, Achuff SC, et al. Acute nifedipine withdrawal: Consequences of preoperative and late cessation of therapy in patients with prior unstable angina. *J Am Coll Cardiol* 1984;4:382-388.

81. Gill JB, Cairns JA, McEwan MP. Improved left ventricular performance during exercise with verapamil or nifedipine in patients with chronic stable angina. *Am Heart J* 1987; 113:700-707.

82. Schurtz CI, Lesbre JP, Kalisa A, et al. Intérêt des inhibiteurs calciques dans l'angor d'effort stable: Diltiazem versus nifedipine. *Ann Cardiol Angeiol* 1983;32:337-341.

83. Chaffman M, Brogden RN. Diltiazem: A review of its pharmacological properties and therapeutic efficacy. *Drugs* 1985;29:387-454.

84. Weiner DA, McCabe CH, Cutler SS, et al. The efficacy and safety of high-dose verapamil and diltiazem in the long-term treatment of stable exertional angina. *Clin Cardiol* 1984;7:648-653.

85. Landmark K. Antihypertensive and metabolic effects of long-term therapy with nifedipine slow-release tablets. *J Cardiovasc Pharmacol* 1985;7:12-17.

86. Feigl EO. Coronary physiology. *Physiol Rev* 1983;63:1-205.

87. Opie LH, Maseri A. Vasospastic angina. In: Krebs R, ed. *Treatment of Cardiovascular Diseases by Adalat^R (nifedipine).* Stuttgart: Schattauer, 1986;231-258.

88. Young MA, Vatner SF. Regulation of large coronary arteries. *Circ Res* 1986;59:579-596.

89. Rapaport RM, Draznin MB, Murad F. Endothelium-dependent relaxation in rat aorta may be mediated through cyclic GMP-dependent protein dephosphorylation. *Nature*

1983;306:174-176.
90. Furchgott RF. Role of endothelium in responses of vascular smooth muscle. *Circ Res* 1983;53:557-573.
91. Rubanyi G, Vanhoutte PM. Inhibitors of prostaglandin synthesis augment beta-adrenergic responsiveness in canine coronary arteries. *Circ Res* 1985;56:117-125.
92. Rapaport RM, Murad F. Endothelium-dependent and nitrovasodilator-induced relaxation of vascular smooth muscle: Role of cyclic GMP. *J Cyclic Nucleotide Protein Phosphor Res* 1983;9:281-296.
93. Yasue H. Coronary artery spasm and calcium ions. In: Opie LH, ed. *Calcium Antagonists and Cardiovascular Disease.* New York: Raven Press, 1984;117-128.
94. Prinzmetal M, Kennamer R, et al. Angina pectoris. I. A variant form of angina pectoris. *Am J Med* 1959;27:375-388.
95. Maseri A, Severi S, De Nes M, et al. "Variant" angina: One aspect of a continuous spectrum of vasospastic myocardial ischemia. Pathogenetic mechanisms, estimated incidence and clinical and coronary arteriographic findings in 138 patients. *Am J Cardiol* 1978;42:1019-1035.
96. Pepine CJ, Feldman RL, Hill JA, et al. Clinical outcome after treatment of rest angina with calcium blockers: Comparative experience during the initial year of therapy with diltiazem, nifedipine and verapamil. *Am Heart J* 1983; 106:1341-1347.
97. Previtali M, Panciroli C, Ardissino D, et al. Spontaneous remission of variant angina documented by Holter monitoring and ergonovine testing in patients treated with calcium antagonists. *Am J Cardiol* 1987;59:235-240.
98. Antman E, Muller J, Goldberg S, et al. Nifedipine therapy for coronary artery spasm. Experience in 127 patients. *N Engl J Med* 1980;302:1269-1273.
99. Kimura E, Kishida H. Treatment of variant angina with drugs: A survey of 11 cardiology institutes in Japan. *Circulation* 1981;63:844-848.
100. Waters DD, Miller DD, Szlachcic J. Factors influencing the long-term prognosis of treated patients with variant angina. *Circulation* 1983;68:258-265.
101. Rich S, Ford LE, Al-Sadir J. The angiographic effect of ergonovine and nifedipine in coronary artery spasm. *Circulation* 1980;62:1127-1130.
102. Tiefenbrunn AJ, Sobel BE, Gowda S, et al. Nifedipine blockade of ergonovine-induced coronary arterial spasm: Angiographic documentation. *Am J Cardiol* 1981;48:184-187.
103. Previtali M, Salerno JA, Tavazzi L, et al. Treatment of angina at rest with nifedipine: A short-term controlled study. *Am J Cardiol* 1980;45:825-830.
104. Shick EC, Liang CS, Heuler FA, et al. Randomized withdrawal from nifedipine: Placebo-controlled study in patients with coronary artery spasm. *Am Heart J* 1982; 104:690-697.
105. Winniford MD, Johnson SM, Mauritson DR, et al. Verapamil therapy for Prinzmetal's variant angina: Comparison with placebo and nifedipine. *Am J Cardiol* 1982; 50:913-918.
106. Prida XE, Gelman JS, Feldman RL, et al. Comparison of diltiazem and nifedipine alone and in combination in patients with coronary artery spasm. *J Am Coll Cardiol* 1987;9:412-419.
107. Waters DD, Theroux P, Szlachcic J, et al. Provocative testing with ergonovine to assess the efficacy of treatment with nifedipine, diltiazem and verapamil in variant angina. *Am J Cardiol* 1981;48:123-130.

108. Ginsburg R, Lamb IH, Schroeder JS, et al. Randomized double-blind comparison of nifedipine and isosorbide dinitrate therapy in variant angina pectoris due to coronary artery spasm. *Am Heart J* 1982;103:44-48.

109. Hill JA, Feldman RL, Pepine CJ, et al. Randomized double-blind comparison of nifedipine and isosorbide dinitrate in patients with coronary arterial spasm. *Am J Cardiol* 1982;49:431-438.

110. Winniford MD, Gabliani G, Johnson SM, et al. Concomitant calcium antagonists plus isosorbide dinitrate therapy for markedly active variant angina. *Am Heart J* 1984;108: 1269-1273.

111. Parodi O, Simonetti I, Michelassi C, et al. Comparison of verapamil and propranolol therapy for angina pectoris at rest: A randomized, multiple crossover, controlled trial in the coronary care unit. *Am J Cardiol* 1986;57:899-906.

112. Tilmant PY, Lablanche JM, Thieuleux FA, et al. Detrimental effect of propranolol in patients with coronary arterial spasm contered by combination with diltiazem. *Am J Cardiol* 1983;52:230-233.

113. Robertson RM, Wood AJ, Vaughan WK, et al. Exacerbation of vasotonic angina pectoris by propranolol. *Circulation* 1982; 65:281-285.

114. Lette J, Gagnon RM, Lemire JG, et al. Rebound of vasospastic angina after cessation of long-term treatment with nifedipine. *Can Med Assoc J* 1984; 130:1169-1171.

115. Moses JW, Wertheimer JH, Bodenheimer MM, et al. Efficacy of nifedipine in rest angina refractory to propranolol and nitrates in patients with obstructive coronary artery disease. *Ann Intern Med* 1981; 94:425-429.

116. Muiesan G, Agabiti-Rosei E, Romanelli G, et al: Adrenergic activity and left ventricular function during treatment of essential hypertension with calcium antagonists. *Am J Cardiol* 1986; 57:44D-49D.

117. Schroeder JS, Walker SD, Skalland L, et al. Absence of rebound from diltiazem therapy in Prinzmetal's variant angina. *J Am Coll Cardiol* 1985; 6:174-178.

118. Yasue H, Omote S, Takizawa A, et al. Circadian variation of exercise capacity in patients with Prinzmetal's variant angina: Role of exercise-induced coronary artery spasm. *Circulation* 1979; 59:938-947.

119. Yasue H, Omote S, Takizawa A, et al. Exertional angina pectoris caused by coronary artery spasm: Effects of various drugs. *Am J Cardiol* 1979; 43:647-652.

120. Opie LH, Jee L, White D. Antihypertensive effects of nifedipine combined with cardioselective beta-adrenergic receptor antagonism by atenolol. *Am Heart J* 1982; 104:606-612.

121. Stone PH. Calcium antagonists for Prinzmetal's variant angina, unstable angina and silent myocardial ischemia. Therapeutic tool and probe for identification of pathophysiologic mechanisms. *Am J Cardiol* 1987; 59:101B-115B.

122. Glazier JJ, Chierchia S, Brown MJ, et al. Importance of generalized defective perception of painful stimuli as a cause of silent myocardial ischemia in chronic stable angina pectoris. *Am J Cardiol* 1986; 58:667-672.

123. Quyyumi AA, Wright C, Fox K. Ambulatory electrocardiographic ST segment changes in healthy volunteers. *Br Heart J* 1983; 50:460-464.

124. Cocco G, Strozzi C, Chu D, et al. Therapeutic effects of pindolol and nifedipine in patients with stable angina pectoris and asymptomatic resting ischemia. *Eur J Cardiol* 1979; 10:59-69.

125. Quyyumi AA, Wright C, Mockus L, et al. Effect of partial

agonist activity in ß-blockers in severe angina pectoris: A double-blind comparison of pindolol and atenolol. *Br Med J* 1984; 289:951-953.

126. Parodi O, Simonetti I, L'Abbate A, et al. Verapamil versus propranolol for angina at rest. *Am J Cardiol* 1982; 50:923-928.

127. Rizzon P, Scrutinio D, Mangini SG, et al. Randomized placebo-controlled comparative study of nifedipine, verapamil and isosorbide dinitrate in the treatment of angina at rest. *Eur Heart J* 1986; 7:67-76.

128. Pepine CJ, Feldman RL, Ludbrook P, et al. Left ventricular dyskinesia reversed by intravenous nitroglycerin: A manifestation of silent myocardial ischemia. *Am J Cardiol* 1986; 58:38B-42B.

129. Gottlieb SO, Weisfeldt ML, Ouyang P, et al. Silent ischemia as a marker for early unfavorable outcomes in patients with unstable angina. *N Engl J Med* 1986;314:1214-1219.

130. Maseri A, Chierchia S, Kaski JC. Mixed angina pectoris. *Am J Cardiol* 1985; 56:30E-33E.

131. Andre-Fouet X, Usdin JP, Gayet CH, et al. Comparison of short-term efficacy of diltiazem and propranolol in unstable angina at rest—randomized trial in 70 patients. *Eur Heart J* 1983; 4:691-698.

132. Parodi O, Maseri A, Simonetti I. Management of unstable angina at rest by verapamil. A double-blind cross-over study in coronary care unit. *Br Heart J* 1979; 41:167-174.

133. Capucci A, Bassein L, Bracchetti D, et al. Propranolol v. verapamil in the treatment of unstable angina. A double-blind cross-over study. *Eur Heart J* 1983; 4:148-154.

134. Moll MG, Dominguez JM, Obrador D, et al. Nifedipine (N) vs. propranolol (P) in unstable angina (UA): A prospective randomized study (abstr). *Eur Heart J* 1984; 5(Suppl 1):238.

135. Rahimtoola SH, Nunley D, Grunkemeier G, et al. Ten year survival after coronary artery bypass surgery for unstable angina. *N Engl J Med* 1983; 308:676-681.

136. Gazes PC, Mobley EM, Faris HM, et al. Preinfarctional (unstable) angina—a prospective study—ten year follow-up. Prognostic significance of electrocardiographic changes. *Circulation* 1973; 48:331-337.

137. Fischl SJ, Herman MV, Gorlin R: The intermediate coronary syndrome. Clinical, angiographic and therapeutic aspects. *N Engl J Med* 1973; 288:1193-1198.

138. Conti, CR, Brawley RK, Griffith LSC, et al. Unstable angina pectoris: Morbidity and mortality in 57 consecutive patients evaluated angiographically. *Am J Cardiol* 1973; 32:745-750.

139. HINT Research Group (Holland Interuniversity Nifedipine/Metroprolol Trial): Early treatment of unstable angina in the coronary care unit: A randomised double-blind placebo-controlled comparison of recurrent ischaemia in patients treated with nifedipine or metoprolol or both. *Br Heart J* 1986; 56:400-413.

140. Theroux P, Taeymans Y, Morissette D, et al. A randomized study comparing propranolol and diltiazem in the treatment of unstable angina. *J Am Coll Cardiol* 1985; 5:717-722.

141. Forrester JS, Litvack F, Grundfest W, et al. A perspective of coronary disease seen through the arteries of living man. *Circulation* 1987; 75:505-513.

142. Opie LH. Metabolism of free fatty acids, glucose and catecholamines in acute myocardial infarction. Relation to myocardial ischemia and infarct size. *Am J Cardiol* 1975; 36:938-953.

143. Hugenholtz PG: Unstable angina pectoris. In: Krebs R, ed. *Treatment of Cardiovascular Diseases by Adalat^R (Nifedipine)*. Stuttgart: Schattauer, 1986;187–229.

144. Muller JE, Turi ZG, Pearle DL, et al: Nifedipine and conventional therapy for unstable angina pectoris: A randomized, double-blind comparison. *Circulation* 1984; 69:728–739.

145. Muller J, Morrison J, Stone PH, et al: Nifedipine therapy for patients with threatened and acute myocardial infarction: A randomized double-blind placebo-controlled comparison. *Circulation* 1984; 69:740–747.

146. Yokoyama M, Koizumi T, Fujitani K, et al. Adverse response to nifedipine in unstable angina pectoris. *Chest* 1982; 81:646–648.

147. Sia STB, MacDonald PS, Triester B, et al. Aggravation of myocardial ischemia by nifedipine. *Med J Aust* 1985; 142:48–50.

148. Gerstenblith G, Ouyang P, Achuff SC, et al. Nifedipine in unstable angina: A double-blind randomized trial. *N Engl J Med* 1982; 306:885–889.

149. Scheidt S, Frishman WH, Packer M, et al. Long-term effectiveness of verapamil in stable and unstable angina pectoris. One-year follow-up of patients treated in placebo-controlled double-blind randomized clinical trials. *Am J Cardiol* 1982; 50:1185–1190.

150. Gordon GD, Mabin TA, Isaacs S, et al: Hemodynamic effects of sublingual nifedipine in acute myocardial infarction. *Am J Cardiol* 1984; 53:1228–1232.

151. Gordon GD, Mabin TA, Lloyd EA, et al. Nifedipine in acute myocardial infarction. In: Lichtlen PR, ed. *Sixth International Adalat Symposium*. Amsterdam: Excerpta Medica, 1986;271–279.

152. Sirnes PA, Overskeid K, Pedersen TR, et al. Evolution of infarct size during the early use of nifedipine in patients with acute myocardial infarction: The Norwegian Nifedipine Multicenter Trial. *Circulation* 1984; 70:638–644.

153. Wilcox RG, Hampton JR, Banks DC, et al. Trial of early nifedipine in acute myocardial infarction: The Trent study. *Br Med J* 1986; 293:1204–1208.

154. Branagan JP, Walsh K, Kelly P, et al. Effect of early treatment with nifedipine in suspected acute myocardial infarction. *Eur Heart J* 1986; 7:858–865.

155. Wolf R, Habel F, Witt E, et al. Wirkung von Verapamil auf die Hemodynamik und Grosse des akuten Myokardinfarkts. *Herz* 1977; 2:110–119.

156. Bussmann WD, Scher W, Grungras M. Reduktion der CK und CKMB-infarktgrosse durch Verapamil. *Deutsche Med Wochschr* 1983; 108:1047–1053.

157. Thuesen L, Jorgenson JR, Kvistgaard HJ, et al. Effect of verapamil on enzyme release after early intravenous administration in acute myocardial infarction: Double-blind randomized trial. *Br Med J* 1983; 286:1107–1108.

158. Danish Study Group on Verapamil in Myocardial Infarction. Verapamil in acute myocardial infarction. *Br J Clin Pharmacol* 1986; 21:197S–204S.

159. Crea F, Deanfield J, Crean P, et al. Effects of verapamil in preventing early postinfarction angina and reinfarction. *Am J Cardiol* 1985; 55:900–904.

160. Gibson RS, Boden WE, Theroux P, et al. Diltiazem and reinfarction in patients with non-Q-wave myocardial infarction. *N Engl J Med* 1986; 315:423–429.

161. Yusuf S, Furberg C. Effect of acute or chronic administration of calcium antagonists on mortality following myocardial infarction (abstr). *J Am Coll Cardiol* 1987; 9:24A.

162. Yusuf S, Peto R, Lewis J, et al. Beta blockade during and after myocardial infarction: An overview of the randomized trials. *Prog Cardiovasc Dis* 1985; 27:335-371.

163. Hearse DJ: Critical distinctions in the modification of myocardial cell injury. In: Opie LH, ed. *Calcium Antagonists and Cardiovascular Disease.* New York: Raven Press, 1984;129-145.

164. Opie LH, Coetzee WA. Are calcium ions involved in the genesis of early ischemic ventricular arrhythmias? In: Hearse D, Manning A, Janse M, eds. *Life-Threatening Arrhythmias During Ischemia and Infarction.* New York: Raven Press, 1987;63-75.

165. Thandroyen FT. Protective action of calcium channel antagonist agents against ventricular fibrillation in isolated perfused rat heart. *J Mol Cell Cardiol* 1982; 14:21-32.

166. Clusin WT, Bristow MR, Bain DS, et al. The effects of diltiazem and reduced serum ionized calcium on ischemic ventricular fibrillation in the dog. *Circ Res* 1982; 50:518-526.

167. Coetzee WA, Dennis SC, Opie LH, et al: Calcium channel blockers and early ischemic ventricular arrhythmias: Electrophysiological versus anti-ischemic effects. *J Mol Cell Cardiol* 1987;19(Suppl 2):77-97.

168. Lubbe WF, Podzuweit T, Daries PS, et al. The role of cyclic adenosine monophosphate in adrenergic effects on vulnerability to fibrillation in the isolated perfused rat heart. *J Clin Invest* 1978; 61:1260-1269.

169. Opie LH, Nathan D, Lubbe WF. Biochemical aspects of arrhythmogenesis and ventricular fibrillation. *Am J Cardiol* 1979; 43:131-148.

170. Opie LH, Muller C, Nathan D, et al. Evidence for role of cyclic AMP as second messenger of arrhythmogenic effects of beta-stimulation. *Adv Cyclic Nucleotide Res* 1980; 12:63-69.

171. Thandroyen FT, Higginson L, Opie LH, et al. The influence of verapamil and its isomers on vulnerability to ventricular fibrillation during acute myocardial ischemia and adrenergic stimulation in isolated rat heart. *J Mol Cell Cardiol* 1986; 18:645-649.

172. Nayler WG, Panagiotopoulos S, Elz JS, et al. Fundamental mechanisms of action of calcium antagonists in myocardial ischemia. *Am J Cardiol* 1987; 59:75B-83B.

173. Sievers RE, Rashid T, Garrett J, et al. Verapamil and diet halt progression of atherosclerosis in cholesterol fed rabbits. *Cardiovasc Drugs Ther* 1987; 1:65-69.

174. Hugenholtz PG, Serruys PW, Fleckenstein A, et al. Why Ca^{2+} antagonists will be most useful before or during early myocardial ischaemia and not after infarction has been established. *Eur Heart J* 1986; 7:270-278.

175. Murakami T, Hess OM, Krayenbuehl HP. Left ventricular function before and after diltiazem in patients with coronary artery disease. *J Am Coll Cardiol* 1985; 5:723-730.

176. Yoon SB, McMillin-Wood JB, Michael LH, et al. Protection of canine cardiac mitochondrial function by verapamil-cardioplegia during ischemic arrest. *Circ Res* 1965; 56:704-708.

177. Bourdillon PD, Poole-Wilson PA. The effects of verapamil, quiescence, and cardioplegia on calcium exchange and mechanical function in ischemic rabbit myocardium. *Circ Res* 1982; 50:360-368.

178. Bersohn MM, Shine KI. Verapamil protection of ischemic isolated rabbit heart: Dependence on pretreatment. *J Mol Cell Cardiol* 1983; 15:659-671.

179. Henry PD, Shuchleib R, Davis J, et al. Myocardial contracture and accumulation of mitochondrial calcium in ischemic rabbit heart. *Am J Physiol* 1977; 233:H677–H684.
180. Cheung JY, Leaf A, Bonventre JV: Mechanism of protection by verapamil and nifedipine from anoxic injury in isolated cardiac myocytes. *Am J Physiol* 1984; 246:C323–C329.
181. Hamm CW, Opie LH. Protection of infarcting myocardium by slow channel inhibitors. Comparative effects of verapamil, nifedipine, and diltiazem in the coronary-ligated, isolated working rat heart. *Circ Res* 1983; 52(Suppl I):129–138.
182. Kenmure ACF, Scruton JH. A double-blind controlled trial of the anti-anginal efficacy of nifedipine compared with propranolol. *Br J Clin Pract* 1980; (Suppl 8):49–52.
183. Humen DP, O'Brien P, Purves P, et al. Effort angina with adequate beta-receptor blockade: Comparison with diltiazem alone and in combination. *J Am Coll Cardiol* 1986; 7:329–335.
184. Khurmi NS, Raftery EB. A comparison of nine calcium ion antagonists and propranolol: Exercise tolerance, heart rate and ST-segment changes in patients with chronic stable angina pectoris. *Eur J Clin Pharmacol* 1987;32:539–548.
185. Oakley GDG, Fox KM, Dargie HJ, et al. Objective assessment of treatment in severe angina. *Br Med J* 1979; i;1540.
186. Mauritson DR, Johnson SM, Winniford MD, et al. Verapamil for unstable angina at rest: A short-term randomized, double-blind study. *Am Heart J* 1983; 106:652–658.
187. Multicenter Diltiazem Postinfarction Trial Research Group. The effect of diltiazem on mortality and reinfarction after myocardial infarction. *N Engl J Med* 1988;319:385–392.

Note added in proof:

In mixed angina, beta-blockade is better than nifedipine or nitrates (Quyyumi et al, *Br Heart J* 1987;57:505-511). Nifedipine may exacerbate angina in nearly half (De Cesare et al, *Chest* 1988;93:485-492). In contrast, in patients already treated by beta-blockade and nitrates, addition of nifedipine is better than placebo (Stone et al, *Am Heart J* 1988;116:961-971). Hence beta-blockade remains the best documented initial therapy for mixed angina.

Prevention of coronary atherosclerosis

The preliminary results of the INTACT trial (International Nifedipine Trial on Antiatherosclerotic Therapy, see first issue of Cardiovascular Drugs and Therapy) claim that nifedipine capsules, 20 mg four times daily, slowed the development of new coronary lesions over a 3-year period (p<0.04). Existing lesions were unchanged.

CALCIUM CHANNEL ANTAGONISTS: PART III: USE AND COMPARATIVE EFFICACY IN HYPERTENSION AND SUPRAVENTRICULAR ARRHYTHMIAS. MINOR INDICATIONS

SUMMARY. The major antihypertensive mechanism of calcium antagonists is by decreasing the systemic vascular resistance, modified by the counter-regulatory responses of the baroreflexes and the renin-angiotensin-aldosterone system. In severe hypertension, the concept that calcium overload of the vascular myocyte could precipitate or aggravate peripheral vasoconstriction provides a logical basis for the use of these agents as first choice therapy; nifedipine, especially, has been well tested. As monotherapy for mild to moderate hypertension each of the three first-generation agents compares well with β-blockers. Calcium antagonists may have a special role in the therapy of certain patient groups (elderly, black) or in those subjects whose life style involves intense physical or mental exertion (hemodynamics better maintained than with β-blockade) or in patients with early end-organ damage such as left ventricular hypertrophy or renal insufficiency. However, the goal blood pressure may not be reached during monotherapy so that drug combinations may be required. Further indications for these compounds are as follows. Verapamil and diltiazem are frequently used in supraventricular tachycardias including acute and chronic atrial fibrillation. In the arrhythmias of the Wolff-Parkinson-White syndrome, there is the potential danger of provocation of anterograde conduction. Further indications for calcium antagonists, still under evaluation, include congestive heart failure (controversial), hypertrophic cardiomyopathy (verapamil), primary pulmonary hypertension (high doses required), Raynaud's phenomenon (nifedipine and diltiazem effective), peripheral vascular disease (proof not yet documented), cerebral insufficiency and subarachnoid hemorrhage (nimodipine promising), migraine, exertional bronchospasm, renal disease, atherosclerosis (experimental), and primary aldosteronism (nifedipine inhibits aldosterone release).

Use and Comparative Efficacy of Calcium Antagonists in Hypertension

Calcium antagonists, having a strong peripheral arteriolar vasodilation (Figure III-1), are all effective in hypertension in addition to their other indications (Table III-1). The major problem is where to place

131

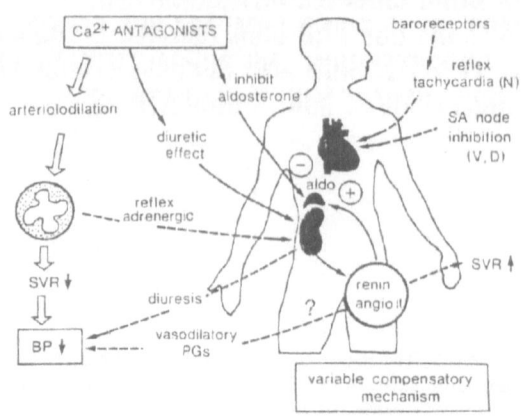

Fig. III-1. Proposed mechanisms whereby calcium antagonists as a class may have an antihypertensive mechanism. Note the major effect is on the peripheral arterioles causing vasodilation and a fall in the systemic vascular resistance (SVR). In response to the hypotension are various compensatory mechanisms such as renin–angiotensin-II– aldosterone release which all tend to increase the blood pressure. Such compensation tends to decrease in time. Aldo, aldosterone; angio II, angiotensin-II; D, diltiazem; vasodilatory PGs, vasodilatory prostaglandins; V, verapamil (see Swartz [11]). Fig. copyright, L.H. Opie.

them in the hierarchy, whether first-, second-, or third-line antihypertensive agents, and whether to use them for severe or mild hypertension. An additional problem is to know how they compare with or combine with established agents such as β-blockers and diuretics.

Physiologic Principles

Role of intracellular calcium overload. Two new findings have drawn attention to the potential role of calcium in hypertension. First, many recent measurements show that calcium levels (free or ionized) are increased in tissues from hypertensive animals or humans (Table III-2). Both the concentrations of sodium and calcium are increased in smooth muscle cells from spontaneously hypertensive rats when compared with normals (Table III-3). The proposal is that in essential hypertension there is a circulating plasma factor that increases cytosolic calcium [1]; possibly this factor may be the same as the sodium-transport inhibitor (natriuretic factor) of DeWardner and MacGregor [2]. Thus, the sodium-calcium exchange in vascular smooth muscle is proposed as the link between the abnormalities of sodium metabolism found in hypertension and the actual vasoconstrictive mechanism [3].

In severe hypertension, abnormalities of calcium regulation may explain the excess peripheral vasoconstriction [4]. An intriguing clinical observation is that verapamil decreased blood pressure (BP) more than did sodium nitroprusside in severe hypertensives. Assuming that top doses of both agents were employed, the "excess hypotensive" effect of verapamil could be plotted against the BP; the higher the BP, the more the excess effect (Figure III-2). This observation agrees with the powerful antihypertensive effect of nifedipine in severe hypertensives (see Severe Hypertension, below).

However, these findings cannot be interpreted as evidence that only calcium antagonists are beneficial in severe hypertension. On the contrary, intracellular calcium in vascular smooth muscle is under complex control (Figure III-3), including the indirect effect of sodium (therefore diuretics may have a vascular relaxing effect), angiotensin [therefore angiotensin converting enzyme (ACE) inhibitors are also concerned with the regulation of calcium], and cyclic nucleotides, with cyclic guanine monophosphate (GMP) the chief vasodilator and a lesser dilator role for cyclic adenosine monophosphate (AMP) (therefore β-adrenoceptor antagonists also modify intracellular calcium). During therapy of hypertension [5], reduction of BP by calcium antagonists, diuretics, or β-blockers all reduce platelet calcium concentration. Nevertheless, the concept of intracellular calcium being the final end trigger to increase vascular smooth muscle tone in hypertension leads directly to the use of calcium antagonist agents in this condition. The concept of the "excess hypotensive" effect of calcium antagonists in severe hypertension [4] makes these agents particularly attractive as therapeutic options.

Role of renin-angiotensin-aldosterone system. In mild to moderate hypertension, the basic mechanism of the antihypertensive action of calcium antagonists is their inhibitory effect on peripheral vascular tone, causing peripheral vasodilation (see Figure III-1). Vasodilation induced by agents such as minoxidil and hydralazine should be followed by a reflex sympathetic stimulation, release of renin and the ultimate formation of angiotensin-II, which in turn stimulates the secretion of aldosterone. The end results are a partial compensatory vasoconstriction tending to offset the vasodilation, and sodium and fluid retention tending to cause edema. Therefore vasodilators such as hydralazine and minoxidil are usually given in combination with a β-blocker and a diuretic to dampen these reflex mechanisms. However, calcium antagonists do not generally lead to a sustained rise of plasma renin levels, although there are reports of a small increase,

Table III-1. *Summary of comparative indications of calcium antagonists including hypertension, angina, and supraventricular arrhythmias*

Condition	Verapamil	Nifedipine	Diltiazem
Severe hypertension[c]	+	++	+
Hypertension (second- or third-line therapy)	+	++	++
Hypertension, monotherapy[c]	+	+	+
Coronary artery spasm (Prinzmetal's)	++	++	++
Chronic stable angina of effort	++	$+/++^a$	++
Angina with hypertension	++	++	++
Angina with heart failure	±	++	+
Angina at rest	++	++	++
Unstable angina (threatened infarction)	++	±	++
Unstable angina already treated by β-blockade	+	++	+
Combination with β-blockade	+	++	++
Supraventricular tachycardia,[c] acute IV use	++	−	++
Supraventricular tachycardia,[d] oral prophylaxis	++	−	++
Chronic atrial fibrillation or flutter[c] (± digitalis)	++	$-^b$	++
Hypertrophy cardiomyopathy[d]	++		+

Adapted from [209] by courtesy of Grune & Stratton.

(++), well tested/frequently used; (+), used; (−), not used or no effect

[a]Careful titration needed.

[b]Contraindicated in obstructive variety.

[c]Only verapamil approved in United States.

[d]Not approved in United States.

Table III-2. Calcium levels (free or ionized) or indices of calcium metabolism in tissues from hypertensive animals or humans

Tissue	Source of Tissue	Change Found	Interpretation/Comment
Free Ca (Quin 2)			
Platelets	Human	+	Rises with BP and falls with therapy by β-blocker, calcium antagonists, or diuretics
Platelets	Human	+	External Ca required to show increase versus normal subjects
Platelets	Human	+	Slight rise of Ca with BP rise (with wide overlap)
Lymphocytes	Milan HR	+	Associated with low cell Na
Free Ca (ionized)			
RBC	Human	+	Associated with low cell Na
VSM, RBC	SHR	+	Elevated Ca but not Na disappears on culture and therefore due to "humoral" factors
RBC	Human	+	Ca changes associated with hypertension, Na changes genetic

(continued)

Table III-2 (continued)

Tissue	Source of Tissue	Change Found	Interpretation/Comment
Ca ATPase			
RBC	Milan HR	−	Explains high Ca
Arteries	SHR	−	Explains high Ca
Platelets	Human	−	Blunted calmodulin stimulation
Ca binding/accumulation			
RBC	SHR	−	Inside-out membrane vesicles
Heart	SHR prehypertensive	−	Differences vs. control eliminated by calmodulin
RBC, heart	SHR	−	Found in prehypertensive rats—genetic
Ca uptake			
Brain synaptosome, platelets	SHR	+	Increased Na^+ permeability in primary hypertension "type of generalized membrane pathology"

From [210] by courtesy *Annals of the New York Academy of Sciences.*
(+), increase; (−), decrease; ATPase, adenosine triphosphatase; HR, hypertensive rat; RBC, red blood cells; SHR, spontaneously hypertensive rat.

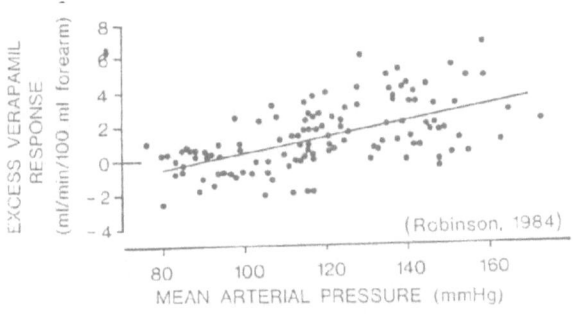

Fig. III-2. The concept of an "excess" calcium-dependent component to hypertension, increasing with the severity of hypertension, is based on the data of Robinson [4] and receives support from MacGregor [68]. The acute dilator response to intravenous verapamil has been compared with that of sodium nitroprusside and the "excess verapamil response" is the amount by which the dilator effect of verapamil exceeds that expected from the regression line for sodium nitroprusside. From [4] by courtesy of Journal of Hypertension *and the author.*

especially in response to acute vasodilation by nifedipine and to a lesser extent in the acute phase of verapamil or diltiazem therapy (Table III-4). During chronic therapy with nifedipine there is only a small increase in plasma renin activity [6] which may not be detectable [7]. Unexpectedly, plasma aldosterone le-

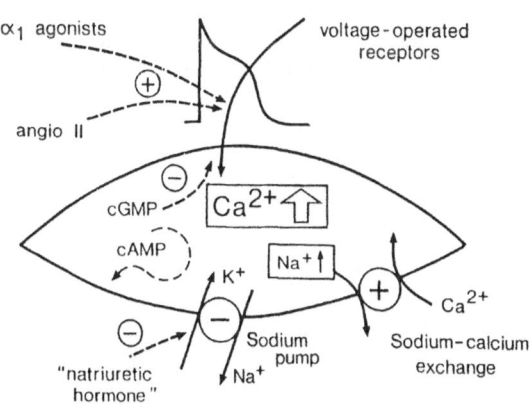

Fig. III-3. Proposed cellular control mechanisms in vascular myocyte. Intracellular cytosolic calcium ion concentration can rise in response to 1) voltage-operated Ca^{2+} entry, which can be facilitated by α_1-agonist activity and/or angiotensin-II; 2) inhibition of the sodium pump by the "natriuretic hormone" with a rise of intracellular sodium and a consequent enhanced activity of the Na^+/Ca^{2+} exchange; and 3) activity of cyclic GMP or cyclic AMP. Cyclic GMP probably acts as a relaxant by inhibiting Ca^{2+} entry or by enhancing Ca^{2+} egress, whereas cyclic AMP may enhance Ca^{2+} uptake into the sarcoplasmic reticulum. Fig copyright, L.H. Opie.

Table III-3. Concentrations of sodium and calcium in smooth muscle cells

Ion	Extracellular Value (Ionized) (mmol/L)	Smooth Muscle Preparation	Value (mmol/L)
Na^+	140	Mesenteric artery	11
		Cultured aortic cells[a]	
		Normal rats	3
		SH rats	15
		Taenia coli	22
Ca^{2+}	1.25	Cultured aortic cells[a]	
		Normal rats	0.016
		SH rats	0.121

From [210] by courtesy of *Annals of New York Academy of Sciences.*
Abbreviations: SH, spontaneously hypertensive.
[a]May not reflect physiologic conditions.

vels do not rise during calcium antagonist therapy, even if renin and angiotensin-II levels do, probably because calcium ions are involved in aldosterone secretion so that the calcium antagonists have an inhibitory effect (Figure III-4).

Plasma catecholamines. In response to peripheral vasodilation, the reflex sympathetic discharge tends to increase plasma norepinephrine levels. The normal levels of epinephrine are low so that the assay is at the bottom limit of its sensitivity and even increases are difficult to measure. In the case of norepinephrine, the general trend is for calcium antagonist therapy to increase plasma levels [8–11] especially during standing [7]. The increase is more consistent with nifedipine than with verapamil [7], and is also found with diltiazem [11].

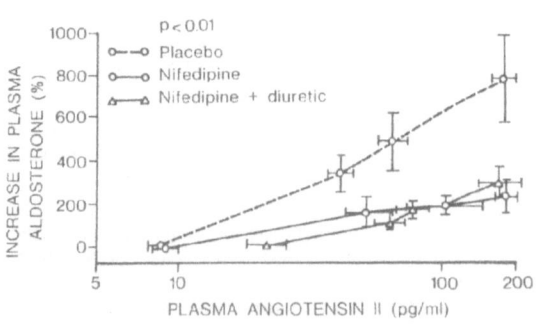

Fig. III-4. The effect of the calcium antagonist nifedipine in inhibiting release of aldosterone in response to angiotensin-II during an infusion of angiotensin-II in patients with mild hypertension. Marone, 1985. Bars are means ± SEM. From [211] by courtesy of Kidney International.

Table III-4. Effects of calcium antagonist agents on the renin-angiotensin-aldosterone system

	PRA	Aldosterone	Plasma NE
Short-term			
Diltiazem	↔	↔	↑
Nifedipine	↑	↔	↑
Nitrendipine	↔	↔	↑
Nicardipine	↔↑	↔	?
Verapamil	↔	↔	↑↔
Long-term			
Diltiazem	↔↑	↔	↑
Nifedipine	↔↑	↔	↑
Nitrendipine	↔↑	↔	—
Nicardipine	↔↑	↔	—
Verapamil	↔	↔	↑
Nisoldipine	↑	—	↑

PRA data adapted from [12] by courtesy of *American Journal of Cardiology* and the authors.
For extra data see [7-9, 11, 44, 102, 200].
Abbreviations: Aldosterone, plasma aldosterone concentration; NE, norepinephrine; PRA, plasma renin activity; ↔, no change.

Role of diuretic effect. Besides inhibiting the secretion of aldosterone, calcium antagonists as a group have an acute diuretic effect (Table III-5), only partially explicable by an increased renal blood flow. The extent of the sodium diuresis appears to be more marked in hypertensive than in normal subjects [9]. This diuretic effect is sustained in some studies, and may contribute to the antihypertensive mechanisms (for other references, see Part I, Renal Effects of Calcium Antagonists). Some reports suggest that calcium antagonists may actually improve glomerular filtration rate [12].

Table III-5. Effects of calcium entry blockers on renal function and hemodynamics

	Urinary Volume and Na$^+$ Loss	GFR	ERPF	RVR
Short-term				
Diltiazem	↑	↔↑	↔↑	—
Nifedipine	↑	↔↑	↔↑	—
Nitrendipine	↑	↔	↔	—
Nicardipine	↑	↔	—	—
Verapamil	↑	↔	—	—
Long-term				
Diltiazem	↔	↔↑	↔↑	↔↓
Nifedipine	↔	↔	↔	—
Nitrendipine	↑↔	↔	↔	↔
Nicardipine	↑↔	↔↑	—	—
Verapamil	↔	↔	—	—

Adapted from [12] by courtesy of *American Journal of Cardiology* and the authors. *Abbreviations:* ERPF, effective renal plasma flow; GFR, glomerular filtration rate; RVR, renal vascular resistance; ↔, no change.

Role of baroreflexes in counter-regulation. In response to acute hypotension, baroreflexes in the aortic arch and carotid body are activated with stimulation of vagal afferent and adrenergic efferent reflexes (Figure III-5). The compensatory adrenergic discharge causes a reflex tachycardia and release of renin, the latter in turn stimulating the formation of angiotensin-II with ultimate vasoconstriction and release of aldosterone. Converting enzyme inhibition buffers this counter-regulatory response [13]. When nifedipine is given to patients with severe hypertension, the acute hypotensive effect is not accompanied by tachycardia (Figures III-6 and III-7), showing inhibition of the baroreflex arc. The explanation is complex and includes the dampening effect of severe hypertension on baroreflexes, possibly as a result of edematous infiltration [14]. Thus, when hypertension is severe, the baroreflex response to an acute fall in BP by any appropriate therapy is diminished. As the BP falls, the baroreflex response is restored [14]. Even in patients with moderate hypertension (mean initial value 173/109 mmHg) nifedipine therapy (10 mg three times daily) is accompanied by an increased baroreceptor sensitivity [15]. The less sensitive the baroreflexes are, the greater the hypotensive response to nifedipine [10], presumably because the reflex vasoconstriction is diminished. Gradual restoration of baroreflex sensitivity [15] may

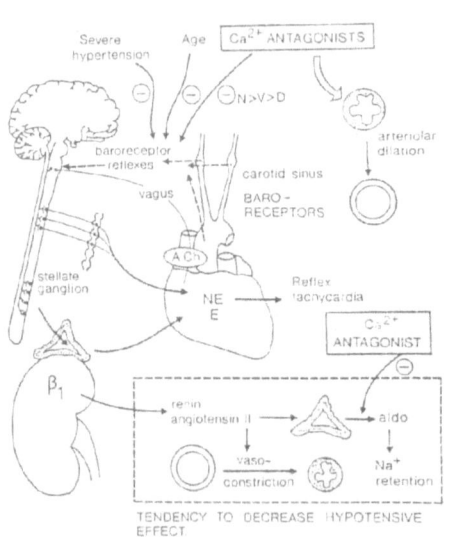

Fig. III-5. *Proposed role of baroreceptors in control of blood pressure, together with effect of severe hypertension, and calcium antagonists in regulating baroreceptor response. Note inhibition of aldosterone secretion by calcium antagonists. Fig. copyright, L.H. Opie.*

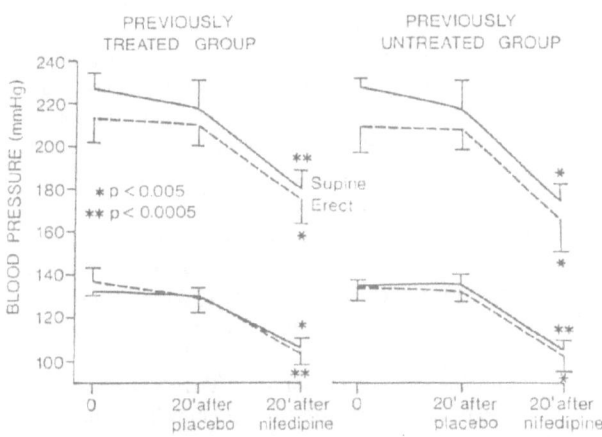

Fig. III-6. Comparison of acute hypotensive response to nifedipine in erect and supine positions. Note that there is a similar response to nifedipine in both previously treated (eight patients) and untreated patients (eight patients), and that nifedipine does not induce acute postural hypotension. * = differences from time zero with $p < 0.005$. ** = differences from time zero with $p < 0.0005$. From [16] by courtesy of American Heart Journal.

explain in part a delayed increased hypotensive effect of nifedipine [16]. If, however, sympathetic activation in response to nifedipine depends at least in part on baroreflexes, then diminished baroreflex activity during chronic nifedipine therapy would have to be postulated to explain the findings of Kiowski et al. [10]. Experimentally the data are confusing. In one study,

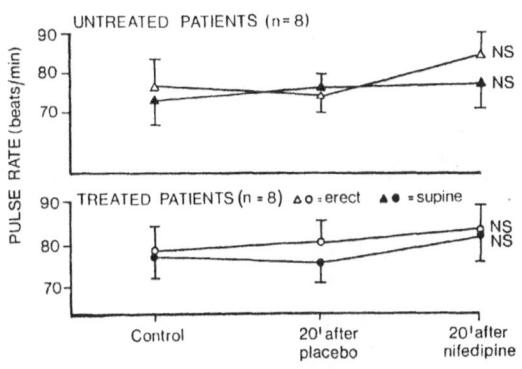

Fig. III-7. Effect of sublingual nifedipine (10 mg) in patients with severe hypertension that was previously untreated (top) compared with those given therapy (bottom) that generally included β-blockade (100 mg atenolol daily). Note the insignificant tendency toward increased heart rate. There were eight patients in each group; comparisons at 20 minutes after nifedipine were nonsignificant. From [223] by courtesy of The Lancet.

nifedipine inhibited the vagally mediated response to an acute BP rise (methoxamine infusion) more so than does verapamil or diltiazem [17], whereas in another study nisoldipine but not nifedipine decreased baroreflex sensitivity [18]. Inhibition of vagal tone should promote sympathetic outflow with tachycardia which is the opposite to what is clinically expected, as shown by the relative absence of tachycardia during the acute nifedipine response (Figure III-7). On the other hand, relative promotion of sympathetic outflow could help to explain the lack of orthostatic hypotension during the acute nifedipine administration (see Figure III-6).

Thus, the situation is complex. Baroreflexes may be blunted by acute hypertension and may have their sensitivity restored by normalization of the blood pressure. On the other hand, acute nifedipine therapy may relatively enhance sympathetic outflow to explain lack of orthostatic hypotension despite a rapid fall of BP. If such activation of baroreflexes occurs, it may explain why elderly patients also avoid postural hypotension in response to nifedipine [19] despite their decreased baroreflex sensitivity (Figure III-8). Thus, there appear to be several conflicting factors at work altering baroreflex sensitivity, including the severity of hypertension, the age of the patient, and the type of calcium antagonist used as well as the stage of therapy, whether acute or chronic.

Hemodynamic changes. From the hemodynamic point of view, the fall in systemic vasular resistance is accompanied by a reflex rise in the cardiac index [20] and the ejection fraction (Figure III-9). However, in

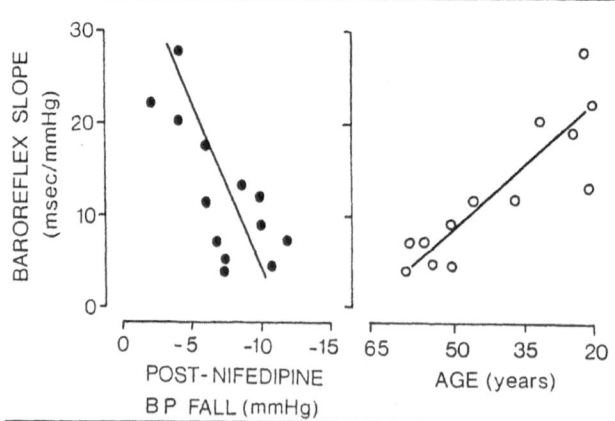

Fig. III-8. As baroreflex sensitivity declines with age, the hypotensive effect of acute nifedipine administration increases. From [10] by courtesy of Journal of the American College of Cardiology *and the authors.*

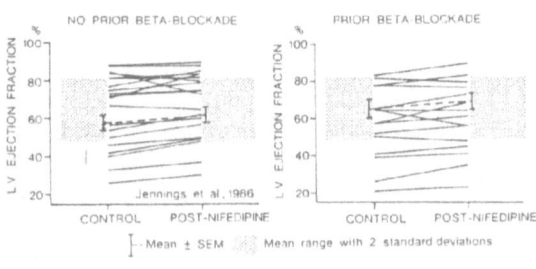

Fig. III-9. Effect of nifedipine (Nif) on LV ejection fraction in patients without prior β-blockade compared with those with prior β-blockade. In both instances, the ejection fraction increases marginally. Note even in patients with low initial ejection fraction, there is an improvement. From [16] by courtesy of American Heart Journal.

patients with myocardial dysfunction, the potential direct negative inotropic effect, especially of verapamil, may become evident (see Side Effects and Contraindications of Calcium Antagonists, below).

Severe Hypertension

Nifedipine. In severe hypertension, the efficacy of sublingual nifedipine is now established (see Figures III-6 and III-7). Nifedipine is now almost standard therapy and reduces BP within 20 to 30 minutes and the effect lasts for 3 to 4 hours or longer [21–26]. The absence of a reflex tachycardia (see Figure III-7) shows that the activity of the baroreceptors is blunted in severe hypertension. In 11 studies reviewed by Sorkin et al. [27], nifedipine reduced BP consistently without inducing hypotension and with apparently no side effects. The absence of any postural hypotension shows that normal compensatory vasoconstriction, presumably α-adrenergic mediated, still occurs on assuming the erect posture, despite the acute hypotension induced by nifedipine (see Figure III-6). As the peripheral resistance falls, the heart rate rises, although not by as much as expected [28] for reasons already analyzed. The hypotensive response is inversely related to the activity of the renin-aldosterone system [29], so that in high-renin patients, there may be no hypotensive effect of nifedipine [30]. Nifedipine has been given acutely to patients with cardiomegaly in whom the ejection fraction improved (see Figure III-9) and to patients with chronic renal failure [31]. Even patients with cerebral manifestations of severe hypertension, including hypertensive encephalopathy and papilledema, have successfully been treated by nifedipine [23, 24, 26]. In addition, nifedipine therapy has also been used successfully for acute left ventricular (LV) failure associated with severe hypertension [32, 33]. However, it must be emphasized that the benefit or risk of the abrupt reduction of severe BP achieved by nifedipine has not been studied [34]. Possibly the presence of a critical coronary or cerebral artery stenosis could precipitate myocardial or cerebral ischemia, or co-therapy with β-blockers or other cardiodepressant drugs could predispose to excessive hypotension when the BP is rapidly lowered by nifedipine or other calcium antagonists. Nonetheless, nifedipine therapy in the "standard" patient with severe or even malignant hypertension appears to be relatively safe [26].

Comparative studies of nifedipine in acute hypertension. Nifedipine is significantly better than placebo [21, 22]. Compared with prazosin 2 mg orally, nifedipine 10 mg orally lowered BP acutely, with prazosin somewhat more effective 2 to 3 hours after the dose at the cost of some postural hypotension [35]. Compared with atenolol 100 mg daily, slow-release nifedipine 40 mg 12-hourly caused a greater initial fall of BP, while the maximum reduction with both agents was similar; atenolol had a more sustained effect [26]. Although these patients had malignant hypertension, no patient developed focal neurologic signs nor heart failure as a result of acute BP reduction. Compared with sodium nitroprusside infusion, nifedipine is quicker and cheaper [36].

Nifedipine failure. In a minority of severely hypertensive patients, nifedipine does not acutely reduce the BP [16]. Logically, nifedipine may then be combined with an ACE inhibitor, because its antihypertensive properties are diminished in high-renin states [30] or with α_1-blockade which potentiates nifedipine action [37, 38].

Verapamil for severe hypertension. Although by custom verapamil is now seldom used in the therapy of acute hypertension, it was probably the first calcium antagonist used for this purpose; 5 mg IV reduced mean BP from 176/116 to 145/110 mmHg within 1 minute in nine hypertensives [39]. Intravenous verapamil was also very effective in 47 patients with severe renal hypertension including some with initial diastolic values of about 135 mmHg [40]. Luna and Carrasco [14] studied the influence of intravenous verapamil on the baroreceptor sensitivity in severe hypertensives (mean initial diastolic BP: 129 mm Hg, 11 patients). Repetitive verapamil infusions improved

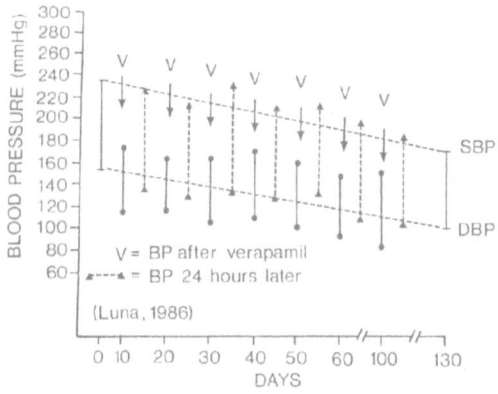

Fig. III-10. Effect of repetitive infusions of verapamil on blood pressure of severely hypertensive patients. V = BP after infusion of verapamil; ▲---▲ = BP 24 hr later. Note progressive fall of systolic BP (SBP) and diastolic BP (DBP) 24 hr after the verapamil infusion, while on constant medication. The authors propose a favorable resetting of baroreceptors as the hypertension is controlled. Adapted from [14] by courtesy of American Journal of Cardiology *and the authors.*

the blunted baroreceptor response in severe hypertensives. The hypotensive effect of verapamil also "sensitized" the patients to their pre-existing therapy to which they had become resistant (Figure III-10), again supporting the proposition that there is a calcium-dependent "excess" BP rise in severe hypertension.

Oral verapamil. Oral verapamil has also been used in severe hypertension. In 16 outpatients with untreated mean BP values of 203/118 mmHg [41], verapamil given in an open-label fashion at a mean oral dose of 500 mg daily was unable to reduce the BP to below 95 mmHg except in combination with captopril (mean dose 55 mg daily). The possible speed of onset of oral verapamil can be assessed by another study in which 22 patients with mild to moderate hypertension (mean initial BP 168/103 mmHg) received 160 mg verapamil orally which reduced the BP maximally at 60 minutes, lasting for at least 4 hours [42]. The hypotensive effects of verapamil in seven other studies on patients with severe hypertension are summarized by Frishman et al. [43].

Diltiazem for severe hypertension. Diltiazem appears not to be have been studied in very severe hypertension [34, 43, 44]. Given intravenously, diltiazem decreases mean BP from 120 mmHg (179/90) to 109 mm Hg (165/81) [45]. Similar data are reported in

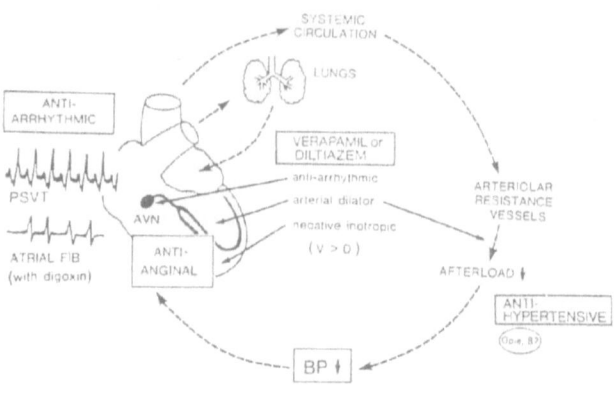

Fig. III-11. Verapamil and diltiazem both have a broad spectrum of therapeutic effects, so that the antihypertensive properties are especially useful when other diseases such as angina or supraventricular tachycardia are present. However, both agents are increasingly used as initial monotherapy. Dilt, diltiazem; PSVT, paroxysmal supraventricular tachycardia; Ver, verapamil. Adapted from [210] by courtesy of Grune & Stratton.

three patients by Bauer and Reams [34]. Given orally, diltiazem 120 mg starts to reduce the BP within 60 to 120 minutes but not to the same degree or speed as nifedipine 20 mg or verapamil 160 mg; these studies by Theroux et al. [46] were, however, on patients with acute myocardial infarction (AMI).

Mild to Moderate Hypertension

As a group, the calcium antagonist agents are uniformly effective in mild to moderate hypertension (for reviews, see Chaffman and Brogden [44], Sorkin et al. [27], and Moser [47]). Because of several extensive existing review articles, only certain aspects will be highlighted here. Some aspects of their antihypertensive properties are summarized in Figures III-11 and III-12.

Verapamil. Verapamil is a "broad-spectrum" therapeutic agent with several indications including hypertension (Figure III-11). Thus, verapamil is especially indicated in the therapy of hypertension when there is coexisting angina or a supraventricular arrhythmia or when β-blockade is contraindicated [48]. As monotherapy for uncomplicated hypertension, verapamil can control the BP over 24 hours [49, 50]. The doses used were 120 to 160 mg three times daily of standard verapamil or 240 to 360-mg sustained-release verapamil (in one or two daily doses, depending on the preparation). At a total daily dose of 480 mg, it is claimed that only 10% of patients are nonresponders [51]. However, at a total maximum dose of 320 mg (160 mg two times daily) no more than 60% of patients responded by a fall of sitting diastolic BP to less than 90 mmHg or with a fall of 10 mmHg or more [52]. Clearly the higher the BP, the less effective verapamil would be so that in severe hypertension (mean diastolic BP 118 mmHg), even an oral daily dose of 500 mg is ineffective [40]. Buhler's group [53] has consistently advocated the use of verapamil in elderly patients and other low-renin groups. However, their analyses appear to be retrospective. There may be a special case for the use of calcium antagonists in black patients with hypertension. Whereas verapamil is equally effective in white and in black patients, propranolol is less effective in blacks [54]. Recently sustained-release verapamil has been approved for use as an antihypertensive agent in the United States, with a usual dose of 240 mg daily, yet with the proviso that sometimes twice daily dosage is required.

Verapamil has also been combined with β-blockade [55], diuretics [56], captopril [41], and reserpine [57] in the therapy of mild to moderate hypertension.

Nifedipine for mild to moderate hypertension. The predominant vasodilator properties of nifedipine (Figure III-12) means that it has been regarded as a third-line agent, suitable for addition to existing dual therapy with β-blockade and diuretics, as for example in the studies of Murphy et al. [58], Opie et al. [22], and Bayley et al. [59]. Nifedipine has also been used as second-line therapy, combined with β-blockade (for review, see Lejeune [60]). In several studies, nifedipine capsules have been used as monotherapy [61–63]. Nifedipine tablets (a slow-release preparation), in a dose of 20 to 120 mg given as monotherapy in two daily doses, have a hypotensive efficacy extending over 24 hours [6, 64–66], although in one study [67] nifedipine tablets only benefited a minority of patients. The relatively high doses of nifedipine required for use in first-line therapy contrast with the low doses required to achieve significant BP decreases when given acutely [60, 68]. The higher the BP, the better the response to nifedipine, as analyzed by MacGregor [68], suggesting a calcium-mediated peripheral vasoconstriction in severe hypertension. In addition to this use in severe hypertension, nifedipine may be particularly effective in patients with low-renin status such as the elderly or black patients [69], thereby suggesting a parallel with verapamil [54]. Nifedipine may also be particularly suitable for patients with hypertension and angina or hypertension associated with heart failure [68].

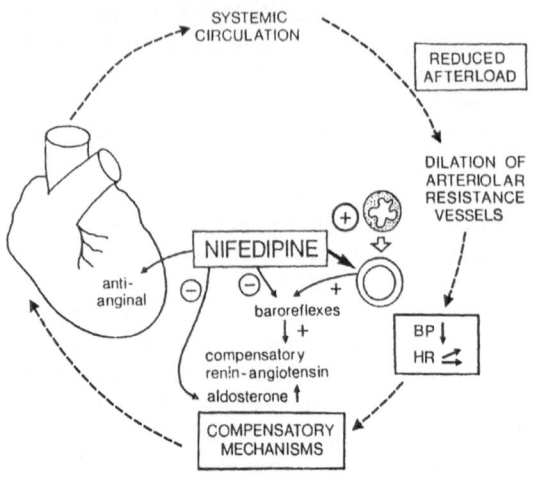

Fig. III-12. Nifedipine has a more limited therapeutic spectrum than verapamil or diltiazem, being without supraventricular antiarrhythmic properties. As the most powerful vasodilator of the three prototypical agents, compensatory mechanisms such as baroreflex activation with renin-angiotensin release are more likely to be powerful. Note inhibitory effect on aldosterone release (see Fig. III-10). Fig. copyright, L.H. Opie.

Subjective side effects in most trials have been modest although frequent and include flushing and lightheadedness. In some trials, pedal edema has been troublesome, occurring in up to 20% of patients [27], and in one study the side effects were intolerable in 7 of 20 patients [70].

Combination therapy has been with β-blockers [60, 62, 63, 67, 71], methyldopa, clonidine, and captopril [27, 68]. Although several studies have shown an added hypotensive effect of nifedipine added to a β-blocker-diuretic combination [22, 58, 72], it is unknown whether the diuretic component in this triple therapy is really effective [68]. The reason may be the weak diuretic effect of nifedipine itself (see Table III-5; see discussion Part I, Renal Effects of Calcium Antagonists).

Nifedipine versus hydralazine. Nifedipine tablets (mean daily dose 70 mg) lowered systolic BP better than hydralazine (mean daily dose 150 mg) in patients already receiving a β-blocker and a diuretic [72].

Diltiazem for mild to moderate hypertension. The pharmacologic properties of diltiazem resemble those of verapamil, except that there is less of a negative inotropic effect (see Figure III-5). Diltiazem *mono-*

therapy has been evaluated in several studies. A multicenter randomized placebo-controlled parallel group study of diltiazem on 77 patients with mild to moderate hypertension showed that a dose of 360 mg daily was required in 85% of patients [73]. Side effects were modest and included dizziness, edema, and headache. There was a suggestion that diltiazem might be more effective in older subjects. Moser [47] gave information on three multicenter studies with diltiazem, one of which included the data of Pool et al. [73] according to the information given by Marion Laboratories, Kansas City, Missouri, and a second of which has now also been published in detail [74]. Diltiazem was somewhat more effective in black patients than in whites. Goal reductions in BP (diastolic BP < 90 mmHg or a decrease of at least 10 mmHg) were achieved in 57% of patients taking diltiazem; about half of the nonresponders then favorably decreased BP on the addition of a thiazide diuretic. Of the diltiazem responders who continued on diltiazem monotherapy, not all maintained the initial response. Therefore, in the end, only about 44% of patients responded to diltiazem monotherapy, while 51% responded to the diuretic.

Comparative studies with diltiazem include several placebo-controlled studies, and comparisons with nifedipine, propranolol, diuretics, and reserpine have been undertaken. For example, diltiazem 180 to 360 mg daily for 8 weeks was equipotent to hydrochlorothiazide 50 to 100 mg daily in mild to moderate hypertension [75]. Diltiazem 240 to 360 mg daily (120 to 180 mg of sustained-release preparation 2 times daily) was compared with hydrochlorothiazide 50 to 100 mg daily in a double-blind parallel study on 40 patients with mild to moderate hypertension [11]. Both agents achieved comparable reductions of BP (with some minor differences). However, only 38% of diltiazem patients achieved goal BP (supine diastolic BP < 90 mmHg) with a mean diltiazem dose of 316 mg daily, whereas 72% of diuretic treated patients (mean dose 82 mg daily) achieved the goal. Such diuretic doses would now probably be rejected by many physicians as being too high. Both diltiazem and diuretic increased plasma renin activity (especially the diuretic) and also the level of the metabolite of the vasodilatory prostaglandin PGE_2 (a metabolite was measured). Diltiazem 90 to 180 mg daily was similar in potency to reserpine 0.1 to 0.3 mg daily in a 12-week randomized double-blind trial [76] with, however, only about half the incidence of side-effects.

Combination therapy of diltiazem with other antihypertensives has not been extensively studied except with diuretics [47, 56, 74] and the new α_1-blocker, alfuzosine [77].

Comparative Studies of Calcium Antagonists Versus Each Other in Mild to Moderate Hypertension

Verapamil versus nifedipine. In 28 patients with mild to moderate hypertension in a double-blind crossover study over 6 weeks, verapamil (160 mg three times daily) was more effective than nifedipine (20 mg slow-release tablets two times daily) and there were fewer subjective side effects except for constipation which occurred more frequently with verapamil [78]. In an open-label study with 24 hour BP recording [49], patients were given either verapamil 120 to 160 mg three times daily or nifedipine tablets 20 to 60 mg two times daily (mean dose 40 mg two times daily). Intra-arterial BPs were recorded at the beginning and at the end of the 6-week therapy period. Somewhat similar BP reductions were achieved. The incidence of side effects was rather similar with constipation being more common with verapamil and pedal edema with nifedipine.

The acute and chronic effects of verapamil and nifedipine on blood pressure, plasma renin activity, and plasma catecholamines have been compared in a single-blinded study [7, 42]. Acutely, verapamil 160 mg and nifedipine 10 mg (sublingually) each appeared to have a similar effect on BP, whereas only nifedipine increased plasma noradrenaline levels. Chronically, in an unblinded study on different groups of patients, verapamil 80 mg three times daily had similar effects on BP to nifedipine 10 mg three times daily except that the heart rate rose with nifedipine and there was more postural hypotension with nifedipine. In the chronic study, neither agent altered plasma renin activity nor aldosterone levels, nor was the emergence of tolerance a problem. Again in the chronic study, nifedipine 10 mg and high-dose verapamil (160 mg three times daily) both increased plasma noradrenaline levels. Thus, nifedipine appears to be a more potent peripheral vasodilator giving a greater baroreflex stimulation (Figure III-5) which, in turn, caused a more sustained increase of plasma noradrenaline concentrations than did verapamil. During chronic therapy with nifedipine the plasma noradrenaline level tends to return toward normal as shown in another study by Kiowski et al. [10], although the data of Agabiti-Rosei et al. [42] are not so definite.

Comparing the two long-acting preparations, Belz

and Spies [79] found an approximately equal hypotensive effect of verapamil slow-release 240 mg two times daily and nifedipine-retard 20 mg two times daily, although verapamil was somewhat more hypotensive with 72% of patients attaining a goal BP of <90 mmHg supine, versus 50% success rate with nifedipine; side effects were chiefly constipation with verapamil (6 of 18 patients) and flushing or headaches with nifedipine (5 each of 18 patients).

Diltiazem versus nifedipine. Klein et al. [80] compared nifedipine capsules 30 to 60 mg daily with diltiazem 180 to 270 mg daily, both doses being titrated over 8 weeks. Similar reductions in BP and systemic vascular resistance were achieved. Both agents increased plasma adrenaline levels, but only nifedipine increased plasma noradrenaline levels at rest. Side effects were somewhat more troublesome with nifedipine. In another study reported only in abstract form [81], slow-release diltiazem 180 to 270 mg daily was compared with slow-release nifedipine 40 to 60 mg daily in a double-blind parallel study. Similar hypotensive effects were obtained. The heart rate increased in patients treated with nifedipine and decreased in those treated with diltiazem.

Comparative trials in hypertension: summary. These trials indicate that diltiazem, verapamil, and nifedipine, all in doses that might be regarded as "high," have somewhat similar effects on mild to moderate hypertension. In some studies the response rate to monotherapy with these agents is disappointing. Heart rate tends not to change with verapamil or to fall, whereas it consistently falls with diltiazem and is unchanged or increases with nifedipine. Nifedipine consistently increases plasma noradrenaline levels as a result of reflex vasodilation, verapamil does so in some studies, and diltiazem causes modest insignificant rises. There are few data to indicate which of these agents remains effective as monotherapy during chronic management of hypertension.

Calcium Antagonists and β-Adrenergic
Blockers in Hypertension:
Combinations and Comparisons

Calcium antagonists have been extensively compared with β-blockers (Tables III-6 to III-8). Furthermore, because the mode of antihypertensive action of calcium antagonists differs from that of β-blockade, combination therapy seems logical. Calcium antagonists act primarily on the periphery as vasodilators and as such they tend to be of greater benefit to patients with low plasma renin levels (such as the elderly or black patients). In contrast, β-blockers act hemodynamically to decrease cardiac output and tend to increase peripheral vascular resistance, at least acutely. By inhibition of the release of renin, they tend to benefit a different group of patients from the calcium antagonists so that it is frequently stated that younger patients and whites benefit preferentially from β-blockade therapy. However, there are many studies with exceptions to the above guidelines. Because nifedipine is a powerful vasodilator, with no clinical effect on heart rate or cardiac conduction, nor on the inotropic state of the myocardium (except when there is prior depression as in congestive heart failure), this agent combines particularly well with β-blockade.

Nifedipine versus or combined with β-adrenergic blockers. Nifedipine (capsular form, 10 mg three times daily) was the approximate equivalent of acebutolol 200 mg three times daily and superior results were obtained with the combination [62]. In a second trial, the same dose of nifedipine in capsular form had similar hypotensive effects to metoprolol 100 mg two times daily [61]. However, the combination of nifedipine 10 mg two times daily and metoprolol 100 mg two times daily was no better than nifedipine 10 mg three times daily. In other trials, slow-release nifedipine tablets have been used. Thus, nifedipine tablets 10 to 30 mg two times daily were better than pindolol 5 to 10 mg two times daily [63]. Again, the combination seemed better yet strictly valid statistics were not obtained. In a recent study from Cape Town, fixed-dose atenolol 100 mg was compared with nifedipine tablets 20 mg two times daily [67]. Although the response rate (erect diastolic BP reduced to <90 mmHg) to atenolol was only 40%, this result was much better than with nifedipine which gave only 25% response. The total response rate was pushed up to 74% by the combination of atenolol (100 mg daily) with nifedipine (20 mg two times daily). This fixed-dose atenolol-nifedipine combination gave few side effects, the most common being tiredness in 5 of 20 patients [67]. Most recently, nifedipine tablets (20 mg two times daily) have been compared with acebutolol (200 mg two times daily); each had similar hypotensive effects to the other and the combination gave enhanced control [71].

Verapamil versus β-blocker. Verapamil 360 mg daily (in three divided doses) was the approximate equivalent of pindolol 15 mg daily (in two divided doses) when both agents were given with a diuretic [82]. Verapamil 160 mg two times daily was about as effective as labetalol 200 mg two times daily and without any of the bronchoconstrictive effects of labetalol [83]. Verapamil 120 mg two times daily was approximately as good as atenolol 100 mg daily in the therapy of 24 patients with initial mean pressures of 154/105 mmHg [84].

Diltiazem versus β-blocker. Diltiazem 180 mg daily was compared with propranolol 60 mg daily for 1 month; both agents produced similar effects on BP and heart rate at rest and during exercise [85]. In a recent study not yet fully published [47], diltiazem 120 to 360 mg daily (mean dose 303 mg) was similar to propranolol 160 to 480 mg daily (mean dose 344 mg), except that diltiazem was more effective in blacks. In a third study, diltiazem 240 mg daily was compared with metoprolol 200 mg daily [86] with similar benefits; however, only metoprolol reduced the maximum increase in systolic BP evoked by exercise. In contrast, a higher dose of diltiazem (mean 307 mg daily) reduced BP at submaximal and maximal exercise, whereas propranolol (mean dose 371 mg daily) did so only at maximal exercise [87]. In the latter study, exercise duration and maximum whole body oxygen uptake during exercise were decreased by propranolol, not by diltiazem, so that diltiazem better maintained normal exercise hemodynamics.

Calcium Antagonists Compared with or Combined with Diuretics in Mild to Moderate Hypertension

Nifedipine. Compared with bendroflumethazide (2.5 mg two times daily), nifedipine (capsules, 10 mg two times daily) gave similar reductions in BP, although standing diastolic pressure fell less with nifedipine [88].

In two other studies, nifedipine was compared with the loop diuretic mefruside. Nifedipine capsules 20 mg two times daily were similar in effect to mefruside 25 mg two times daily [88]. Nifedipine tablets 20 mg two times daily were as effective as mefruside 25 mg daily [90].

Three studies suggest that diuretics combined with nifedipine are not much better than nifedipine alone. In one study, only marginal added effects were achieved [88]. Second, MacGregor [68] found that the addition of bendroflumethazide 5 mg to patients already controlled by nifedipine (tablets, 20 mg two times daily) gave little added benefit. Third, nifedipine-mefruside was no better than nifedipine itself [89].

Verapamil. There appear to be no studies comparing verapamil with diuretic therapy for hypertension in

Table III-6. *Effects of verapamil compared with β-blockers in patients with mild to moderate essential hypertension*

Author (No.)	Trial Design	Patients (N)	Drug test period (wk)	Verapamil Daily Dose	β-blocker Daily Dose	Antihypertensive Result (drug doses in mg)
Anavekar et al. [82]	Placebo, double-blind, randomized cross-over, washout	17	6	360 mg + thiazide	Pin 15 mg + thiazide	V 360 = Pin 15 on resting BP
Anavekar et al. [83]	Randomized, double-blind, cross-over	9	6	320 mg	L 400 mg	V 320 = L 400 for resting BP, patients with COAD V 320 > L 400 lung function, COAD
Leonetti et al. [20]	Placebo, unblinded, randomized, cross-over	31	6	360–480 mg	P 180–240 mg	V = P, rest BP falls with both doses of V and P
McInnes et al. [213]	Placebo, double-blind, randomized (including placebo), cross-over	14	4	360 mg	P 240 mg	V 360 = P 240; V + P best yet more side effects

Hornung et al. [214]	Open, cross-over, washout, 24-hr intra-arterial BP, isometric and dynamic exercise	18	8-12	240-480 mg	P 80-480 mg	V = P, rest and exercise
Escudero et al. [84]	Placebo, double-blind, cross-over, washout	24	4	240 mg	A 100 mg	V 240 = A 100
Cubeddu et al. [54][a]	Placebo (single-blind), randomized, double-blind, parallel	138	4	240-480 mg (mean 339 mg)	P 160-360 mg (mean 222 mg)	V 339 > P 222 P less effective in whites than in blacks, V equally effective
Mooy et al. [101]	Placebo, single-blind, crossover	8	—	Mean 450 mg	P 160 mg mean	V 450 = P 160; P not V decreases exercise capacity

Abbreviations: A, atenolol; BP, blood pressure; COAD, chronic obstructive airways disease; L, labetalol; P, propranolol; Pin, pindolol; V, verapamil; >, better than.
[a]Includes patients of [224].

Table III-7. Effects of nifedipine compared with β-blockers in patients with mild to moderate essential hypertension

Author (No.)	Trial Design	Patients (N)	Drug Test Period (wk)	Nifedipine Daily Dose	β-blocker Daily Dose	Antihypertensive Result (drug doses in mg)
Eggertsen and Hansson [61]	Randomized, double-blind, parallel, placebo	22	12	30 mg	M 200 mg	N 30 < M 200
De Divitiis et al. [62]	Randomized, double-blind, crossover, placebo	15	4	30 mg	Ac 600 mg	N 30 = Ac 600 N + Ac best
Tsukiyama et al. [63]	Open, parallel	25	6	20–60 mg	Pin 5–10 mg	N = Pin or N > Pin
Daniels and Opie [67]	Placebo, run-in, double-blind, randomized, crossover after washout	35	4	40 mg (slow-release)	A 100 mg	N 40 ≪ A 100

Abbreviations: A, atenolol; Ac, acetubolo; M, metoprolol; Pin, pindolol; <, worse than; >, better than.

Table III-8. Effects of diltiazem compared with β-blockers in patients with mild to moderate hypertension

Author (No.)	Trial Design	Patients (N)	Drug Test Period (wk)	Diltiazem Daily Dose	β-blocker Daily Dose	Antihypertensive Result (drug doses in mg)
Yamakado et al. [85]	Placebo-controlled, not blinded, sequential, no washout	16	4	180 mg	P 60 mg	D 180 = P 60 at rest and exercise DBP D 180 < P 60 for exercise SBP
Trimarco et al. [86]	Randomized, double-blind	20	4	240 mg	M 200 mg	D 240 = M 200 at rest D 240 < M 200 for exercise SBP
Moser [47]	Multicenter, placebo-controlled, dose titration, parallel	196	18	120–360 mg (mean 303 mg)	P 160–480 mg (mean 344 mg)	D 303 = P 344 at rest In 8-week follow-up, 35% responded to D monotherapy (45% to P)
Szlachcic et al. [87]	Placebo-controlled, double-blinded, parallel	23	4 (after 12 wk titration)	120–360 mg (mean 307 mg)	P 160–480 mg (mean 307 mg)	D 307 = P 307 at rest Exercise hemodynamics better maintained with D

Abbreviations: DBP, diastolic blood pressure (mmHg); M, metoprolol; P, propranolol; SBP, systolic blood pressure; <, better than.

a double-blind and randomized fashion. Buhler et al. [53] found that verapamil (average dose 427 mg daily) was the approximate equivalent of prior diuretic therapy with hydrochlorothiazide 50 mg and amiloride 5 mg (i.e., one Moduretic tablet daily). In an open-label study [91], 15 patients with mild to moderate hypertension who had been receiving hydrochlorthiazide (25 to 50 mg daily) were given verapamil 80 to 160 mg two times daily. Equivalent BP control was achieved but 1) heart rate was lower with verapamil, 2) body weight was about 1 kg higher with verapamil, 3) serum uric acid and calcium were lower with verapamil and the urinary calcium higher, and 4) serum potassium rose with verapamil. Verapamil caused a transient rise in total blood cholesterol. In a single-blind comparison with indapamide (2.5 mg daily), verapamil slow-release (120 mg two times daily) was more effective than the diuretic; however, patients in each treatment group still had diastolic values above 95 mmHg, so they were given the combination with a good control of BP.

Diltiazem. In an open-label study [75], diltiazem 360 mg daily gave approximately the same antihypertensive effect as hydrochlorothiazide 50 to 100 mg daily (9 of 13 patients received 100 mg). In a double-blind, parallel multicentered trial, diltiazem was titrated to 240 to 360 mg daily and compared with hydrochlorothiazide 50 to 100 mg daily [47, 74] with similar BP reductions; possibly the diuretic achieved somewhat better control, yet at a "high" dose of hyrochlorothiazide 100 mg daily which would not presently be chosen by many as first-choice antihypertensive therapy because of the dose. Only about half the patients responded well to monotherapy with either agent to decrease the diastolic BP to 90 mmHg or by 10 mmHg. The combination diltiazem-diuretic gave a good response in about half of the nonresponders to monotherapy, so that the total response rate to combination therapy was about 75%.

Comparisons Between Calcium Antagonists and Other Vasodilators in Hypertension

Nifedipine. Nifedipine is more effectively antihypertensive than prazosin in patients with mild to moderate hypertension [92] but there was no careful dose-titration of both agents, so that the comparison between nifedipine 10 mg and prazosin 1 mg both given three times daily hardly seems appropriate. Comparisons between nifedipine and hydralazine have only been carried out in patients with congestive heart failure and may not be applicable to hypertension.

Verapamil. There appear to be no comparisons available between verapamil and conventional vasodilators.

Diltiazem versus dihydralazine. Patients with mean BPs of approximately 180/90 mmHg and mean age 43 years were given either 0.1 mg/kg dihydralazine or 0.1 mg/kg diltiazem followed by 0.1 mg/kg over 25 minutes. The doses were calculated to bring down BP in an equivalent way so that the mean BP after dihydralazine was 158/73 mmHg and after diltiazem 165/81 mmHg. Total peripheral resistance fell modestly with diltiazem but much more with dihydralazine and the cardiac index and heart rate rose with dihydralazine but not with diltiazem. However, the arterial diameter of the brachial artery fell after dihydralazine but increased after diltiazem. Thus, while both agents must have achieved arteriolar dilation (of the resistance vessels), only diltiazem increased the diameter of large vessels. Diltiazem avoided the tachycardia that is sometimes an irritating side effect of dihydralazine. This study also shows that diltiazem very acutely, within 2 minutes, can increase the heart rate and cardiac index before these revert to normal at 25 minutes.

Comparisons Between Calcium Antagonists and Centrally Active Agents

Verapamil has been compared with methyldopa [93]. In these 15 previously untreated black hypertensive patients, verapamil 120 to 360 mg total daily dose had similar hypotensive effects to methyldopa 750 to 1500 mg total daily dose. *Nifedipine* has been combined with methyldopa [94] with an addictive effect. Guazzi et al. [95] followed up their patients for 3 years and found that the combination was still effective and furthermore there was a reduction in cardiomegaly and decreased electrocardiographic signs of LV strain. Brief interrruptions in nifedipine therapy were tested at 2, 8, and 24 months which invariably caused BP to rise and which led Guazzi et al. [95] to suppose that tolerance to nifedipine did not occur. *Diltiazem* has been compared with reserpine. In a randomized double-blind trial [76], diltiazem 90 to 180 mg daily was the approximate equivalent of reserpine 0.1 to 0.3 mg daily except that the higher diltiazem dose was more effective than the higher reserpine dose and side effects were less frequent.

Combinations Between Calcium Antagonists and Agents Other than Diuretics or β-Blockers

Nifedipine. There is an added hypotensive effect when nifedipine is combined with clonidine [96].

Nifedipine and captopril have also been combined with benefit [41, 97, 98]. However, MacGregor [68] notes that the combination nifedipine-captopril may have to be given three to four times daily.

Verapamil. Verapamil has also been combined with captopril. In patients with diastolic BPs >95 mm Hg resistant to monotherapy with verapamil 500 mg daily, the further combination with captopril (average dose 53 mg daily) achieved the goal diastolic BP of <95 mm Hg in 15 of 16 patients [41].

Diltiazem does not appear to have been studied in combination with agents other than diuretics, as already referred to.

Calcium antagonists for special patient groups (elderly, black patients, physically or mentally active patients).As vasodilators with a mild tendency to increase plasma renin, calcium antagonists should be beneficial in the therapy of hypertension of low-renin groups (Table III-9) such as elderly or black patients, as confirmed [47, 53, 54, 93, 99, 100]. Nevertheless, there are few data strictly comparing effects in young versus old subjects or in blacks versus whites, nor is there proof that the proposed beneficial effects in these groups can be related to the renin status. In the case of diltiazem, an acute infusion causes more of a hypotensive effect in the elderly (mean age 68 years) than in the young (mean age 30 years); diltiazem is also cleared more slowly. Yet, the hypotensive response to a single oral dose of 120 mg diltiazem was similar in both age groups. Unexpectedly, the P-R interval on the electrocardiogram (ECG) was less prolonged in the elderly than in the young.

For physically active hypertensive patients, first principles suggest that calcium antagonists, which reduce systemic vascular resistance and increase cardiac output, should allow better exercise tolerance than β-blockers which decrease cardiac output. This expectancy has been confirmed by a recent single-blinded crossover study in which verapamil (mean daily dose 450 mg) was equally hypotensive to propranolol (mean daily dose 160 mg) while propranolol but not verapamil decreased the endurance time during exercise [101]. Similarly, exercise time was better with diltiazem than with metoprolol [86] or propranolol [87]. However, in one other study neither diltiazem nor propranolol decreased exercise time [85]. In evaluating these apparently conflicting results, it should be noted, first, that most studies show a benefit for calcium antagonists with enhanced excercise time and, second, that the end-points of the different studies vary, some involving short-term acute exercise

Table III-9. Special situations favoring use of calcium antagonists at first-line antihypertensive agents

	Rationale	Author (reference no.)
Patient category		
Black	Low-renin and/or primary vasoconstriction	Cubeddu et al. [54]
		Moser [47]
		M'Buyamba-Kabangu et al. [99, 100]
		Frishman et al. [23]
Elderly	Low-renin and/or increased arterial wall stiffness	Buhler et al. [53]; Muller et al. [215]
		Ben-Ishay et al. [19]
Physically active	Normal hemodynamics	Mooy et al. [101]
Intense mental activity	Better hemodynamics than with β-blockade	Schmieder et al. [102]
		Floras et al. [103]
Associated conditions		
Angina, vasospastic	Coronary vasodilation	Stone [225]
Angina, β-blocker C/I	Effective antianginal mechanisms	Johnston et al. [216]
Exercise-induced asthma	Bronchodilator effect	Patel [200]
Renal disease	Renal hemodynamics improved	Isshiki et al. [201]
Raynaud's disease[a]	Peripheral vasodilation	Aldoori et al. [180]
		Kahan et al. [183]
Left ventricular hypertrophy	Regression of LV mass	Frohlich [108]
		Muiesan et al. [106]

Abbreviations: C/I, contraindicated; LV, left ventricular.
[a]Therapeutic effect not yet shown for verapamil (see Vayssairat et al. [184]).

with exercise times over minutes [85], whereas others assess the endurance time which is nearly 1 hour in normal subjects [101].

Intense mental activity, like exercise, involves a hypertensive response (Figure III-13). Logically it might be supposed that β-blockade should be the therapy of choice, yet calcium antagonist therapy normalized the hemodynamic response more than did β-blockade [102]. β-blockade by either selective or non-selective agents is unable to reduce the hypertensive response to mental arithmetic or isometric exercise; only during intense bicycle exercise did β-blockade reduce the BP, when cardioselective agents were better, presumably because of unopposed α-mediated vasoconstriction resulting from β_2-vascular blockade by the nonselective agents [103].

Hypertensive Complications

Left ventricular hypertrophy and left ventricular function. The arrhythmogenic potential of LV hypertrophy with concentric hypertrophy has been contrasted with that of LV hypertrophy combined with dilation, both defined echocardiographically [104]. Patients with LV dilation had many more ventricular premature beats and 6 of 28 patients had salvoes of ventricular tachycardia. In patients treated by nifedipine (10 mg four times daily) but not verapamil (120 mg three times daily), there was a remarkable reduction of circumferential wall stress with an obvious decrease in ventricular extrasystoles (note that there is an error in Figure 4 of the article of Loaldi et al.; the figure in panel 3 labeled "verapamil" is in fact "nifedipine" according to text).

Left ventricular hypertrophy itself is decreased by nifedipine both in rats and in humans ([15]; for review, see Fouad-Tarazi and Libson [105]) and by verapamil [105] and diltiazem [107, 108]. In the case of diltiazem, Frohlich [108] has recently claimed that there is good evidence that it can revert LV hypertrophy.

There are suggestions that the acute administration of calcium antagonists improves both LV systolic function [16, 109] and also diastolic function in myocardial hypertrophy. There is improved early diastolic filling after nitrendipine and the addition of atenolol causes further improvement [110].

Renal function. Calcium antagonists appear to have a role in preserving or possibly improving renal function in hypertension (see Renal Disease, below).

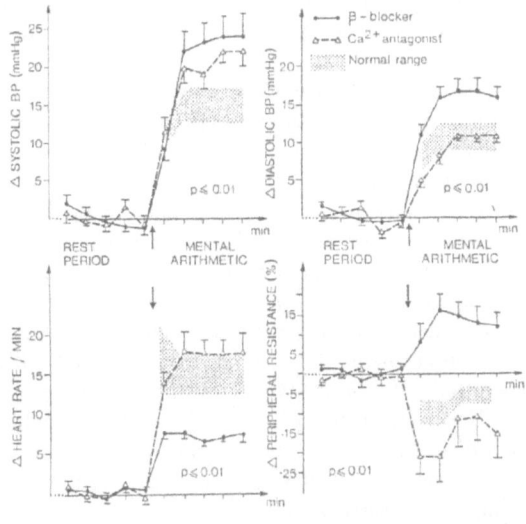

Fig. III-13. During mental arithmetic, systolic BP (SBP) and diastolic BP (DBP) both increase in patients with mild essential hypertension, to values beyond those found in nonhypertensives (shaded areas). Therapy by calcium antagonists (nitrendipine) maintains a more normal cardiovascular hemodynamic profile than therapy by a β-blocker (oxprenolol). Adapted from [102] by courtesy of American Journal of Medicine and the authors.

Calcium Antagonists for Hypertension: Principles of Choice

Calcium antagonists compare well in their hypotensive effect with the established first-line agents, diuretics or β-blockers. Calcium antagonists act primarily to reduce peripheral vascular resistance, aided by an initial diuretic effect. Even in the case of verapamil, no negative inotropic effect can be detected in patients with actively normal myocardial function. All three prototypical calcium antagonists, especially nifedipine, tend modestly to increase plasma catecholamines with a borderline elevation of plasma renin activity. There are no long-term outcome studies available on calcium antagonists in hypertension. As a group, calcium antagonists and especially nifedipine and verapamil are well tested in patients with severe hypertension. Evidence for a hypotensive effect when given as first-line agents to black patients is also accumulating. Although calcium antagonists are effective in hypertension of the elderly, there is at present no proof that this benefit is specially related to the lower renin status found in the elderly. Calcium antagonists may be selected as initial monotherapy, especially if there are other indications for these agents such as angina pectoris or Raynaud's phenomenon (all three agents) or supraventricular tachycardia (verapamil and diltiazem).

Compared with diuretics (also advocated for elderly or black patients), calcium antagonists are more expensive and most need multiple daily doses; however, calcium antagonists cause little or no metabolic disturbances in potassium, glucose, uric acid, or lipid metabolism, nor does aldosterone increase, while renin rises only slightly or not at all. Patients on calcium antagonists do not require intermittent blood chemistry checks. There is no evidence that calcium antagonists cause impairment of renal function as found with thiazide diuretics; rather they may improve renal function. However, when hypertension is caused by chronic renal disease it is frequently volume dependent and diuretics are more logical therapy than calcium antagonists. For further comparisons between diuretics and calcium antagonists, see Sowers and Mohanty [111].

Compared with β-blockers, calcium antagonists cause less fatigue and little or no interference with normal cardiovascular dynamics, especially during exercise. Calcium antagonists have fewer contraindications and can, for example, be used safely in asthmatics, cause little or no interference with diabetic control and are not contraindicated in peripheral vascular disease nor in borderline heart failure (especially not nifedipine). However, β-blockers have established once-a-day administration and ultralong-acting agents such as nadolol and sotalol are already available. β-blockers are particularly well tested for the "quality of life" (kept better with atenolol than with propranolol, pindolol, or metoprolol). In the case of propranolol, long-term outcome trials are available showing a reduction of coronary events in nonsmokers [112]; however, stroke was not reduced.

The *response rate* to each of these three groups of agents—calcium antagonists, diuretics, and β-blockers—may be no more than about 50% depending on the criteria used and the dose given. Of the combinations, calcium antagonist–β-blocker therapy has been studied and is especially safe in the case of nifedipine. Calcium antagonist-diuretic therapy is not so well studied, though reported effective for diltiazem-thiazide. Logically, calcium antagonists are thought to be most effective in the same groups as diuretics (elderly patients, blacks) and calcium antagonists may have inherent diuretic properties. Therefore the combination of calcium antagonists with β-blockers seems more ideal than that of calcium antagonists with diuretics. Currently little information is available about the long-term effects of calcium antagonists on cardiac and renal complications of hypertension, although preliminary data are promising. There are no comparative outcome studies in which calcium antagonists have been put against β-blockers or diuretics. Such considerations may become critical when choosing between calcium antagonists and other potential first-line agents in the therapy of hypertension.

Likewise, considerably more information is needed on the comparison between calcium antagonists and ACE inhibitors and their possible use in combination. Theoretically they should combine very well, without the hemodynamic disadvantages of β-blockade or the metabolic disadvantages of diuretics.

Use and Comparative Efficacy of Calcium Antagonists in Supraventricular Arrhythmias

Physiologic Principles

The depolarization pacemaking current in the sino-atrial node is particularly calcium-dependent, with another prominent part caused by a decaying outward potassium current. In the atrioventricular (AV) node, both Ca^{2+} and Na^+ inward currents play a role in depolarization, with the calcium current dominant in the mid-nodal zone. The calcium current itself consists of two components, the early part probably dependent on the T channels (see Part I of this series) and the latter part on the L channels, so that even complete inhibition of that part of the calcium current sensitive to calcium antagonists (L channels–mediated activity) would be unlikely to cause asystole, unless there is pre-existing sick sinus syndrome or excess therapy with β-blockade.

Effects on the sinoatrial node. The calcium antagonists have a direct inhibitory effect on the sinus node thereby causing bradycardia. There are, however, complex reflex changes involved whereby the peripheral vasodilatory effect of the calcium antagonists stimulates the sinus node via the sympathetic nervous system. With nifedipine there is a net tachycardia, whereas with verapamil the sinus rate is variable, acutely rising for a short time and then being unchanged or even falling. With diltiazem the sinus rate more consistently decreases. The varying contributions of these effects to the antianginal mechanisms of the calcium antagonists have been discussed in Part II. In addition, during electrophysiologic studies, none of the three primary agents when given acutely alters the sinus nodal recovery time nor the sinoatrial conduction time (for review, see Mitchell et al. [113]). In patients with the *sick sinus syndrome,* verapamil may severely decrease the heart rate [112A, 112B], so that it is contraindicated in this condition. Diltiazem can cause the heart rate of patients with the sick sinus syndrome to fall up to 24%, so that like verapamil it is contraindicated [113]. Nifedipine, although potentially having a direct depressant effect on the sinus node, in practice causes a reflex stimulation tending to increase the heart rate so that it can usually be given to patients who have a sick sinus syndrome.

Effects on the atrioventricular node (Table III-10). The critical qualities altered by verapamil and diltiazem are AV nodal conduction time (A-H interval measured by anterograde conduction during the paced rhythm) and AV nodal refractoriness (the V-A interval during retrograde conduction). "Despite an equivalent depression of AV nodal conduction, verapamil affects AV nodal refractoriness to a greater degree than does verapamil" [113]. These changes explain why both verapamil and diltiazem could be clinically effective in slowing AV nodal conduction as in atrial fibrillation [114–116]. Theoretically, verapamil could be more effective than diltiazem in the therapy of supraventricular tachycardia with rapid re-entry through the AV node; however, there are no direct studies to prove this expectancy. Nonetheless, both the agents decrease the ventricular rate in atrial fibrillation and may result in "regularization" of the ventricular rate.

Chronic Atrial Fibrillation

Intravenous verapamil. Historically, one of the first indicators of the effect of verapamil on the AV node was in the classical study of Schamroth [114]. He was asked by Knoll Pharmaceutical Company to test a compound regarded as a β-blocker. He found a rapid effect of intravenous verapamil in reducing the ventricular response rate in atrial fibrillation and in "regularizing" the ventricular response. Schamroth relates how the article ensuing from this observation was turned down by the American journal *Chest* and later accepted by the British journal, *Cardiovascular Research* [114]. Since then intravenous verapamil has come to be standard therapy when the ventricular rate in rapid atrial fibrillation needs urgent control; when used for uncontrolled atrial fibrillation combined with myocardial disease, verapamil is infused at a very low dose (0.0001 mg/kg/min) and titrated against the ventricular response, especially if the patient has already received β-blockade or when digitalis toxicity is suspected. In the absence of these relative contraindications, verapamil may safely be given at a higher rate

Table III-10. Comparative electrophysiologic effects of calcium antagonists on the atrioventricular node

	A-H interval (%)	V-A interval (%)	A-V FRP (%)	A-V ERP (%)	Wenckebach Cycle Length (%)
Verapamil	24-31	Delayed	12-15	21-35	17-24
Diltiazem	7-24	Delayed	6-18	10-25	10-20
Nifedipine	NS	Not measured	11-13	13-17	7

Data adapted from [113] by courtesy American Journal of Cardiology.
Abbreviations: A-H interval, atrial-His interval; A-V ERP, atrial-ventricular effective refractory period; A-V FRP, atrial-ventricular functional refractory period; NS, not significant; V-A interval, ventricular-atrial interval.

(0.005 mg/kg/min, increasing) or as an IV bolus of 5 mg (0.075 mg/kg) followed by double the dose if needed [117].

Oral verapamil. Oral verapamil may be used instead of digoxin as first-line therapy for chronic atrial fibrillation and has been claimed to be more effective in controlling ventricular rate and in improving exercise tolerance [118, 119]. These results can be criticized because the studies were not blinded. In a more recent double-blind study on 12 patients with chronic atrial fibrillation and without overt heart failure, verapamil was titrated from 120 to 360 mg daily (three divided doses) with end-points exercise testing on a treadmill with a Bruce protocol and using a Borg score to quantify the severity of the perceived exertion [120] together with a visual analog score for side effects. Compared with digoxin (therapeutic plasma levels), verapamil 1) decreased postexercise heart rate more than did digoxin and in an optimal dose of 240 mg daily, 2) did not change exercise duration, and 3) gave increased constipation and lower "physical activity" scores with similar "well-being" scores. The apparently lesser effect of the higher dose of verapamil (360 vs. 240 mg daily) was surprising but could perhaps be explained by an excess peripheral vasodilatory effect. Thus, verapamil and digoxin seem to be approximately similar in their effects at the optimal verapamil dose of 240 mg daily.

Verapamil plus digoxin for chronic atrial fibrillation. Because digoxin inhibits AV nodal conduction by enhanced vagal tone and verapamil acts by calcium channel inhibition, the effects of these agents should be additive [121]. When digoxin alone fails to give an optimal response, it is better to double the dose of digoxin or to add verapamil [122]. In 14 patients with chronic atrial fibrillation, the majority with congestive heart failure (dyspnea in 11, diuretic therapy in 8) and mostly with mitral valve disease (9 of 14 patients), ambulatory monitoring and walking tests were used in a randomized crossover and then a single observer-blinded study. Doubling the digoxin dose increased plasma levels from 1.15 to 1.8 µg/L of digoxin, which in five patients came to lie in the toxic range, whereas adding verapamil 120 mg daily only increased the digoxin levels to 1.3 µg/L [not significant (NS) versus digoxin alone]. Both regimes reduced the sensation of palpitations, especially digoxin plus verapamil without any decrease of breathlessness. The combination digoxin and verapamil gave some better findings on ambulatory recording such as less variability of ventricular rate and less nighttime bradycardia, yet neither doubling the dose of digoxin nor adding verapamil could be translated into obvious patient symptomatic benefit. A defect of this study is that there was a fixed "low" dose of verapamil of 120 mg daily and higher doses might have given better improvement when combined with digoxin.

Diltiazem for chronic atrial fibrillation. Like verapamil, diltiazem slows AV conduction and may regularize the ventricular response, reducing exercise and resting heart rates [115, 116, 123].

Diltiazem plus digoxin for chronic atrial fibrillation. Roth et al. [123] showed that diltiazem (optimal dose 240 mg daily) added to digoxin in patients with chronic rheumatic heart disease reduced exercise and resting ventricular rates; diltiazem itself also had benefit. Best results were obtained with the combination diltiazem-digoxin. The optimal dose of diltiazem was 240 mg daily, whereas 360 mg daily caused side effects such as edema and constipation in 9 of 12 patients. Steinberg et al. [124] also improved the control of ventricular rate when diltiazem 240 to 360 mg was added to digoxin, yet maximal exercise time was unexpectedly not prolonged. Subjective improvement in symptoms, including fewer palpitations, occurred in 11 of 16 patients. High-dose diltiazem again caused more side effects, although not as clearly documented as in the study of Roth et al. [123]. Steinberg's study was not blinded nor placebo-controlled making the assessment of some of the results problematic. Thus, diltiazem, like verapamil, improves 1) symptoms in patients with chronic atrial fibrillation and 2) decreases the ventricular rate at rest and during exercise. Yet, unexpectedly, diltiazem does not increase the exercise time when added to digoxin.

Diltiazem versus verapamil for chronic atrial fibrillation. In a preliminary report on 25 patients with stable chronic atrial fibrillation, Ochs et al. [124A] compared verapamil with diltiazem, both in doses of 180 to 480 mg daily. Here the end-point was conversion to sinus rhythm and only 1 patient in each group did so; however, another 14 of the verapamil group converted when quinidine 750 mg daily was added. This study may appear to favor the use of verapamil but had an impractical end-point so that little can be read into it. A second study also does not solve the problem. Diltiazem 120 mg given acutely to ten patients with stable chronic atrial fibrillation reduced the mean ventricular rate by 30%; subsequent long-term therapy with verapamil 270mg daily reduced the rate by 21% [116]. It needs emphasis that 8 of 10 patients were already receiving digoxin.

Atrial Flutter

Neither verapamil nor diltiazem alters the atrial flutter rate, but both can inhibit conduction through the AV node to reduce the ventricular response rate. *Verapamil* increases the degree of AV block, occasionally restoring sinus rhythm, especially in acute myocardial infarction [124B] and sometimes the rhythm changes to atrial fibrillation [125]; note that in the latter study most of the patients were receiving digoxin which might have contributed to the development of atrial fibrillation.

Diltiazem has actions similar to verapamil, increasing AV block, decreasing LV response rate, and occasionally reverting to atrial fibrillation [126]; diltiazem therapy may safely be followed by cardioversion with DC counter-shock.

Paroxysmal Supraventricular Tachycardia

Verapamil. This agent is particularly well studied in the therapy of paroxysmal supraventricular tachycardia (PSVT). An IV bolus of 5 to 10 mg verapamil restores sinus rhythm in 75% or more of cases [125]. Thereafter, oral prophylactic therapy against recurrent PSVT may be either by verapamil [127] or by verapamil-propranolol [128]. Oral prophylactic verapamil by itself is about as effective as digoxin or propranolol [129]. Intravenous verapamil should not be used as a diagnostic test to distinguish supraventricular tachycardia with aberrant conduction from ventricular tachycardia because of the risk of acute hypotension in patients with ventricular tachycardia [130].

Diltiazem. Like verapamil, diltiazem may be used either intravenously or orally, but in most countries the intravenous preparation is not available. The usual intravenous dose is 0.25 mg/kg [115, 131, 132], although Betriu et al. [126] used 0.15 mg/kg. In each case the majority of episodes were converted within 15 to 150 seconds (over 200 seconds required at the lower dose). A particularly useful therapy for termination of PSVT is a single oral dose of diltiazem (120 mg) with propranolol (160 mg) which usually works within 20 to 40 minutes [133]. Diltiazem can also prevent recurrent supraventricular tachycardias including those of the Wolff-Parkinson-White variety [134]. Fifteen of the 36 patients studied by Yeh et al. [134] received diltiazem follow-up therapy (mean dose 270 mg daily); 13 of those responding to acute therapy also benefitted by chronic prophylactic therapy with diltiazem.

Verapamil versus diltiazem. In an acute electrophysiologic comparative study, verapamil 0.15 mg/kg was the equivalent of diltiazem 0.25 mg/kg [131].

Wolff-Parkinson-White Arrhythmias

Verapamil. This agent usually has no effects on the accessory pathway but depresses the AV node and inhibits the reciprocating re-entry tachycardias at the site of the AV node. Verapamil does not work and may be dangerous when there is anterograde (antegrade) conduction down the anomalous bundle with atrial flutter or fibrillation. In this situation verapamil, like digoxin, may accelerate the ventricular response and is contraindicated [135].

Diltiazem. The principles of therapy with diltiazem in Wolff-Parkinson-White syndrome are similar to those of verapamil. Diltiazem acts to inhibit re-entry at the site of the normal anterograde pathway [136]; there may also be an additional effect on the fast retrograde pathway [134]. However, as in the case of verapamil, in patients with anterograde conduction who develop atrial fibrillation, there is the potential danger of enhanced conduction down the anterograde pathway with increased risk of ventricular fibrillation. This risk is much greater with intravenous than with oral diltiazem [136]. Diltiazem, like verapamil, can also cause atrial fibrillation to be sustained in patients with the Wolff-Parkinson-White syndrome [136].

Minor Indications for Calcium Antagonists

Congestive Heart Failure Including Dilated Cardiomyopathy

Although nifedipine has been extensively tested in patients with congestive heart failure (Table III-11), two general reservations have been expressed about the use of nifedipine and other calcium antagonist compounds in this condition. First, neurohumoral activation (proven in the case of nisoldipine) may increase plasma renin and norepinephrine levels [137]. Second, the intrinsic negative inotropic effect of calcium antagonists as a group may account for the adverse hemodynamic effects found in a sizeable minority (10% to 40%) of patients thus treated [138].

Nifedipine. Because of the powerful afterload reducing and mild diuretic properties, nifedipine is also being evaluated for hemodynamic effects in various types of LV failure [139, 140], including those of acute

Table III-11. Acute effects of nifedipine on left ventricular function in congestive heart failure

Nif Dose	LV Filling Pressure		Cardiac Index		Mean BP		Comments	Author (No.)
	C	Nif	C	Nif	C	Nif		
Reports of improvement								
20 mg SL	25	17^a	2.12	3.11^a	95	75^a	10 of 11 patients with COCM	Klugmann et al. [139]
20 mg SL	11	12	3.51	4.06^a	85	76^a	Mixed patient group of 8 patients	Matsumoto et al. [148]
10 mg SL	26	23^a	1.67	1.99^a	87	77^a	7 patients, 5 with CAD	Kubo et al. [217]
20 mg SL	17	16	2.4	3.3^a	104	94^a	10 patients, COCM	Margorien et al. [144]
20 mg SL	27	18^a	2.5	3.5^a	157	90^a	15 patients, hypertensive CHF	Guazzi et al. [161]
10 mg SL	28	18^b	2.5	3.4^a	150	122^a	7 patients, pulmonary edema, hypertension	Polese et al. [33]
10 mg SL	26	17^b	2.5	3.5^b	99	85^b	7 patients, COCM	Polese et al. [33]
10 mg SL	31	23^a	2.8	3.6^b	102	81^a	7 patients, mitral regurgitation	Polese et al. [33]
10–20 mg SL	23	24	2.4	3.2^a	90	75^a	7 or 9 patients, CAD; dP/dt fell	Fifer et al. [218]

10 mg SL	17	11^b	2.8	3.6^a	103	89^a	9 patients, COCM	Miller et al. [219]
20 mg SL	23	20	2.1	2.4^a	94	80^b	6/11 patients CAD; 3 of 8 decreased SVI	Elkayam et al. [220]
20 mg SL	20	17	2.6	2.8^a	85	68^a	18 patients, COCM, no long-term benefit	Agostoni et al. [150]
Report of mixed effects								
1. 10 mg SL	29	31	2.1	2.5	96	91	7 of 12 patients CAD; 3 COCM; 2 AMI. 8 of 12 patients improve; 4 of 12 patients deteriorate, especially those with high plasma renin	Lefkowitz et al. [221]
Reports of deterioration								
1. 30 mg SL	34	25	2.77	1.68	102	35	Single patient with COCM	Brooks et al. [151]
2. 20 mg SL	35	22	2.37	1.79	80	50	Single patient with CAD	Brooks et al. [151]

Abbreviations: AMI, acute myocardial infarction; BP, blood pressure (mmHg); C, control; CAD, coronary artery disease; cardiac index (L/m^2/min); CHF, congestive heart failure; COCM, congestive cardiomyopathy; dp/dt = differentiated pressure increase per unit time; I.V, left ventricular; Nif, nifedipine; SVI, stroke volue index. a = $p < 0.01$; b = $p < 0.05$ versus control. Units for I.V filling pressure and mean BP = mmHg.

pulmonary edema of ischemic heart disease [32, 33, 141], aortic regurgitation [142, 143], and idiopathic congestive cardiomyopathy [144].

The peripheral vasodilating effect of nifedipine usually offsets the direct negative inotropic effect [145], so that mild degrees of congestive heart failure are not a contraindication to the therapy of angina by nifedipine [146]. Rather, the beneficial oxygen-sparing hemodynamic effects of nifedipine in patients with an increased end-diastolic volume and pressure argue for the use of nifedipine [140]. In contrast, severe aortic stenosis is a contraindication to arteriolar dilation with nifedipine [147] as in the case of other vasodilating agents. A major advantage of nifedipine as a vaso-dilator for congestive heart failure [148] is that, com-pared with hydralazine, there is no risk of a secondary systemic lupus erythematosus. Also, in contrast to prazosin, tachyphylaxis does not develop with nifed-ipine [149].

Following recent studies showing the beneficial ef-fects of ACE inhibitors on mortality in patients with congestive heart failure, these agents are now receiving a lot of preferential usage in congestive heart failure. In a direct comparison with captopril 50 mg three times daily [150], nifedipine 20 mg three times daily also de-creased systemic vascular resistance, but only captopril relieved the enhanced wall stress. Because of the vari-able hemodynamic status of patients with congestive heart failure, the response to nifedipine is variable and sometimes unpredictable [151]. Packer et al. [138] pro-posed that most patients with congestive heart failure need preload as well as afterload reduction, so that calcium antagonists were not appropriate therapy. In their view, the beneficial effects of ACE inhibitors and nitrates-hydralazine on mortality could be explained as the result of the combined unloading of the right ventricle and left ventricle. However, 1) there are no long-term outcome studies with calcium antagonists; and 2) there are still good arguments for the use of calcium antagonists even in severe LV failure; es-pecially when caused by hypertension or valvular regurgitation.

Recent attention has turned to the possible effects of nifedipine on the regional circulation in congestive heart failure including kidneys [152] and skeletal mus-cle [153]. Thus far a beneficial redistribution of cardiac output has not been found. An increase of cardiac out-put must be distinguished from a true improvement in exercise tolerance.

Hence effects of nifedipine on LV function (see Table III-3) cannot directly be extrapolated to an im-provement in symptoms nor of prognosis in patients with chronic congestive heart failure.

Other dihydropyridines are also being evaluated in

congestive heart failure, including nisoldipine, nicardipine, and felodipine. Especially the latter appears to be promising (see Dihydropyridines in Second-Generation Calcium Antagonists).

Verapamil, with its prominent negative inotropic effect, is usually held to be contraindicated in the presence of myocardial failure, although when given very carefully the reduction of afterload can beneficially outweigh the potential for myocardial depression [154], especially in patients with valvular regurgitation [155]. Experimentally, verapamil may protect from alcoholic dysfunction of the myocardium and from the hereditary cardiomyopathy of Syrian hamsters [156]; the relevance of such models to human disease is still an open question.

Diltiazem, with its relative lack of negative inotropic effect, should theoretically be an attractive agent for afterload reduction in congestive heart failure. In eight patients, intravenous diltiazem (100 to 200 µg/min infusion) decreased afterload and improved cardiac index and stroke work without altering dP/dt [157]. Oral diltiazem (120 mg three times daily) caused similar effects. However, in three of eight patients and one of eight patients given intravenous and oral diltiazem respectively, transient junctional arrhythmias occurred. Lower oral doses of diltiazem (60 and 90 mg as single doses) do little in patients with severe LV failure [158]. Materne et al. [159] also safely administered diltiazem (0.5 mg/kg at 5 mg/min) to eight patients with congestive heart failure with a fall in systemic vascular resistance and a rise in stroke volume and ejection fraction; however, marked bradycardia below 50 beats per min occurred as a side effect in two of the patients. Diltiazem requires further appraisal in congestive heart failure. Its relative lack of a negative inotropic potential on the normal myocardium may not hold for the failing heart [160].

Nifedipine versus verapamil. These agents have been compared in congestive heart failure caused by hypertension. Nifedipine was better [161]. Over a period of 1 month both agents had similar vasodilating effects yet only nifedipine reduced LV diastolic diameter and the pulmonary capillary wedge pressure.

Summary. The use of calcium antagonists as LV unloading agents in congestive heart failure remains controversial. Some authors find good acute hemodynamic benefit, while others counsel against the use of these agents unless heart failure occurs with well-maintained LV systolic function as in hypertension or valvular regurgitation. At present nifedipine seems to be the best tested agent in congestive heart failure. Other dihydropyridines, such as nicardipine and felodipine, thought by some workers to have less negative inotropic effect than nifedipine, are also being evaluated (see Part IV—Drug Interactions and Combinations). Calcium antagonists are especially used in congestive heart failure if there is coexisting angina and/or hypertension. If there is prominent tachycardia, diltiazem should logically be preferred to the nifedipine group. There is, unfortunately, relatively little experience with diltiazem in the therapy of congestive heart failure. If there is pre-existing bradycardia, then the nifedipine group appears a logical choice. Long-term outcome trials with these agents are not available, although the experience with nifedipine over 2 months in patients with dilated cardiomyopathy was disappointing [150].

Hypertrophic Cardiomyopathy

Another potentially important use of calcium antagonists and especially *verapamil* is for hypertrophic cardiomyopathy. Potentially verapamil has two benefits, that of the negative inotropic effect which, if sufficiently marked, may lead to chamber enlargement with improvement in wall stress, and secondly verapamil may benefit diastolic function [162]. A theoretical problem is that the mild afterload reduction caused by verapamil can in patients with an obstructive component to the cardiomyopathy increase the gradient across the obstruction and thereby worsen the symptoms. However, if patients are carefully selected and monitored, then verapamil can improve obstructive features in about half of the patients [163] with, however, adverse hemodynamic effects in 12%. Kaltenbach and Hopf [164] have reported a large series of patients studied with verapamil over a prolonged period with apparent symptomatic benefit. However, the study was not placebo-controlled.

In a placebo-controlled short-term study of verapamil (80 or 120 mg four times daily), in hypertrophic obstructive cardiomyopathy, Rosing et al. [165] found only a benefit of 15 to 26% on indices of LV function which was sustained in a follow-up period of 3.5 to 6 months [166]; subjective benefit was, however, only modest. It should be noted that 17 of 19 patients had LV outflow tract obstruction. In a recent acute study, the question was asked whether intravenous verapamil (20 mg over 2 minutes) could be beneficial to patients with hypertrophic obstructive cardiomyopathy [167]. There were no consistent benefits on myocardial metabolism nor on hemodynamics with acute administration, yet it is possible that intravenous administration of such a high dose of verapamil is not optimal in this condition. Previous studies with intravenous verapamil used lower doses [165].

Nifedipine has been safely given to 15 patients with hypertrophic cardiomyopathy with improved diastolic myocardial function [168]. However, in hypertrophic obstructive cardiomyopathy it is contraindicated because it may exaggerate the pressure gradient across the obstruction [169] unless combined with propranolol. In contrast, *nifedipine plus propranolol* seems to be a beneficial combination in hypertrophic obstructive cardiomyopathy [170]; long-term studies have, however, not been reported.

Diltiazem gives acute hemodynamic benefits in patients with hypertrophic cardiomyopathy [171] with improvement of the impaired diastolic filling found in this condition [172]. Systolic function did not change. Benefit was maintained for 2 weeks [172].

Primary Pulmonary Hypertension

All three agents have been tested with varying results. Benefit has especially been found in hypoxic, vasoconstrictive pulmonary hypertension [173]. Experimentally, this type of pulmonary hypertension in dogs responds best to nifedipine [174]. In patients with pulmonary vasoconstriction, nifedipine increases cardiac output and reduces hypoxia [175]. In primary pulmonary hypertension, long-term benefit of calcium antagonists is best found at high doses such as nifedipine 240 mg daily or diltiazem 720 mg daily, after lower initial test doses [176].

Raynaud's Phenomenon

The subjective success rate for verapamil and diltiazem is high, with approximately 60 to 80% of patients benefiting. However, a minority of patients may not respond to either of these agents. At least four studies with *nifedipine* used in a double-blind crossover design, showed that the majority of patients improved symptomatically [177–180]. However, side effects were frequent, occurring in up to 30% of patients. Nifedipine is considerably more effective than is prazosin [181] and can be given sublingually before cold exposure to avoid attacks [182]. *Diltiazem* 360 mg daily also benefits the subjective aspects of Raynaud's phenomenon [183]. An intriguing feature, not studied in the case of nifedipine, is that secondary Raynaud's phenomenon (caused by scleroderma or rheumatoid arthritis) responds considerably less well than primary Raynaud's phenomenon. In the case of *verapamil*, only one study is available; doses of 160 to 320 mg/day were ineffective [184]. It should be noted that in all studies the benefit of nifedipine and diltiazem was subjective and not objective, for reasons which are obscure [185].

Peripheral Vascular Disease

Like coronary artery disease, peripheral vascular disease may be accompanied by arterial spasm to aggravate the severity of tissue ischemia. Hence, calcium antagonists should be logical therapy. A theoretical problem is vasodilation in the nonischemic muscle so that blood can "shunt" away from the ischemic area. Thus far, therapy of peripheral[70] vascular disease by calcium antagonists has not gained widespread acceptance except in the case of Raynaud's phenomenon. Di Perri et al. [186] describe the vasodilating effects of intra-arterial and intravenous nifedipine and diltiazem on normal subjects; effects on those with peripheral vascular disease are not reported.

Cerebral Insufficiency and
Subarachnoid Hemorrhage

Thus far, the standard agents—verapamil, nifedipine, and diltiazem—appear not to have been studied in these conditions. In contrast, nimodipine [187–189] improves the outcome in subarachnoid hemorrhage, and is also effective in early stroke [190]. Because nifedipine is also a powerful cerebral vasodilator [23], it could be that the standard calcium antagonists were equieffective with nimodipine in cerebral insufficiency, and comparative studies are required.

Migraine

Migraine has both vasoconstrictive and vasodilatory phases. Therefore, it is perhaps not surprising that both vasoconstrictive agents, such as propranolol, and vasodilatory agents, such as calcium channel antagonists, have been used as prophylaxis with therapeutic success. Of the classical calcium antagonists, only verapamil (80 mg four times daily) has been well studied in a double-blind placebo-controlled manner [191]; it reduced migraine frequency by about half. However, the series was small, with only 12 patients. As reported in a letter, diltiazem (240 to 360 mg daily) was successful in a small open study on nine patients who had failed to respond to nadolol [192]. Diltiazem (180 mg daily) helped to prevent migraine in a double-blind study of 150 patients, yet the study is at present only available in abstract form [193]. Nifedipine (10 mg three times daily) improved eight patients with both Raynaud's disease and migraine; although double-blinded, the study was only reported in letter form [194] and the patient population may have a somewhat unusual combination of symptoms. Therefore, further studies are required with the three prototypical agents before general acceptance for their use in migraine, especially in the case of nifedipine which is least well studied and most likely to have headaches as a side-effect (see Table IV-2). In the case of the proposed "cerebroselective agents" such as nimodipine [195] and flunarizine [196] the studies are more substantial and the arguments for their use correspondingly stronger.

Bronchospasm

Because of the widespread effects of calcium antagonists in relieving smooth muscle spasm, including coronary spasm and Raynaud's phenomenon, tests have been undertaken in patients with bronchoconstriction and asthma. *Nifedipine* has been used with benefit in patients with chronic obstructive lung disease [197], but is really only a mild bronchodilator as judged by the response to 10 to 30 mg nifedipine given acutely [198]. It is especially effective in exercise-induced asthma [199]. *Verapamil,* given by inhalation (a special preparation not normally available), is about as effective as sodium cromoglycate in the therapy of exercise-induced asthma [200].

Renal Disease

Calcium antagonists generally exert their antihypertensive effect with minimal alterations in the renin-angiotensin-aldosterone system. An exception is the acute stimulation of renin secretion found in some studies after the administration of nifedipine, but during chronic administration no sustained change is found [27]. Glomerular filtration rate is sustained, or possibly increased [12]. In the case of diltiazem, the filtration fraction falls as a result of improved intra-renal hemodynamics [201]. In addition, early experimental evidence suggests that verapamil and dihydropyridines protect against the progression of chronic experimental renal failure [202, 203]. For these reasons, the use of calcium antagonists in hypertension with renal involvement or in primary progressive renal disease warrants further appraisal. However, when chronic renal failure is accompanied by volume-dependent hypertension, calcium antagonists may be less effective than anticipated as antihypertensive agents. Likewise when there is chronic anemia, peripheral vasodilation may detract from the antihypertensive effect of calcium antagonists. These questions need further detailed study.

Atherosclerosis

In view of the promising experimental data showing that the rate of development of atherosclerosis can be slowed, a large-scale study in humans is now under way, comparing nifedipine (15 to 80 mg daily in three to four divided doses) with placebo [204]. Besides preventing experimental atherosclerosis [205], verapamil reduces cholesteryl ester deposits in macrophages; the latter effect is not, however, shared by diltiazem so that the mechanism cannot be by calcium entry antagonism [206].

Primary Aldosteronism (Conn's Syndrome)

Nifedipine (20 mg followed by 30 to 50 mg daily) acutely reduced hypertension within 60 minutes and aldosterone levels within 120 minutes [207]. During the chronic study, plasma K^+ was normalized and plasma aldosterone remained reduced. Nicardipine also reduces plasma aldosterone in volunteers [13]. It is proposed that transmembrane Ca^{2+} influx is required for aldosterone secretion and that nifedipine therapy may be beneficial in primary aldosteronism. Other dihydropyridines such as nitrendipine [208] are also likely to be effective in this condition.

References

1. Lindner A, Kenny M, Meacham AJ. Effects of a circulating factor in patients with essential hypertension on intracellular free calcium in normal platelets. *N Engl J Med* 1987; 316:509-513.

2. DeWardener HE, MacGregor GA. The relation of a circulating sodium transport inhibitor (the natriuretic hormone?) to hypertension. *Medicine (Baltimore)* 1983; 62: 310-326.

3. Blaustein MP, Ashida T, Goldman WF, et al. Sodium/calcium exchange in vascular smooth muscle: A link between sodium metabolism and hypertension. *Ann NY Acad Sci* 1986; 488:199-216.

4. Robinson BF. Altered calcium handling as a cause of primary hypertension. *J Hypertens* 1984; 2:453-460.

5. Erne P, Bolli P, Burgisser E, et al. Correlation of platelet calcium with blood pressure. Effect of antihypertensive therapy. *N Engl J Med* 1984; 310:1084-1088.

6. Landmark K. Antihypertensive and metabolic effects of long-term therapy with nifedipine slow-release tablets. *J Cardiovasc Pharmacol* 1985; 7:12-17.

7. Muiesan G, Agabiti-Rosei E, Castellano M, et al. Antitihypertensive and humoral effects of verapamil and nifedipine in essential hypertension. *J Cardiovasc Pharmacol* 1982; 4:S325-S329.

8. Petru MA, Crawford MH, Sorensen SG, et al. Short- and long-term efficacy of high-dose oral diltiazem for angina due to coronary artery disease: A placebo-controlled, randomized, double-blind crossover study. *Circulation* 1983; 68:139-147.

9. Laederach K, Weidmann P, Lauener F, et al. Comparative acute effects of the calcium channel blockers tiapamil, nisoldipine and nifedipine on blood pressure and some regulatory factors in normal and hypertensive subjects. *J Cardiovasc Pharmacol* 1986; 8:294-302.

10. Kiowski W, Erne P, Bertel O, et al. Acute and chronic sym-

pathetic reflex activation and antihypertensive response to nifedipine. *J Am Coll Cardiol* 1986; 7:344-348.

11. Swartz SL. Endocrine and vascular responses in hypertensive patients to long-term treatment with diltiazem. *J Cardiovasc Pharmacol* 1987; 9:391-395.

12. Bauer JH, Reams GP. Short- and long-term effects of calcium entry blockers on the kidney. *Am J Cardiol* 1987; 59:66A-71A.

13. Bellet M, Sassano T, Guyenne P, et al. Converting-enzyme inhibition buffers the counter-regulatory response to acute administration of nicardipine. *Br J Clin Pharmacol* 1987; 24:465-472.

14. Luna RL, Carrasco RM. Efficacy of verapamil in patients resistant to other antihypertensive therapy. *Am J Cardiol* 1986; 57:64D-68D.

15. McLeay RAB, Stallard TJ, Watson RDS, et al. The effect of nifedipine on arterial pressure and reflex cardiac control. *Circulation* 1983; 67:1084-1090.

16. Jennings AA, Jee LD, Smith JA, et al. Acute effect of nifedipine on blood pressure and left ventricular ejection fraction in severely hypertensive outpatients: Predictive effects of acute therapy and prolonged efficacy when added to existing therapy. *Am Heart J* 1986; 111:557-563.

17. Millard RW, Lathrop DA, Grupp G, et al. Differential cardiovascular effects of calcium channel blocking agents: Potential mechanisms. *Am J Cardiol* 1982; 49:499-506.

18. Warltier DC, Zyvoloski MG, Gross GJ, et al. Comparative actions of dihydropyridine slow channel calcium blocking agents in conscious dogs: Alterations in baroreflex sensitivity. *J Pharmacol Exp Ther* 1984; 230:376-382.

19. Ben-Ishay D, Leibel B, Stessman J. Calcium channel blockers in the management of hypertension in the elderly. *Am J Med* 1986; 81(Suppl 6A):30-34.

20. Cody RJ. The hemodynamics of calcium-channel antagonists in hypertension: vascular and myocardial responses. *Circulation* 1987; 75(Suppl I):I-175-I-79.

21. Beer N, Gallegos I, Cohen A, et al. Efficacy of sublingual nifedipine in the acute treatment of systemic hypertension. *Chest* 1981; 79:571-574.

22. Opie LH, Jee L, White D. Antihypertensive effects of nifedipine combined with cardioselective beta-adrenergic receptor antagonism by atenolol. *Am Heart J* 1982; 104:606-612.

23. Bertel O, Conen D, Radu EW, et al. Nifedipine in hypertensive emergencies. *Br Med J* 1983; 286:19-21.

24. Huysmans FT, Sluiter HE, Thien TA, et al. Acute treatment of hypertensive crisis with nifedipine. *Br. J Clin Pharmacol* 1983; 16:725-727.

25. Haft JI, Litterer WE. Chewing nifedipine to rapidly treat hypertension. *Arch Intern Med* 1984; 144:2357-2359.

26. Isles CG, Johnson OC, Milne FJ. Slow-release nifedipine and atenolol as initial treatment in Blacks with malignant hypertension. *Br J Clin Pharmacol* 1986; 21:377-383.

27. Sorkin EM, Clissold SP, Brogden RN. Nifedipine. A review of its pharmacodynamic and pharmacokinetic properties, and therapeutic efficacy, in ischemic heart disease, hypertension and related cardiovascular disorders. *Drugs* 1985; 30:182-274.

28. Pedersen OL, Mikkelsen E. Acute and chronic effects of nifedipine in arterial hypertension. *Eur J Clin Pharmacol* 1978; 14:375-381.

29. Resnick LM, Sealy JE, Laragh JH. Calcium metabolism and the renin-aldosterone system determine the acute blood pressure response to calcium channel blockade. *Cir-*

culation 1982; 66(Suppl II):II-107.

30. Erne P, Bolli P, Bertel O, et al. Factors influencing the hypotensive effects of calcium antagonists. *Hypertension* 1983; 5(Suppl II):II-97-II-102.

31. Ambroso GC, Como G, Scalamogna A, et al. The treatment of arterial hypertension with nifedipine in patients with chronic renal insufficiency. *Clin Nephrol* 1985; 23:41-45.

32. Guazzi M, Olivari MT, Polese A, et al. Nifedipine, a new antihypertensive with rapid action. *Clin Pharmacol Ther* 1977; 22:528-532.

33. Polese A, Fiorentini C, Olivari MT, et al. Clinical use of a calcium antagonistic agent (nifedipine) in acute pulmonary edema. *Am J Med* 1979; 66:825-830.

34. Bauer JH, Reams GP. The role of calcium entry blockers in hypertensive emergencies. *Circulation* 1987; 75(Suppl V): V174-V180.

35. Yagil Y, Kobrin I, Stessman J, et al. Effectiveness of combined nifedipine and propranolol treatment in hypertension. *Hypertension* 1983; 5(Part II):II-113-II-117.

36. Franklin C, Nightingale S, Mamdani B: A randomized comparison of nifedipine and sodium nitroprusside in severe hypertension. *Chest* 1986; 90:500-503.

37. Jee LD, Opie LH. Acute hypotensive response to nifedipine added to prazosin in treatment of hypertension. *Br Med J* 1983; 287:1514-1516.

38. Sluiter HE, Huysmans FThM, Thien ThA, et al. The influence of alpha$_1$-adrenergic blockade on the acute antihypertensive effect of nifedipine. *Eur J Clin Pharmacol* 1985; 29:263-267.

39. Bender VF. Die Behandlung der Tachycarden Arrhythmien und der arteriellen Hypertonie mit Verapamil. *Drug Res* 1970; 20:1310-1316.

40. Brittinger WD, Schwarzbeck A, Wittenmeier KW, et al. Klinisch-experimentalle Untersuchungen uber die blutdrucksendkende Wirkung von Verapamil. *Dtsch Med Wochenschr* 1970; 37:1871-1877.

41. Brouwer RML, Bolli P, Erne P, et al. Antihypertensive treatment using calcium antagonists in combination with captopril rather than diuretics. *J Cardiovasc Pharmacol* 1985; 7(Suppl 1):S88-S91.

42. Agabiti-Rosei E, Muiesan ML, Romanelli G, et al. Similarities and differences in the antihypertensive effect of two calcium antagonist drugs, verapamil and nifedipine. *J Am Coll Cardiol* 1986; 7:916-924.

43. Frishman WH, Weinberg P, Peled HB, et al. Calcium entry blockers for the treatment of severe hypertension and hypertensive crisis. *Am J Med* 1984; 77:35-45.

44. Chaffman M, Brogden RN. Diltiazem: A review of its pharmacological properties and therapeutic efficacy. *Drugs* 1985; 29:287-454.

45. Safar ME, Simon AC, Levenson JA, et al. Hemodynamic effects of diltiazem in hypertension. *Circ Res* 1983; 52(Suppl 1):169-173.

46. Theroux P, Waters DD, Debaisieux JC, et al. Hemodynamic effects of calcium ion antagonists after acute myocardial infarction. *Clin Invest Med* 1980; 3:81-85.

47. Moser M. Calcium entry blockers for systemic hypertension. *Am J Cardiol* 1987; 59: 115A-121A.

48. Lewis GRJ, Morley KD, Lewis BM, et al. The treatment of hypertension with verapamil. *NZ Med J* 1978; 87:351-354.

49. Gould BA, Hornung RS, Mann S, et al. Slow channel inhibitors verapamil and nifedipine in the management of

hypertension. *J Cardiovasc Pharmacol* 1982; 4(Suppl III):S369-S373.

50. Zachariah PK, Sheps SG, Schirger A, et al. Verapamil and 24-hour ambulatory blood pressure monitoring in essential hypertension. *Am J Cardiol* 1986; 57:74D-79D.

51. Midtbo K, Hals O, van der Meer J, et al. Instant and sustained-release verapamil in the treatment of essential hypertension. *Am J Cardiol* 1986; 57:59D-63D.

52. Frishman W, Charlap S, Kimmel B, et al. Twice-daily administration of oral verapamil in the treatment of essential hypertension. *Arch Intern Med* 1986; 146:561-565.

53. Buhler FR, Hulthen U, Kiowski W, et al. The place of the calcium antagonist verapamil in antihypertensive therapy. *J Cardiovasc Pharmacol* 1982; 4:S350-S357.

54. Cubeddu LX, Aranda J, Singh B, et al. A comparison of verapamil and propranolol for the initial treatment of hypertension. Racial differences in response. *JAMA* 1986; 256:2214-2221.

55. Dargie H, Cleland J, Findlay I, et al. Combination of verapamil and beta-blockers in systemic hypertension. *Am J Cardiol* 1986; 57:80D-82D.

56. Corea L, Bentivoglio M, Verdecchia P, et al. Calcium antagonists and diuretics in arterial hypertension: A useful combination. In: Reid JL, Pickup AJ, eds. *Calcium Antagonists and the Treatment of Hypertension.* London: Royal Society of Medicine, 1984;23-30.

57. Leary WP, Asmal AC. Treatment of hypertension with verapamil. *Curr Ther Res* 1979; 25: 747-752.

58. Murphy MB, Scriven AJI, Dollery CT. Role of nifedipine in treatment of hypertension. *Br Med J* 1983;287:257-259.

59. Bayley S, Dobbs RJ, Robinson BF. Nifedipine in the treatment of hypertension: Report of a double-blind controlled trial. *Br J Clin Pharmacol* 1982; 14:509-512.

60. Lejeune PO. Nifedipine and beta-blocking agents. In: Krebs R, ed. *Treatment of Cardiovascular Diseases by Adalat (Nifedipine).* Stuttgart-New York: Schattauer, 1986;259-278.

61. Eggertsen R, Hansson L. Effects of treatment with nifedipine and metoprolol in essential hypertension. *Eur J Clin Pharmacol* 1982; 21:389-390.

62. De Divitiis O, Petitto M, Di Somma S, et al. Acebutolol and nifedipine in the treatment of arterial hypertension: Efficacy and acceptability. Arzneimittelforsch 1984; 34:710-715.

63. Tsukiyama H, Otsuka K, Yamamoto Y. Effect on pindolol and nifedipine alone and in combination on haemodynamic parameters/variables in essential hypertension. *J Intern Med Res* 1984; 12:154-162.

64. Hornung RS, Gould BA, Jones RI, et al. Nifedipine tablets for hypertension: a study using continous ambulatory intra-arterial recording. *Am J Cardiol* 1983; 51:1323-1327.

65. Gould BA, Hornung RS, Mann S, et al. Nifedipine or verapamil as sole treatment of hypertension. An intra-arterial study. *Hypertension* 1983; 5(Suppl II):II-91-II-96.

66. Bonaduche D, Canonico V, Mazza F, et al. Evaluation of the efficacy of slow-release nifedipine in systemic hypertension by ambulatory intraarterial blood pressure monitoring. *J Cardiovasc Pharmacol* 1985; 7:145-151.

67a. Daniels AR, Opie LH. Effect of slow-release nifedipine on glucose tolerance. In: Lichtlen PR, ed. *Sixth International*

Adalat Symposium. Amsterdam: Excerpta Medica, 1986;495–496.

67b. Daniels AR, Opie LH. Atenolol plus nifedipine for mild to moderate systemic hypertension after fixed doses of either agent alone. *Am J Cardiol* 1986; 57:965–970.

68. MacGregor GA. Hypertension. In: Krebs R, ed. *Treatment of Cardiovascular Diseases by Adalat (Nifedipine).* Stuttgart: Schattauer, 1986; 231–258.

69. Fadayomi MO, Akinroye KK, Ajoe RO, et al. Monotherapy with nifedipine for essential hypertension in adult blacks. *J Cardiovasc Pharmacol* 1986; 8:466–469.

70. Brennan F, Flanagan M, Blake S, et al. Nifedipine in the treatment of hypertension. *Eur J Clin Pharmacol* 1983; 25:713–715.

71. Singer DRJ, Markandu ND, Shore AC, et al. Nifedipine and acebutolol in combination for the treatment of moderate to severe essential hypertension. *J Hum Hypertens* 1987; 1:31–37.

72. Myers MG, Leenen FHH, Burns R, et al. Nifedipine tablets vs hydralazine in patients with persisting hypertension who receive combined diuretic and beta-blocker therapy. *Clin Pharmacol Ther* 1986; 39:409–413.

73. Pool PE, Massie BM, Venkararaman K, et al. Diltiazem as monotherapy for systemic hypertension: A multicenter, randomized, placebo-controlled trial. *Am J Cardiol* 1986; 57:212–217.

74. Frishman W, Zawada ET, Smith K, et al. Comparison of hydrochlorothiazide and sustained-release diltiazem for mild to moderate systemic hypertension. *Am J Cardiol* 1987; 59:615–623.

75. Inouye IK, Massie BM, Benowitz N, et al. Antihypertensive therapy with diltiazem and comparison with hydrochlorothiazide. *Am J Cardiol* 1984; 53:1588–1592.

76. Ogawa K, Ban M, Ito T, et al. Diltiazem for treatment of essential hypertension: A double-blind controlled study with reserpine. *Clin Ther* 1984; 6:844–853.

77. Menasche S, Elkik F, Cocco G, et al. Synergistic antihypertensive effect of diltiazem combined with the alphaadrenoceptor blocker alfuzosine (abstr). Presentation to NY Acad Sci, Feb 1987.

78. Midtbo K, Hals O, van der Meer J. Verapamil compared with nifedipine in the treatment of essential hypertension. *J Cardiovasc Pharmacol* 1982; 4(Suppl 3):363–368.

79. Belz GG, Spies G. Kontrollierte Studie zur Behandlung der Hypertonie mit Verapamil in Retardform. *Z Cardiol* 1985; 74:453–459.

80. Klein W, Brandt D, Vrecko K, et al. Role of calcium antagonists in the treatment of essential hypertension. *Circ Res* 1983; 52(Suppl 1): 174–181.

81. Schulte K-L, Meyer-Sabellek WA, Distler A, et al. Longterm treatment with diltiazem and nifedipine in essential hypertension. *J Hypertens* 1984;2:93.

82. Anavekar SN, Christophidis M, Louis WJ, et al. Verapamil in the treatment of hypertension. *J Cardiovasc Pharmacol* 1981; 3:287–292.

83. Anavekar SN, Barter C, Adam WR, et al. A double-blind comparison of verapamil and labetalol in hypertensive patients with coexisting chronic obstructive airways disease. *J Cardiovasc Pharmacol* 1982; 4:S374–S377.

84. Escudero J, Hernandez H, Martinez F. Comparative study of the antihypertensive effect of verapamil and atenolol. *Am J Cardiol* 1986; 57:54D–58D.

85. Yamakado T, Oonishi N, Kondo S, et al. Effects of diltiazem on cardiovascular responses during exercise in

systemic hypertension and comparison with propranolol. *Am J Cardiol* 1983; 52: 1023-1027.

86. Trimarco B, DeLuca N, Ricciardelli B, et al. Diltiazem in the treatment of mild or moderate essential hypertension. Comparison with metoprolol in a crossover double-blind trial. *J Clin Pharmacol* 1984; 24:218-227.

87. Szlachcic J, Hirsch AT, Tubau JF, et al. Diltiazem versus propranolol in essential hypertension: Responses of rest and exercise blood pressure and effects on exercise capacity. *Am J Cardiol* 1987; 59:393-399.

88. Hallin L, Andren L, Hansson L. Controlled trial of nifedipine and bendroflumethiazide in hypertension. *J Cardiovasc Pharmacol* 1983; 5:1083-1085.

89. Douglas-Jones AP, Mitchell AD. Comparison of nifedipine (retard formulation) and mefruside in the treatment of mild to moderate hypertenion—a prospective randomized double-blind crossover study in general practice. *Postgrad Med J* 1984; 60:529-532.

90. Rosenthal J. Antihypertensive effects of nifedipine, mefruside and a combination of both substances in patients with essential hypertensions. In: Kaltenbach M. Neufeld HM, eds. *New Therapy of Ischaemic Heart Disease and Hypertension.* Amsterdam: Excerpta Medica, 1982;175-181.

91. Lehtonen A, Gordin A. Metabolic parameters after changing from hydrochlorothiazide to verapamil treatment in hypertension. *Eur J Clin Pharmacol* 1984; 27:153-157.

92. Corea L, Bentivoglio M, Cosmi F. Nifedipine versus prazosin in essential hypertension: a double-blind study. *Curr Ther Res* 1981; 30:698-670.

93. Olowoyeye JO, Giwa LO, Araoye MA. A controlled clinical trial of verapamil in the treatment of hypertension: Comparison with alpha methyldopa. *Curr Ther Res* 1983; 34:523-530.

94. Guazzi MD, Fiorentini C, Olivari MT, et al. Short- and long-term efficacy of a calcium antagonist agent (nifedipine) combined with methyldopa in the treatment of severe hypertension. *Circulation* 1980; 61:913-919.

95. Guazzi MD, Polese A, Fiorentini C, et al. Treatment of hypertension with calcium antagonists: Review. *Hypertension* 1983; 5:II-85-II-90.

96. Imai Y, Abe K, Otsuka Y, et al. Management of severe hypertension with nifedipine in combination with clonidine or propranolol. *Arzneimeimittelforsch* 1980; 30: 674-678.

97. Guazzi MD, De Cesare N, Galli C, et al. Calcium-channel blockade with nifedipine and angiotensin converting-enzyme inhibition with captopril in the therapy of patients with severe primary hypertension. *Hypertension* 1984; 70:279-284.

98. Mimran A, Ribstein J. Effect of chronic nifedipine in patients inadequately controlled by a converting enzyme inhibitor and a diuretic. *J Cardiovasc Pharmacol* 1985; 7(Suppl 1):S92-S95.

99. M'Buyamba-Kabangu JR, Lepira B, Fagard R, et al. Relative potency of a beta-blocking and a calcium entry blocking agent as antihypertensive drugs in black patients. *Eur J Clin Pharmacol* 1986; 29:523-527.

100. M'Buyamba-Kabangu JR, Fagard R, Lijnen P, et al. Calcium entry blockade or beta-blockade in long-term management of hypertension in blacks. *Clin Pharmacol Ther* 1987; 41:45-54.

101. Mooy J, van Baak M, Bohm R, et al. The effects of verapamil and propranolol on exercise tolerance in hyper-

tensive patients. *Clin Pharmacol Ther* 1987; 41: 490–495.

102. Schmieder RE, Rueddel H, Neus H, et al. Disparate hemodynamic responses to mental challenge after antihypertensive therapy with β-blockers and calcium entry blockers. *Am J Med* 1987; 82:11–16.

103. Floras JS, Hassan MO, Jones JV, et al. Cardioselective and nonselective beta-adrenoceptor blocking drugs in hypertension: A comparison of their effect on blood pressure during mental and physical activity. *J Am Coll Cardiol* 1985; 6:186–195.

104. Loaldi A, Pepi M, Agostoni PG, et al. Cardiac rhythm in hypertension assessed through 24 hour ambulatory electrocardiographic monitoring. Effects of load manipulation with atenolol, verapamil, and nifedipine. *Br Heart J* 1983; 50:118–126.

105. Fouad-Tarazi FM, Libson PR: Echocardiographic studies of regression of left ventricular hypertrophy in hypertension. *Hypertension* 1987; 9(Suppl II):II-65–II-68.

106. Muiesan G, Agabiti-Rosei E, Romanelli G, et al. Adrenergic activity and left ventricular function during treatment of essential hypertension with calcium antagonists. *Am J Cardiol* 1986; 57:44D–49D.

107. Amodeo C, Kobrin I, Ventura HO, et al. Immediate and short-term hemodynamic effects of diltiazem in patients with hypertension. *Circulation* 1986; 73:108–113.

108. Frohlich ED. Correction of physiological alterations of hypertension (editorial). *Cardiovasc Drugs Ther* 1987; 1:345–348.

109. Ortiz J, Matsumoto A, Monaco CAF, et al. Left ventricular function after a single large dose of verapamil. *Am J Cardiol* 1986; 57:30D–34D.

110. De Kock M, Melin JA, Nannan ME, et al. Alteration of left ventricular diastolic filling in hypertensive patients: Effects of nitrendipine and atenolol. *Eur Heart J* 1986; 7:792–799.

111. Sowers JR, Mohanty PK. Comparison of calcium-entry blockers and diuretics in the treatment of hypertensive patients. *Circulation* 1987; 75(Suppl V):V170–V173.

112. MRC trial of treatment of mild hypertension: Principal results. *Br Med J* 1985; 291:97–104.

113. Mitchell LB, Schroeder JS, Mason JW. Comparative clinical electrophysiologic effects of diltiazem, verapamil and nifedipine: A review. *Am J Cardiol* 1982; 49: 629–635.

114. Schamroth L. Immediate effects of intravenous verapamil on atrial fibrillation. *Cardiovasc Res* 1971; 5:419–424.

115. Rozanski JJ, Zaman L, Castellanos A. Electrophysiologic effects of diltiazem hydrochloride on supraventricular tachycardia. *Am J Cardiol* 1982; 49:621–628.

116. Theisen K, Haufe M, Peters J, et al. Effect of the calcium antagonist diltiazem on atrioventricular conduction in chronic atrial fibrillation. *Am J Cardiol* 1985; 55: 98–102.

117. Talano JV, Tommaso C. Slow channel calcium antagonists in the treatment of supraventricular tachycardia. *Prog Cardiovasc Dis* 1982; 25:141–156.

118. Lang R, Klein HO, Di Segni E. Verapamil improves exercise capacity in chronic atrial fibrillation: Double-blind crossover study. *Am Heart J* 1983; 105:820–825.

119. Lang R, Klein HO, Weiss E, et al. Superiority of oral verapamil therapy to digoxin in treatment of chronic atrial fibrillation. *Chest* 1983; 83:491–499.

120. Lewis R, Lakhani M, Moreland TA, et al. A comparison of verapamil and digoxin in the treatment of atrial fibrilla-

tion. *Eur Heart J* 1987; 8:148-153.
121. Beasley R, Smith DA, McHaffie DJ. Excess heart rates at different serum digoxin concentrations in patients with atrial fibrillation. *Br Med J* 1985; 290:9-11.
122. Channer KS,Papouchado M, James MA, et al. Towards improved control of atrial fibrillation. *Eur Heart J* 1987; 8:141-147.
123. Roth A, Harrison E, Mitani G, et al. Efficacy and safety of medium- and high-dose diltiazem alone and in combination with digoxin for control of heart rate at rest and during exercise in patients with chronic atrial fibrillation. *Circulation* 1986; 73:316-324.
124. Steinberg JS, Katz RJ, Bren GB, et al. Efficacy of oral diltiazem to control ventricular response in chronic atrial fibrillation at rest and during exercise. *J Am Coll Cardiol* 1987; 9:405-411.
125. Singh BN, Ellrodt G, Peter CT. Verapamil: A review of its pharmacological properties and therapeutic use. *Drugs* 1978; 15:169-197.
126. Betriu A, Chaitman BR, Bourassa MG, et al. Beneficial effect of intravenous diltiazem in the acute management of paroxysmal supraventricular tachyarrhythmias. *Circulation* 1983; 67:88-94.
127. Mauritson DR, Winniford MD, Walker WS, et al. Oral verapamil for paroxysmal supraventricular tachycardia. A long-term, double-blind randomized trial. *Ann Intern Med* 1982; 96:409-412.
128. Yee R, Gulamhusein SS, Klein GJ. Combined verapamil and propranolol for supraventricular tachycardia. *Am J Cardiol* 1984; 53:757-763.
129. Winniford MD,Gabliani G, Johnson SM, et al. Concomitant calcium antagonist plus isosorbide dinitrate therapy for markedly active variant angina. *Am Heart J* 1984; 108:1269-1273.
130. Buxton AE, Marchlinski FE,Doherty JU, et al. Hazards of intravenous verapamil for sustained ventricular tachycardia. *Am J Cardiol* 1987; 59:1107-1110.
131. Rowland E, McKenna WJ, Gulker H, et al. Comparative effects of diltiazem and verapamil on atrioventricular conduction and atrioventricular reentry tachycardia. *Circ Res* 1983; 52(Suppl 1):163-168.
132. Hung J, Yeh S, Lin F, et al. Usefulness of intravenous diltiazem in predicting subsequent electrophysiologic and clinical responses to oral diltiazem. *Am J Cardiol* 1984; 54:1259-1262.
133. Yeh S-J, Lin F-C, Chou Y-Y, et al. Termination of paroxysmal supraventricular tachycardia with a single oral dose of diltiazem and propranolol. *Circulation* 1985; 71:104-109.
134. Yeh S-J, Kou H-C, Lin F-C, et al. Effects of oral diltiazem in paroxysmal supraventricular tachycardia. *Am J Cardiol* 1983; 52:271-278.
135. Gulamhusein S, Ko P, Carruthers SG, et al. Acceleration of the ventricular response during atrial fibrillation in the Wolff-Parkinson-White syndrome after verapamil. *Circulation* 1982; 65:348-354.
136. Shenasa M, Fromer M, Faugere G, et al. Efficacy and safety of intravenous and oral diltiazem for Wolff-Parkinson-White syndrome. *Am J Cardiol* 1987; 59: 301-306.
137. Barjon J-N, Rouleau J-L, Bichet D, et al. Chronic renal and neurohumoral effects of the calcium entry blocker nisoldipine in patients with congestive heart failure. *J Am Coll Cardiol* 1987; 9:622-630.
138. Packer M, Kessler PD, Lee WH. Calcium-channel block-

ade in the management of severe chronic congestive heart failure: A bridge too far. *Circulation* 1987; 75(Suppl V):V56–V64.

139. Klugmann S, Salvi A, Camerini F. Haemodynamic effects of nifedipine in heart failure. *Br Heart J* 1980; 43:440–446.

140. Ludbrook PA, Tiefenbrunn AJ, Sobel BE. Influence of nifedipine on left ventricular systolic and diastolic function. *Am J Med* 1981; 71:683–692.

141. Gordon GD, Mabin TA, Isaacs S, et al. Hemodynamic effects of sublingual nifedipine in acute myocardial infarction. *Am J Cardiol* 1984; 53:1228–1232.

142. Fioretti P, Benussi B, Scardi S, et al. Afterload reduction with nifedipine in aortic insufficiency. *Am J Cardiol* 1982; 49:1728–1732.

143. Shen WF, Roubin GS, Hirasawa K, et al. Noninvasive assessment of acute effects of nifedipine on rest and exercise hemodynamics and cardiac function in patients with aortic regurgitation. *J Am Coll Cardiol* 1984; 4: 902–907.

144. Magorien RD, Leier CV, Kolibash AJ, et al. Beneficial effects of nifedipine on rest and exercise myocardial energetics in patients with congestive heart failure. *Circulation* 1984; 70:884–890.

145. Joshi PI, Dalal JJ, Ruttley MSJ, et al. Nifedipine and left ventricular function in beta-blocked patients. *Br Heart J* 1981; 45:457–459.

146. Terry RW. Nifedipine therapy in angina pectoris: Evaluation of safety and side-effects. *Am Heart J* 1982; 104:681–689.

147. Gillmer DJ, Kark P. Pulmonary oedema precipitated by nifedipine. *Br Med J* 1980; 280:1420–1421.

148. Matsumoto S, Ito T, Sada T, et al. Hemodynamic effects of nifedipine in congestive heart failure. *Am J Cardiol* 1980; 46:476–480.

149. Olivari MT, Bartorelli C, Polese A, et al. Treatment of hypertension with nifedipine, a calcium antagonistic agent. *Circulation* 1979; 59:1056–1062.

150. Agostoni PG, De Cesare N, Doria E, et al. Afterload reduction: a comparison of captopril and nifedipine in dilated cardiomyopathy. *Br Heart J* 1986; 55:391–399.

151. Brooks N, Cattell M, Pidgeon J, et al. Unpredictable response to nifedipine in severe cardiac failure (Letter). *Br Med J* 1980; 281:1324.

152. Elkayam U, Weber L, Campese VM, et al. Renal hemodynamic effects of vasodilation with nifedipine and hydralazine in patients with heart failure. *J Am Coll Cardiol* 1984; 4:1261–1267.

153. Choong CYP, Roubin GS, Shen W-F, et al. Effects of nifedipine on systemic and regional oxygen transport and metabolism at rest and during exercise. *Circulation* 1985; 71:787–796.

154. Ferlinz J, Citron PD. Hemodynamics and myocardial performance characteristics after verapamil use in congestive heart failure. *Am J Cardiol* 1983; 51:1339–1345.

155. Butman SM, Eagan J, Olson HG. Hemodynamic effects of verapamil in left ventricular valvular volume overload. *Am Heart J* 1985; 110:416–426.

156. Garrett JS, Wikman-Coffelt J, Sievers R, et al. Verapamil prevents the development of alcoholic dysfunction in hamster myocardium. *J Am Coll Cardiol* 1987; 9: 1326–1331.

157. Walsh RA, Porter CB, Starling MR, et al. Beneficial effects of intravenous and oral diltiazem in severe congestive heart failure. *J Am Coll Cardiol* 1984; 3: 1044–1050.

158. Kulick DL, McIntosh N, Campese VM, et al. Central and renal hemodynamic effects and hormonal response to diltiazem in severe congestive heart failure. *Am J Cardiol* 1987; 59:1138-1143.

159. Materne P, Legrand V, Vandormael M, et al. Hemodynamic effects of intravenous diltiazem with impaired left ventricular function. *Am J Cardiol* 1984; 54: 733-737.

160. Porter CB, Walsh RA, Badke FR, et al. Differential effects of diltiazem and nitroprusside on left ventricular function in experimental chronic volume overload. *Circulation* 1983; 68:685-692.

161. Guazzi MD, Cipolla C, Della Bella P, et al. Disparate unloading efficacy of the calcium channel blockers, verapamil and nifedipine, on the failing hypertensive left ventricle. *Am Heart J* 1984; 108:116-123.

162. Bonow RO, Ostrow HG, Rosing DR, et al. Effects of verapamil on left ventricular systolic and diastolic function in patients with hypertrophic cardiomyopathy: Pressure-volume analysis with a nonimaging scintillation probe. *Circulation* 1983; 68:1062-1073.

163. Rosing DR, Condi JR, Maron BJ, et al. Verapamil therapy: A new approach to the pharmacologic treatment of hypertrophic cardiomyopathy. III. Effects of long-term administration. *Am J Cardiol* 1981; 48:545-553.

164. Kaltenbach M, Hopf R. Treatment of hypertrophic cardiomyopathy: Relation to pathological mechanisms. *J Mol Cell Cardiol* 1985; 17(Suppl 2):59-68.

165. Rosing DR, Kent KM, Borer JS, et al. Verapamil therapy: A new approach to the pharmacologic treatment of hypertrophic cardiomyopathy. I. Hemodynamic effects. *Circulation* 1979; 60:1201-1207.

166. Rosing DR, Kent KM, Maron BJ, et al. Verapamil therapy: A new approach to the pharmacologic treatment of hypertrophic cardiomyopathy. II. Effects on exercise capacity and symptomatic status. *Circulation* 1979; 60:1208-1213.

167. Wilmhurst PT, Thompson DS, Juul SM, et al. Effects of verapamil on haemodynamic function and myocardial metabolism in patients with hypertrophic cardiomyopathy. *Br Heart J* 1986; 56:544-553.

168. Lorell BH, Paulus WJ, Grossman W, et al. Modification of abnormal left ventricular diastolic properties by nifedipine in patients with hypertrophic cardiomyopathy. *Circulation* 1982; 65:499-507.

169. Betocchi S, Cannon RO, Watson RM, et al. Effects of sublingual nifedipine on hemodynamics and systolic and diastolic function in patients with hypertrophic cardiomyopathy. *Circulation* 1985; 72:1001-1007.

170. Landmark K, Sire S, Thaulow E, et al: Haemodynamic effects of nifedipine and propranolol in patients with hypertrophic obstructive cardiomyopathy. *Br Heart J* 1982; 48:19-26.

171. Nagao M, Yasue H, Omote S, et al: Diltiazam-induced decrease of exercise elevated pulmonary arterial diastolic pressure in hypertrophic cardiomyopathy patients. *Am Heart J* 1981; 102:789-790.

172. Suwa M, Hirota Y, Kawamura K: Improvement in left vetricular diastolic function during intravenous and oral diltiazem therapy in patients with hypertrophic cardiomyopathy: An echocardiographic study. *Am J Cardiol* 1984; 54:1047-1053.

173. Simonneau G, Escourrou P, Duroux P, et al: Inhibition of hypoxic pulmonary vasoconstriction by nifedipine. *New Engl J Med* 1981; 304:1582-1585.

174. Young TE, Lundquist LJ, Chesler E, et al: Comparative effects of nifedipine, verapamil and diltiazem on experimental pulmonary hypertension. *Am J Cardiol* 1983; 51:195-200.

175. Singh H, Ebejer MJ, Higgins DA, et al: Chronic cor pulmonale. Acute haemodynamic and neurohumoral effects of nifedipine at rest and on maximal exercise. In: Lichtlen PR, ed. 6th International Adalat® Symposium. Amsterdam: Excerpta Medica, 1986, 537-542.

176. Rich S, Brundage BH: High-dose calcium channel-blocking therapy for primary hypertension: evidence for long-term reduction in pulmonary arterial pressure and regression of right ventricular hypertrophy. *Circulation* 1987; 76:135-141.

177. Smith CD, McKendry RJR: Controlled trial of nifedipine in the treatment of Raynaud's phenomenon. *Lancet* 1982; ii:1299-1301.

178. Rodeheffer RJ, Rommer JA, Wigley F, et al: Controlled double-blind trial of nifedipine in the treatment of Raynaud's phenomenon. *New Engl J Med* 1983; 308:880-883.

179. Gjorup T, Kelbaek H, Hartling OJ, et al: Controlled double-blind trial of the clinical effect of nifedipine in the treatment of idiopathic Raynaud's phenomenon. *Am Heart J* 1986; 111:742-745.

180. Aldoori M, Campbell WB, Dieppe PA. Nifedipine in the treatment of Raynaud's syndrome. *Cardiovasc Res* 1986; 20:466-470.

181. Kahan A, Foult JM, Weber S. Nifedipine and α_1-adrenergic blockade in Raynaud's phenomenon. *Eur Heart J* 1985; 6:702-705.

182. Gush RJ, Taylor LJ, Jayson MIV. Acute effects of sublingual nifedipine in patients with Raynaud's phenomenon. *J Cardiovasc Pharmacol* 1987; 9:628-631.

183. Kahan A, Amor B, Menkes CJ. A randomized double-blind trial of diltiazem in the treatment of Raynaud's phenomenon. *Ann Rheum Dis* 1985; 44:30-33.

184. Vayssairat M, Captron L, Flessinger J-N, et al. Calcium channel blockers and Raynaud's disease. *Ann Intern Med* 1981; 95:243.

185. Smith CR, Rodeheffer RJ. Raynaud's phenomenon. Pathophysiologic features and treatment with calcium-channel blockers. *Am J Cardiol* 1985; 55:154B-157B.

186. Di Perri T, Pasini FL,Pecchi S, et al. Clinical pharmacology of calcium entry blockers. Peripheral circulation changes. In: Godfraind T, et al., eds. *Calcium Entry Blockers and Tissue Protection.* New York: Raven Press, 1985;203-214.

187. Towart R. The selective inhibition of serotonin-induced contractions of rabbit cerebral vascular smooth muscle by calcium antagonistic dihydropyridines. An investigation of the mechanism of action of nimodipine. *Circ Res* 1981; 48:650-657.

188. Allen GS, Ahn HS, Preziosi TJ, et al. Cerebral arterial spasm—a controlled trial of nimodipine in patients with subarachnoid hemorrhage. *N Engl J Med* 1983; 308: 619-624.

189. Auer LM. Acute operation and preventive nimodipine improve outcome in patients with ruptured cerebral aneurysms. *Neurosurgery* 1984; 15:57-66.

190. Gelmers HJ. The effects of nimodipine on the clinical course of patients with acute ischemic stroke. *Acta Neurol Scand* 1984; 69:232-239.

191. Solomon GD, Steel G, Spaccavento LJ. Verapamil prophylaxis of migraine. A double-blind, placebo-controlled study. *JAMA* 1983; 250:2500-2502.

192. Smith R, Schwartz A. Diltiazem prophylaxis in refractory migraine. *N Engl J Med* 1984; 310:1327-1328.

193. Paterna S, Campisi D, Montaina G, et al. The role of diltiazem in the prophylaxis of essential headaches (abstr). Presentation to NY Acad Sci, Feb 1987.

194. Kahan A, Weber S, Amor B, et al. Nifedipine in the treatment of migraine in patients with Raynaud's phenomenon. *N Engl J Med* 1983; 308:1102-1103.

195. Gelmers HJ. Nimodipine, a new calcium antagonist, in the prophylactic treatment of migraine. *Headache* 1983; 23:106-109.

196. Spierings ELH. Calcium entry blockers in the treatment of migraine. In: Godfraind T, et al., eds. *Calcium Entry Blockers and Tissue Protection.* New York: Raven Press, 1985;245-254.

197. Elmslander HP, Sauer E, Munteanu J, et al. The acute effect of nifedipine on airways resistance in patients with chronic obstuctive lung disease. In: Lichtlen PR, ed. *Sixth International Adalat Symposium.* Amsterdam: Excerpta Medica, 1986;497-503.

198. Townley RG, Cheng J, Bewtra AK. The role of calcium channel blockers in reactive airway disease. *Ann NY Acad Sci* 1988;522:732-746.

199. Raftery P, Varley JG, Edwards JS, et al. Inhibition of exercise-induced asthma by nifedipine: A dose-response study. *Br J Clin Pharmacol* 1987; 24:479-484.

200. Patel KR. Calcium antagonists in exercise-induced asthma. *Br Med J* 1981; 282:932-933.

201. Isshiki T, Amodeo C, Messerli FH, et al. Diltiazem maintains renal vasodilation without hyperfiltration in hypertension: Studies in essential hypertensive man and the spontaneously hypertensive rat. *Cardiovasc Drugs Ther* 1987; 1:359-366.

202. Harris DCH, Hammond WS, Burke TJ, et al. Verapamil protects against progression of experimental chronic renal failure. *Kidney Int* 1987; 31:41-46.

203. Garthoff B, Hirth C, Federmann A, et al. Renal effects of 1,4-dihydropyridines in animal models of hypertension and renal failure. *J Cardiovasc Pharmacol* 1987; 9(Suppl 1):S8-S13.

204. Lichtlen PR, Nellessen U, Rafflenbeul W, et al. International nifedipine trial on antiatherosclerotic therapy (INTACT). *Cardiovasc Drugs Ther* 1987; 1:71-79.

205. Sievers RE, Rashid T, Garrett J, et al. Verapamil and diet halt progression of atherosclerosis in cholesterol fed rabbits. *Cardiovasc Drugs Ther* 1987; 1:65-69.

206. Daugherty A, Rateri DL, Schonfeld G, et al. Inhibition of cholesteryl ester deposition in macrophages by calcium entry blockers: An effect dissociable from calcium entry blockade. *Br J Pharmacol* 1987; 91:113-118.

207. Nadler JL, Hsueh W, Horton R. Therapeutic effect of calcium channel blockade in primary aldosteronism. *J Clin Endocrinol Metab* 1985; 60:896-899.

208. Scriabine A, Anderson CL, Janis RA, et al. Some recent pharmacological findings with nitrendipine. *J Cardiovasc Pharmacol* 1984; 6(Suppl 7):S937-S943.

209. Opie LH, Singh BN. *Drugs for the Heart. III. Calcium Antagonists.* Orlando: Grune & Stratton, 1987;34-53.

210. Opie LH, Davey DA. Biological membranes in hypertension: Is control of intracellular calcium and other ions mediated by a membrane defect. *Ann NY Acad Sci* 1986; 488:154-173.

211. Ventura HO, Messerli FH, Ojgman W, et al. Immediate hemodynamic effects of a new calcium-channel blocking agent (nitrendipine) in essential hypertension. *Am J Cardiol* 1983; 51:783–786.

212. Leonetti G, Pasotti C, Ferrari GP, et al. Verapamil and propranolol: A comparison of two antihypertensive agents. *Acta Med Scand* 1984; Suppl 681:137–141.

213. McInnes GT, Findlay IN, Murray G, et al. Cardiovascular responses to verapamil and propranolol in hypertensive patients. *J Hypertens* 1985; 3(Suppl 3):S219–S221.

214. Hornung RS, Jones RI, Gould BA, et al. Twice-daily verapamil for hypertension: A comparison with propranolol. *Am J Cardiol* 1986; 57:93D–98D.

215. Muller FB, Bolli P, Erne P, et al. Calcium antagonism—a new concept for treating essential hypertension. *Am J Cardiol* 1986; 57:50D–53D.

216. Johnston DL, Lesoway R, Humen DP, et al. Clinical and hemodynamic evaluation of propranolol in combination with verapamil, nifedipine and diltiazem in exertional angina pectoris: A placebo-controlled, double-blind, randomized, crossover study. *Am J Cardiol* 1985; 55:680–687.

217. Kubo SH, Fox SC, Prida XE, et al. Combined hemodynamic effects of nifedipine and nitroglycerin in congestive heart failure. *Am Heart J* 1985; 110:1032–1034.

218. Fifer MA, Colucci WS, Lorell BH, et al. Inotropic, vascular, and neuroendocrine effects of nifedipine in heart failure: Comparison with nitroprusside. *J Am Coll Cardiol* 1985; 5:731–737.

219. Miller AB, Conetta DA, Bass TA. Sublingual nifedipine: Acute effects in severe chronic congestive heart failure secondary to idiopathic dilated cardiomyopathy. *Am J Cardiol* 1985; 55:1359–1362.

220. Elkayam U, Weber L, Torkan B, et al. Acute hemodynamic effect of oral nifedipine in severe congestive heart failure. *Am J Cardiol* 1983; 52:1041–1045.

221. Lefkowitz CA, Moe GW, Armstrong PW. A comparative evaluation of hemodynamic and neurohumoral effects of nitroglycerin and nifedipine in congestive heart failure. *Am J Cardiol* 1987; 59:59B–63B.

222. Marone C, Luisoli S, Bomio F, et al. Body sodium-blood volume state, aldosterone, and cardiovascular responsiveness after calcium entry blockade with nifedipine. *Kidney Int* 1985; 28:658–665.

223. Opie LH, Jennings AA. Sublingual captopril versus nifedipine in hypertensive crises (Letter). *Lancet* 1985;555.

224. Halperin AK, Gross KM, Rogers JF et al. Verapamil and propranolol in essential hypertension. *Clin Pharmacol Ther* 194; 36:750–758.

225. Stone PH. Calcium antagonists for Prinzmetal's variant angina, unstable angina and silent myocardial ischemia. Therapeutic tool and probe for identification of pathophysiologic mechanisms. *Am J Cardiol* 1983; 59: 101B–115B.

CALCIUM CHANNEL ANTAGONISTS: PART IV: SIDE EFFECTS AND CONTRAINDICATIONS DRUG INTERACTIONS AND COMBINATIONS

SUMMARY. With the correct selection of drug and patient, the calcium antagonists as a group can be remarkably effective at relatively low cost of serious side effects. Almost all side effects are dose related. Minor side effects include those caused by vasodilation (flushing and headaches), constipation (verapamil), and ankle edema. Serious side effects are rare and result from improper use of these agents, as when intravenous verapamil (or diltiazem) is given to patients with sinus or atrioventricular nodal depression from drugs or disease, or nifedipine to patients with aortic stenosis. The potential of a marked negative inotropic effect is usually offset by afterload reduction, especially in the case of nifedipine which actually has the most marked negative inotropic effect. Yet caution is required when even calcium antagonists, especially verapamil, are given to patients with myocardial failure unless caused by hypertensive heart disease. Drug interactions of calcium antagonists occur with other cardiovascular agents such as α-adrenergic blockers, β-adrenergic blockers, digoxin, quinidine, and disopyramide. The most marked interaction with digoxin is that with verapamil, which may raise digoxin levels by over 50%. Combination therapy of calcium antagonists with β-blockers is increasingly common, and is probably safest in the case of dihydropyridines. Other combinations being explored are those with angiotensin-converting enzyme inhibitors and diuretics.

Side Effects and Contraindications of Calcium Antagonists

Class Side Effects of Calcium Antagonists

All the three major calcium antagonists have a direct negative inotropic effect, as already discussed (Section 1) with nifedipine having the most powerful action (Table IV-1). In normal clinical practice, this myocardial effect is adequately offset by peripheral vasodilation and consequent reflex sympathetic activation. However, in the presence of severe myocardial failure, these negative inotropic effects could become dangerous (see Congestive Heart Failure Including Dilated Cardiomyopathy). In addition, all the agents have vasodilatory side effects such as flushing and ankle edema, the latter being caused by precapillary vasodilation and not by general salt and water retention [1]. Ankle edema is more likely to occur in patients with varicose veins or lower leg paresis [1].

193

Table IV-1. Comparative contraindications of β-adrenergic blocking agents, verapamil, nifedipine, and diltiazem

Contraindications	β-blockade	Verapamil	Nifedipine	Diltiazem
Absolute				
Sinus bradycardia	++	0/+	0	0/+
Sick sinus syndrome	++	+	0	+
AV conduction defects	+	++	0	++
Digitalis toxicity with AV block[a]	+	++	0	++
Asthma	+++	0	0	0
Bronchospasm	++	0	0	0
Heart failure	++	+	0	+
Hypotension	+	+	++	+
Coronary artery spasm	+	0	0	0
Raynaud's and active peripheral vascular disease	+	0	0	0
Severe mental depression	+	0	0	0
Severe aortic stenosis	+	+	++	+
Obstructive cardiomyopathy	0	0/+	++	0/+

Relative			
Adverse blood lipid profile	Care	0	0
Digitalis without toxicity	Care	Care	Care
β-blockade	0	Care	Care
Verapamil therapy	Care	0	Avoid
Quinidine therapy	Care	Care/avoid[b]	Care
Disopyramide therapy	Care	Care/avoid[b]	Care
Angina at rest (threatened myocardial infarction)	0	Query	0
		Hypotension	
		Hypotension	
		Care[c]	
		0	
		$++^d$	

From [12] by courtesy of Grune & Stratton.

Abbreviations: AV, atrioventricular.

[a]Contraindication to rapid intravenous administration.

[b]However, the combination can be effective in antiarrhythmic therapy.

[c]Nifedipine depresses blood quinidine levels with rebound upon nifedipine withdrawal.

[d]As monotherapy; may be used in combination with a β-blockade.

Verapamil Side Effects

Relatively *minor side effects* are those of vasodilation—headaches and dizziness, with occasional palpitations and hypotension [2]. Ankle edema may also result (Table IV-2). The side effect causing trouble, especially in elderly patients, is constipation. Straining at stool can in turn cause cardiovascular problems such as syncope. The incidence of constipation occurs in 25% to 40% of patients [2, 3]. With a higher mean dose (416 mg daily), constipation occurred in 10 of 16 patients, i.e., 63% [4]. The minor side effects of verapamil, apart from constipation, are somewhat less than those of nifedipine when both are used in doses equipotent for chronic stable angina [5] or hypertension [6].

Severe side effects with verapamil were initially stressed by reports of fatality when intravenous verapamil was abruptly given to isolated patients with pre-existing atrioventricular AV inhibition by disease or β-adrenergic blockade [7]. In addition to individual case reports of fatalities, largely resulting from asystole, there have been several "near-misses" [3]. The thrust of Fleckenstein's [8] original experiments in defining myocardial depression as a basic property of calcium channel antagonists led to the view that calcium channel antagonists must be negative inotropic agents. Logically, the combination of therapy by calcium channel antagonists and β-blockade was feared [9]. It is now becoming apparent that calcium channel antagonists, when correctly used, seldom induce a serious negative inotropic state [10]. Furthermore, careful patient selection has diminished the possibility of severe side effects. In the case of verapamil, sick sinus syndrome, pre-existing AV nodal disease, excess therapy with β-adrenergic blockade or digitalis or quinidine, and myocardial depression, are all still contraindications (Figure IV-1) especially in the intravenous therapy of supraventricular tachycardias [3, 11, 12]. In the rarer type of Wolff-Parkinson-White syndrome with anterograde (= antegrade) conduction through the bypass tract, the risk of verapamil is that atrial fibrillation can be too rapidly conducted to the ventricles with fear of ventricular fibrillation. Nonetheless, verapamil can be safely used in the vast majority of patients with supraventricular tachycardias and narrow QRS complexes.

In the average patient with angina pectoris, verapamil therapy is probably as safe as or safer than β-adrenergic blockade [3]. Two extreme reactions reported for β-blockade—fatal bronchospasm and gangrene—have thus far not been found with verapamil, nor can they be expected. Cardiovascular collapse, occasionally found in patients with bor-

Table IV-2. Some side effects of the three prototypical calcium antagonists

	Verapamil (%)	Nifedipine (%)	Diltiazem (%)
Facial flushing	6–7	6–25	0–3
Headaches	6	1–34	4–9
Tachycardia	0	low–25	0
Lightheadedness, dizziness	7	3–12	6–7
Constipation	34	0	4
Rash	0–3	Rare	Rare, can be severe
Ankle edema, swelling	6	1–8	6–10
Provocation of angina	0	low–14	0
Withdrawal rebound	Rare but possible	Rare but possible	Rare

Verapamil data from [2] and Subramanian et al. (1983) quoted in [3], [97], and [98].
Nifedipine data from [3], [15], [16], [99], and [100]. See also [101].
Diltiazem data from [35], [102], and [103]. See also [17], [36], [38], [39], and [102].
[a]Side effects are dose related; no strict comparisons exist except for nifedipine vs. diltiazem [17].

derline heart failure given β-adrenergic blockade, has also been found when intravenous verapamil is given in the presence of overt cardiomegaly [11].

Pharmacokinetic factors predisposing to verapamil toxicity include the delayed hepatic clearance in the elderly [3, 13], in renal impairment, and in hepatic disease [3].

Rare side effects include hepatotoxicity [14], occasional rashes, and transient mental confusion [3].

Nifedipine Side Effects

Minor side effects are dose dependent [2]. In the majority of patients without serious pre-existing myocardial disease, nifedipine has been given with only a few side effects (see Table IV-2) such as facial flushing, headaches, heat sensations, ankle edema, and exaggeration of varicose veins [15, 16]. However, with high-dose nifedipine (120 mg daily), 12 of 15 patients complained of side effects [17]. Muscle cramps [18] are among a number of unusual and probably rare side effects, several of which have been described in the unrefereed report section of the *British Medical Journal* in 1984 (excessive diuretic effect, complete heart block, periorbital edema) and in 1986 (generalized fixed drug eruption, photosensitivity, unilateral gynecomastia). Profound muscular weakness was found in 1 of 32 patients by Subramanian [2]. Sometimes light headedness or dizziness prevents continuation of nifedipine therapy. With high doses, side effects are more frequent [2]. Although the powerful hypotensive effect of nifedipine could have been expected to cause frequent tachycardia and orthostatic hypotension, such effects are usually absent [19]. Myocardial ischemia can be precipitated [20, 21] so that in the therapy of angina pectoris, dose titration of nifedipine is required. No instance of exaggeration or precipitation of cerebrovascular symptoms has yet been reported, possibly because nifedipine may also act as a cerebral vasodilator [22]. *Ankle swelling* is a local phenomenon, not well understood and possibly the result of a greater precapillary rather than venular dilation [1]. Nifedipine may also interfere with capillary autoregulation [1]. Although ankle swelling does not indicate edematous fluid retention [23], careful balanced studies have shown that nifedipine administration is accompanied by an overall sodium retention, presumably in the extravascular space [24]. If ankle swelling does occur, associated therapy with captopril is helpful [25]. *Slow-release nifedipine* tablets may reduce the incidence of vasodilating side effects of the ordinary nifedipine capsules, because the blood level of nifedipine rises more slowly. However, more strict comparisons between these preparations are required.

Serious side effects of nifedipine are rare, probably because clinical effects on the AV node are absent and the peripheral vasodilation prevents overt heart failure in patients with borderline failure. *Aortic stenosis and hypertrophic obstructive cardiomyopathy* are containdications to any vasodilator therapy (Figure IV-2). One patient with aortic stenosis [26] given nifedipine for acute pulmonary edema developed severe heart failure. Nifedipine has caused *excess hypotension or cardiovascular depression* only in a few seriously ill patients [9, 10]. One retrospective report suggests that nifedipine may induce *renal dysfunction* in elderly patients, possibly as a result of altered renal blood flow [27]. This case against nifedipine is not yet proven. Although occasional reports suggest a *diabetogenic effect* [28, 29], the effects on glucose tolerance are variable and controversial [3]. Sometimes glucose tolerance may actually improve [28]. When glucose tolerance does deteriorate, it may be the result of reflex sympathetic stimulation [28]. *Hypokalemia*, although found in one study when nifedipine was combined with a diuretic and β-blocker [30], could not be found in another study when a similar combination was made [31]. Perhaps the use of a relatively high dose of a thiazide diuretic (bendrofluazide 5 mg daily) combined with very high doses of nifedipine (up to 30 mg three times daily) caused hypokalemia in the study of Murphy et al. [30]. In general, hypokalemia is not frequently ascribed to nifedipine therapy [32](see also Part I, Metabolic Effects of Calcium Antagonists).

Diltiazem Side Effects

Subjective or relatively minor side effects. When diltiazem is given for angina, the incidence of side effects seems to be remarkably low [2]. In the United States, the package insert claims that side effects of oral therapy are similar to those of placebo, but lists nausea (3%), pedal edema (2%), headache (2%), and heart block (0.4%), and in two trials diltiazem for stable angina was "remarkably free of adverse effects" in doses of 240 mg daily [33] and all doses (up to 360 mg daily) were "extremely well tolerated" [34]. The true incidence of side effects will clearly depend on the severity of underlying myocardial or conduction system disease, the skill of the prescribing physician, and the dose of diltiazem.

Recent data suggest that high-dose diltiazem may cause troublesome side effects incuding edema and constipation (see Table IV-2). For example, in a comparative study with propranolol (both given for hypertension), diltiazem (up to 360 mg daily) caused edema in nearly 10%, asthenia in 7%, and impotence in 4%, whereas propranolol caused asthenia in 12%, bradycardia in 10%, and edema in 6% [35]. In another study, diltiazem failure in 5 of 12 patients treated for 20 weeks [36], 2 patients needed additional diuretic therapy. In another multicenter study, diltiazem for hypertension(usually 360 mg daily) caused a somewhat similar incidence of dizziness, edema, and headaches [37]. High dose diltiazem (360 mg daily) given in the therapy of coronary artery spasm, caused side effects in 5 of 15 patients, including a rash that required drug withdrawal [17].

Two other studies on high-dose diltiazem were on patients with atrial fibrillation. Diltiazem 360 mg daily given instead of digoxin caused side effects in 9 of 12 patients (75%) with atrial fibrillation; 11 of these patients had mitral valve disease [38]. The most common symptom was leg edema, accompanied in one patient by periorbital edema. Constipation was noted in three patients (25%). Only two patients developed severe headaches. In one patient, congestive heart failure occurred as the digoxin was replaced by diltiazem. Edema and constipation and other subjective side effects were reduced in all but one patient by decreasing the diltiazem dose to 240 mg daily. In the second study, diltiazem was added to digoxin with the production of side effects in 8 of 16 patients [39], 4 of whom were older than 70 years or receiving diltiazem 360 mg daily.

Double-blind comparisons of the incidence of side effects of high-dose diltiazem versus verapamil, both titrated against their efficacy in angina or hypertension, would be particularly instructive. (For side effects of diltiazem versus nifedipine, see Side Effects of Diltiazem Versus Nifedipine, and Diltiazem Combined with Nifedipine, below.)

Potentially serious nodal and myocardial side effects of diltiazem. Because experience with the intravenous form has been limited to carefully controlled studies, the type of serious negative chronotropic or inotropic side effect previously found with verapamil has not yet been reported. Furthermore, the general impression (supported by animal data; see Table I-6) is that diltiazem is less negatively inotropic than verapamil. However, few or no careful comparative clinical studies with these end points appear to exist. Even the oral drug can inhibit AV and/or sinus nodal tissue with AV dissociation and severe sinus bradycardia, as shown by the three patients with angina or coronary artery spasm reported by Ishikawa et al. [40]. Such side effects can especially be expected when the patients selected for diltiazem therapy have pre-existing sinus or AV nodal disease or when there is co-therapy with β-blockade or during digitalis toxicity [12]. With due care such side effects should therefore be rare. First-degree AV block can be expected in about one-fifth of patients with angina treated with diltiazem up to 360 mg daily [34].

Drug interactions predisposing to diltiazem side effects. Additive effects of β-blockade and diltiazem may predispose to bradycardia [41], AV conduction block, or even to congestive heart failure [42].

Metabolic effects of diltiazem. In the chronic therapy of hypertension, diltiazem caused only a small rise in triglycerides, considerably less than did propranolol [35].

Skin reactions with diltiazem. In the United Kingdom the annual report on side effects of new drugs noted in 1985 that there were some cases of serious skin reactions such as exfoliative dermatitis and epidermal necrolysis [43].

Hypotension. One case of unexpected hypotension has been reported following diltiazem [44]. However, insufficient details are provided in this abstract for any evaluation.

Side effects of diltiazem versus nifedipine. In a double-blind study on patients with coronary artery spasm [17], diltiazem 360 mg daily caused fewer side effects than did nifedipine 120 mg daily (5 of 15 patients complained about diltiazem vs. 12 of 15 for nifedipine, $p < 0.05$), although similar clinical benefit was achieved.

Q-T Interval Prolongation with Class B Calcium Antagonists

Such side effects have not been reported with the three prototypical calcium antagonists but only with *prenylamine, lidoflazine, and bepridil* which may all prolong the Q-T interval with potential for precipitation of atypical ventricular tachycardia [45]. Electrocardiograms should, therefore, be monitored during therapy with these agents. Serum potassium and magnesium also require monitoring. Diuretic therapy should be given with caution. Other drugs likely to prolong the Q-T interval such as sotalol, amiodarone, quinidine, disopyramide, and tricyclic antidepressants should not be used concomitantly. Bradycardia predisposes to Q-T interval lengthening, so that the combination of lidoflazine and propranolol should be avoided [46].

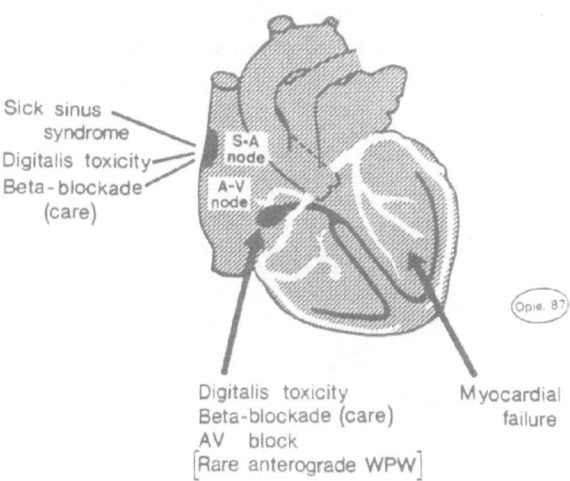

Fig. IV-1. Contraindications to verapamil and diltiazem. In patients already receiving a β-blocker, verapamil or diltiazem should seldom or never be given intravenously. Neither agent may be given to patients with digitalis toxicity. Successful combination during oral use of these agents is reported in atrial fibrillation, watching for excess effects. SA, sinoatrial; WPW, Wolff-Parkinson-White syndrome.

Contraindications to Calcium Antagonists

The contraindications to therapy with calcium channel antagonists are significantly fewer than in the case of β-adrenoceptor antagonists (see Table IV-1). For *verapamil* (Figure IV-1), the contraindications are sick sinus syndrome, overt AV disease or block, or myocardial failure, with caution in the presence of β-adrenoceptor blockade, quinidine, or disopyramide. Heart failure remains a contraindication to verapamil, even though this drug has been successfully given with care to such patients [47]. It should be emphasized that chronic asthma and bronchitis are not contraindications. In practice, two important relative contraindications in the elderly are constipation and pre-existing bradycardia or sick sinus syndrome.

For *nifedipine* (Figure IV-2), the major contraindications are severe aortic stenosis and hypertrophic obstructive cardiomyopathy. These are contraindications to any form of arteriolar vasodilation; acute vasodilation in the presence of aortic stenosis with left ventricular failure may be especially dangerous. There may be drug interactions of nifedipine with β-blockade and with α_1-adrenergic blockade (excess hypotension).

For *diltiazem,* the contraindictions are not clear; presumably depression of the sinus or AV node is a potential danger as in the case of verapamil (see Figure IV-1). There may be a greater risk of sinus bradycardia [41] and a lesser risk of a negative inotropic effect than with verapamil (see Table I-6).

In the Wolff-Parkinson-White syndrome, suspicion of anterograde conduction or detection thereof at elec-

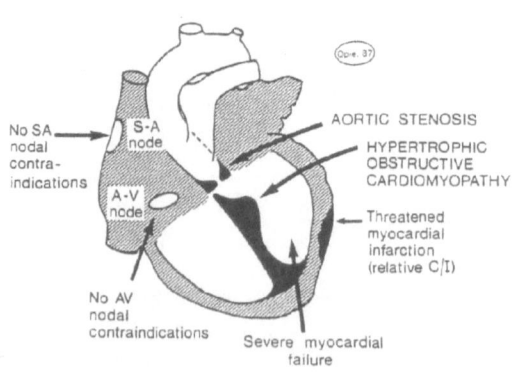

Fig. IV-2. Nifedipine contraindictations are chiefly obstructive lesions such as aortic stenosis or hypertropic obstructive cardiomyopathy. Unstable angina (threatened infarction) is a relative contraindication (C/I) to nifedipine unless caused by coronary spasm.

trophysiologic testing contraindicates the use of verapamil or diltiazem unless these agents have been carefully tested by electrophysiologic techniques.

The possible interactions of *combinations of calcium channel antagonists* have not been well studied; such combination therapy is theoretically possible because the nifedipine group of agents bind differently to the sarcolemma than do the verapamil and diltiazem groups (see discussion above).

Side Effects: Conclusions

All in all, bearing in mind the very powerful cardiovascular effects of the calcium channel antagonists, the spectrum and severity of side effects reported thus far is surprisingly reassuring and favorable, especially when compared with β-blockade [10]. Nevertheless, it remains appropriate to be very careful and vigilant in the use of all calcium channel antagonists and to be sure that they are used in the absence of contraindications and in the appropriate dose. Careful note should be made of all drug co-therapy, with extra care required when the pre-existing drugs are likely to cause hypotension or inhibition of the sinus or AV nodes (particularly in the case of verapamil and diltiazem).

Drug Interactions and Combinations

An overall review of drug interactions with calcium antagonists is given in Table IV-3, modified from Piepho et al. [48]. Most clinical interest has centered on the interaction and combination with β-adrenoceptor antagonists and with digoxin, but there are several other interactions of clinical significance.

Interaction and Combination of Calcium Antagonists with α_1-adrenoceptor Antagonists

Nifedipine sometimes interacts with prazosin so that excess hypotension develops (Figure IV-3); hence nifedipine or prazosin should both be added cautiously and in low dose to the therapy of patients already receiving the other agent [49]. An additive therapeutic benefit of prazosin pretreatment (2 mg) to the hypotensive effect of nifedipine has been reported [50]. *Verapamil* has also been used combined with prazosin in hypertension, with added and possibly synergistic effects [51]; the latter may be partially explained by pharmacokinetic interactions [52]. *Diltiazem* has also been combined with α_1-adrenergic blockade by alfuzosine [53].

Table IV-3. Side effects of nisoldipine compared with placebo and hydrochlorothiazide-amiloride in a double-blinded randomized study on patients with mild to moderate hypertension—number of side effects per visit[a]

Side Effect	Placebo $(N = 32)$	Nisoldipine $(N = 32)$	Hydro-chloro-thiazide $(N = 32)$	Combina-nation $(N = 9)$
Headache	7.3	12.5*	8.5	4
Flushing	3.5	9.0^b	3.0	1
Swollen ankles	2.8	6.5^b	2.0	0
Tiredness	3.0	2.0	2.0	0
Dizziness	1.0	1.5	2.5	0
Palpitations	3.0	1.0	1.0	0
CNS (irritability)	1.3	2.5	4.0^b	0
Constipation/ nausea	1.2	0.5	1.5	0
Breathlessness	0.5	1.5	0.5	0
Cold extremities	0.2	2.5	0	0
Total	24	40	25	5

From [94] by courtesy of *American Journal of Cardiology.*
Abbreviations: CNS, central nervous system.
[a]Incidence of patients with side effects of population sample of 32 patients, with 9 studied in combination phase.
[b]Significant only with Student's paired t-test.
*$p < 0.05$ vs. placebo, hydrochlorothiazide-amiloride using analysis of variance.

Interaction and Combination of Calcium Antagonists with β-adrenoceptor Antagonists

Because of the different hemodynamic and electrophysiologic properties of the three prototypical agents, each combines with β-blockade to give different potential end-results (see Figure III-13).

Verapamil. Special care is required when verapamil is acutely added by intravenous injection in the presence of pre-existing β-adrenergic blockade [54]. Also in patients with angina pectoris already receiving propranolol or metoprolol, intravenous [55] or oral verapamil [56] can reduce contractility [56], increase heart size [57], and cause symptomatic sinus bradycardia [58]. Depending on the dose, the combination may be well tolerated [57] or not tolerated [41]. Johnston et al. [57] showed that propranolol-verapamil versus propranolol-diltiazem versus propranolol-nifedipine are all about equally effective in patients with angina pectoris, but propranolol-verapamil depressed left ventricular function most (as expected). An unexpected interaction has been shown between verapamil and metoprolol, verapamil raising the blood level of metoprolol but not of atenolol, probably because of the hepatic metabolism of metoprolol, whereas atenolol is a strictly hydrophilic agent [59].

Nifedipine. Potentially the indirect positive inotropic effect of nifedipine, acting via afterload reduction, is capable of offsetting the negative effects of β-adrenoceptor blockade [57, 60]. Theoretically this should not be so, because β-adrenoceptor blockade would inhibit the reflex β-adrenergic sympathetic stimulation. An alternate explanation is that nifedipine may be considerably more powerful than verapamil or diltiazem in decreasing vagal tone [61], although the experimental data are in conflict [62]. Even among various dihydropyridines, an equal degree of hypotension does not elicit the same "reflex" tachycardia so that other ill-understood factors must be at work [62]. The combination of nifedipine and β-blockade is relatively safe because of 1) the complementary qualities of these agents [19, 63, 64]; and 2) the relatively few contraindications to nifedipine. Sometimes combined nifedipine and propranolol therapy can lead to hypotensive symptoms [57]. Some hypotensive interactions between nifedipine and β-adrenoceptor blockers have also been documented in some patients with either excess hypotension [9] or severe heart failure [65] as a result. Furthermore, the potential direct inhibitory effect of nifedipine on the sinus and AV nodes may become apparent when

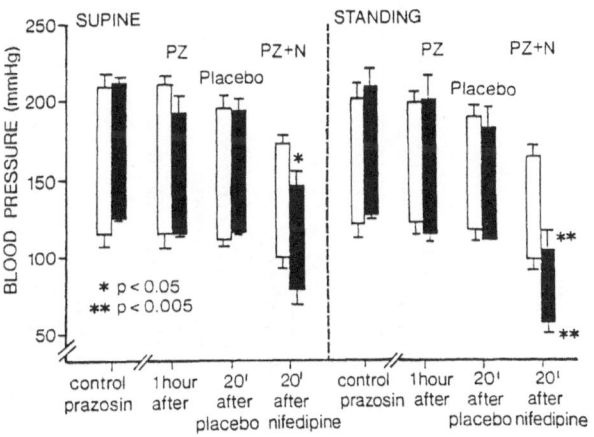

Fig. IV-3. *Evidence for excessive hypotensive interaction between prazosin and nifedipine in one of eight patients. In other patients, note added beneficial hypotensive effect. Mean (SEM) blood pressures in eight patients (open columns) receiving prazosin (P) 5 mg and nifedipine (N) 10 mg compared with results of repeated challenge with 10 mg nifedipine after 5 mg prazosin in one patient (solid columns) with severe hypertension who was already receiving long-term prazosin therapy. Note the postural hypotension caused by additive therapy in the one patient who was sensitive. For beneficial therapeutic combination of prazosin and nifedipine, see Sluiter et al. [50]. Reproduced from [49] by courtesy of the* British Medical Journal.

Table IV-4. Comparative effects of combinations of various calcium antagonists with propranolol (propranolol combined with verapamil, nifedipine, or diltiazem) in a double-blind randomized study on 19 patients with effort angina

	Placebo	Propranolol 160 mg Daily	Propranolol-Verapamil 300 mg Daily	Propranolol-Nifedipine 60 mg Daily	Propranolol-Diltiazem 240 mg Daily
Subjective data					
Angina attacks per week	10	6	3*	4*	3*
Chest pain during exercise test	13/19	No data	4/19	2/19	5/19
Patient preference	No data	2/19	3/19	5/19	7/19
Adverse effects	5	8	20	14	7
Most common side effects	Various	Dreams	Constipation Dyspnea	Dizziness Leg edema	Fatigue Constipation
Objective data					
P-R interval (sec)	0.16	0.17	0.19	0.17	0.19**
Exercise heart rate (beats/min)	107	93**	88**	92**	86*
Exercise ST segment depression (to nearest mm)	1.8	1.5	1.3*	1.1**	1.3*

Exercise systolic blood pressure (mmHg)	154	148	144**	138**	137**
Exercise rate-pressure product (mmH $\times$ 10^3)	164	137*	127**	127**	117**
Exercise cardiac index (L/m^2)	6.7	6.0**	5.8**	6.4*	6.1**
End-diastolic volume (to nearest 5 ml/m^2)					
Rest	90	90	100*	90	100*
Exercise	105	115	120*	115	120*
LV segmental function (%)					
Rest	59	71*	68*	70*	70*
Exercise	52	59	62	65**	62
Increase in systolic volume^a (to nearest 5%)	30	25	15*	15*	15*

Data from [57] by courtesy of the *American Journal of Cardiology*.
Abbreviations: LV, left ventricular.
^{a}The consequence of exercise-induced angina.
*p < 0.05 vs. placebo.
**p < 0.001 vs. placebo.

nifedipine and propranolol are given together in high doses to anesthetized dogs[66].

There is a complex hepatic *pharmacokinetic interaction* between nifedipine and propranol which may lead to additive effects on blood pressure control [67]. Thus, it is simpler to combine nifedipine with atenolol which undergoes no first-pass liver metabolism and does not alter nifedipine kinetics [68].

Diltiazem. The addition of diltiazem to propranolol may cause excess bradycardia or hypotension [41], however, the combination is better tolerated from the subjective point of view than propranolol-nifedipine [57]. Besides additive effects on nodal tissue and additive negative inotropic effects, diltiazem can displace propranolol from plasma binding sites thereby elevating free propranolol levels [69]. When propranolol is ineffective in patients with coronary artery spasm, then the combination of diltiazem-propranolol becomes effective although without any advantage over diltiazem alone [70].

Comparison of verapamil or nifedipine or diltiazem, each combined with a β-blocker. Only one study (Table IV-5) compares these three drugs in a double-blind randomized pattern in combination with propranolol and in comparison with placebo (see Table IV-5). The combination propranolol-diltiazem (160 to 240 mg, respectively) caused less symptomatic side effects than the combination propranolol-verapamil (160 to 360 mg, respectively) while having approximately equal therapeutic efficacy, whereas propranolol-nifedipine was somewhat in between [57]. Although the authors recommend the combination propranolol-diltiazem provided that there are no conduction problems, there would still appear to be substantial arguments favoring the combination propranolol-nifedipine: 1) the major subjective side effect with propranolol-nifedipine was orthostatic hypotension which should presumably have been avoided by blood pressure measurements in the erect position and a subsequent reduction in the nifedipine dose to say 10 mg three times daily (30 mg total); 2) objectively, propranolol-nifedipine gave the "best values" for P-R interval, ST segment depression, exercise cardiac index, end-diastolic volume, and left ventricular segmental function when compared with propranolol-verapamil or propranolol-diltiazem (see Table IV-1). None of these differences among the combinations appears to be statistically significant (exact statistics are not given by the authors), yet the trend is in every case for the combination propranolol-nifedipine to benefit most. A justifiable conclusion is that from the hemodynamic point of view propranolol-nifedipine is marginally better than the combinations and should be the first choice if tolerated (watching for orthostatic hypotension). Propranolol-diltiazem is hemodynamically similar to propranolol-verapamil, yet subjectively much better (see Table IV-1).

New dihydropyridines plus β-blockers. Intravenous *nicardipine* (5 mg) given to patients with coronary artery disease without heart failure, already receiving large doses of propranolol, decreased the systemic vascular resistance and increased cardiac output [71]. Hence nicardipine counteracted the adverse hemodynamic effects of propranolol.

When *felodipine* plus atenolol was given to patients with coronary artery disease and no heart failure, the systemic vascular resistance fell, the cardiac index rose, but there was no negatively inotropic effect as assessed by first derivative of left ventricular pressure (dP/dt) [72].

Nisoldipine with propranolol has been studied in pigs [73]. Myocardial blood flow, reduced by propranolol, may be reversed to normal by high-dose intravenous nisoldipine (1.0 µg/kg/min). However, the relatively depressed endocardial blood flow did not increase (the endocardial/epicardial ratio was unchanged).

Diltiazem combined with nifedipine. Theoretically, because of the different binding sites and the different modes of action, these agents should be useful in combination, especially because diltiazem may enhance nifedipine binding to its site (see Figure I-1). However, a recent open-label study [17] suggests that the combination of both in high doses (diltiazem 360 mg plus nifedipine 120 mg daily) is likely to cause significant side effects in almost all patients even though some added subjective benefit is obtained in the therapy of coronary spasm. In three of nine patients tested by Prida et al. [17], dizziness during combination diltiazem-nifedipine therapy was severe enough to cause drug withdrawal. In a small open series [74], nifedipine plus diltiazem appears to be effective in all patients with vasospastic variant angina; however, this possible added benefit of the nifedipine-diltiazem combination has not been subject to rigorous testing. In lower doses (diltiazem 120 mg plus nifedipine 40 to 120 mg daily) the combination improved effort tolerance while plasma nifedipine rose as a result of a drug interaction [75]. There appears to be considerable scope for evaluating diltiazem in combination with nifedipine in hypertension.

Table IV-5. Clinical significance of reported drug interactions with calcium-entry blockers

Drug	Verapamil	Nifedipine	Diltiazem
Cardiac glycosides			
Digoxin	3(+)	1(+)	1(+)
Digitoxin	2(+)	0	0
β-adrenergic blockers	2(+)	1(+)	2(+)
α-adrenergic blockers	2(+)	3(+)	NA
Antiarrhythmic drugs			
Quinidine	2(+)	1(−)	1(+)
Disopyramide	3(+)	0	1(+)
Nitrates	0/1(+)	1(+)	0/1(+)
H_2-receptor antagonists			
Cimetidine	3(+)	3(+)	3(+)
Ranitidine	0	0	0
Anticonvulsants			
Phenobarbital	3(−)	0	NA
Phenytoin	NA	2(+)	NA
Carbamazepine	3(+)	NA	NA
Lithium carbonate	NA	NA	2(+)
General anesthetics			
Halothane	3(+)	3(+)	NA
Isoflurane	3(+)	NA	NA
Cytostatic agents	3(−)	NA	NA
Theophylline	1(+)	NA	NA
Enzyme inducers			
Rifampin	3(−)	NA	NA
Sulfinpyrazone	3(−)	NA	NA
Social drugs			
Cigarettes	3(−)	3(−)	3(−)
Ethanol	NA	1(+)	NA

Adapted from [48] by courtesy of the American Heart Association. The following changes have been made: 1) α-blocker–verapamil interaction added according to the section Drug Interactions and Combinations; 2) antiarrhythmic drugs specified according to Table IV-1 and degree of interaction reduced; 3) significance of nifedipine–β-blocker and digoxin-diltiazem interaction downgraded.

Abbreviations: −, decreased effect of either drug; +, enhanced effect of either drug; 4, relative contraindications; 3, significant interaction—commonly observed; 2, significant interaction—only seen in a limited number of cases; 1, reported interaction—questionable clinical significance; 0, no contraindications; NA, no data available on specific interaction.

Interaction and Combination of Calcium Antagonists with Digoxin

Verapamil may interact with digitalis. The mechanism is not fully known but may include decreased renal and extrarenal clearance of digoxin thereby increasing blood digoxin levels [76] by up to 60% to 90% [77]. An advantage of nifedipine and diltiazem is that such major interactions with digoxin have not yet been established [78, 79], although relatively small increases have also been reported [80, 81]. In some studies there is no interactive effect of diltiazem with digoxin (e.g., Roth et al. [38]). In the case of nifedipine and nitrendipine, blood digoxin levels may increase by

20% [82] and in the case of nisoldipine, greater increases up to doubling have been reported [83]. Of interest is the possibility of combination digoxin-nifedipine therapy for congestive heart failure, with nifedipine reducing systematic and pulmonary vascular resistance values when given after digoxin [84]. Afterload reduction by nifedipine could be of special benefit in patients with mitral or aortic regurgitation. However, the long-term benefit of such combined nifedipine-digoxin therapy remains to be established.

Interaction and Combination of Calcium with Antiarrhythmic Agents

Quinidine. Verapamil may adversely interact with quinidine, presumably due to the combined effect on peripheral α-receptors causing hypotension [85]. Nevertheless verapamil-quinidine may be used with care in the therapy of some reentrant supraventricular arrythmias. The negative inotropic potential of verapamil should also give rise to concern when combined with disopyramide although such an adverse interaction has not yet been reported.

Verapamil plus disopyramide. In dogs given intravenous verapamil and disopyramide, there was intense sinus node depression, leading to concern that this interaction may be harmful in patients [86].

Verapamil plus carbamazepine. Verapamil 360 mg daily added to carbamazepine, an agent used in the therapy of epilepsy, caused blood concentrations of the latter to rise with side effects of excess carbamazepine (diplopia, headache, dizziness)[87]. Therefore the dose of carbamazepine should be halved when verapamil is added. Diltiazem may likewise interact.

Combination of Calcium Antagonists with Nitrates

Calcium channel antagonists are freely combined with nitrates in the therapy of angina pectoris. Sometimes additive therapy leads to syncope or tachycardia (depending on the calcium channel antagonist).

Because calcium channel antagonists are as effective as isosorbide dinitrate in the therapy of patients with angina already receiving propranolol [88], and because of the problems with nitrate tolerance recently raised, the combination of calcium channel antagonist-β-blocker is being increasingly used.

A question frequently asked is whether "maximal" therapy combination calcium channel antagonist, β-

blocker, and nitrates is necessarily the best for angina. One study says "no," probably because of the problem of hypotension [89]. In another study, nifedipine 80 to 120 mg was added to patients already receiving both β-blockers and nitrates [90]. Ventricular filling improved as did the duration of exercise in patients given nifedipine. However, it should be noted that only the study of Tolins et al. [89] was double-blinded and randomized.

Combination of Calcium Antagonists with ACE Inhibitors

Angiotensin-converting enzyme inhibitors (ACE inhibitors) are being used increasingly as antihypertensive agents. Theoretically, they could be expected to act better in high-renin hypertension, whereas calcium channel antagonists might be expected to act better in low-renin hypertension. In severe hypertension, the combination of nifedipine (10 mg four times daily) and captopril (25 mg four times daily) gave better blood pressure control than either agent singly [25]. However, the observers were unblinded and each study period was only 7 days. In another unblinded study, not placebo-controlled, nifedipine tablets 20 mg twice daily and captopril 25 mg three times daily had an additive hypotensive effect, wearing off 12 hours after the tablets were given [91]. In a third open-label study, enalapril (mean daily dose about 30 mg) was added to verapamil (slow-release, mean daily dose 460 mg) again with additive hypotensive effects [92]. Further blinded and controlled assessment of the efficacy of the combination is required.

Combination of Calcium Antagonists with Diuretics

A logical combination in the therapy of hypertension would be diuretics plus calcium antagonists, because diuretics activate the renin-angiotensin system, whereas calcium antagonists vasodilate without causing prominent renin-angiotensin activation which is only a temporary phenomenon with nifedipine and hardly found with the other primary agents. Yet the mild diuretic effect of calcium antagonists has led to the supposition that the addition of diuretics may be less effective than anticipated [93], especially in the case of nifedipine. This concept needs further testing. Nonetheless we found that the combination nisoldipine-diuretics [94] was highly effective in the treatment of mild to moderate hypertension and more so than nisoldipine monotherapy. Likewise, the combination diltiazem-diuretic is more effective than diltiazem alone in the therapy of hypertension [35].

Interaction with H_2-receptor Antagonists

Cimetidine inhibits the liver enzymes that mediate drug metabolism, and not unexpectedly it decreases the rate of nifedipine elimination, so that the area under the curve increases and there are increased blood nifedipine levels during chronic dosing [95]. Furthermore, nifedipine is more antihypertensive in the presence of cimetidine co-therapy [96]. Ranitidine has no such kinetic effects [95]. Therefore, in general, ranitidine rather than cimetidine should be the H_2-blocker of choice during co-therapy with all calcium antagonists because they are all metabolized in the liver.

References

1. Gustafsson D. Microvascular mechanisms involved in calcium antagonist edema formation. *J Cardiovasc Pharmacol* 1987; 10(Suppl 1):S121–S131.
2. Subramanian VB. *Calcium Antagonists in Chronic Stable Angina Pectoris.* Amsterdam: Excerpta Medica, 1983;97–116, 152–156, 217–229.
3. Lewis JG. Adverse reactions to calcium antagonists. *Drugs* 1983; 25:196–222.
4. Pepine CJ, Feldman RL, Hill JA, et al. Clinical outcome after treatment of rest angina with calcium blockers: Comparative experience during the initial year of therapy with diltiazem, nifedipine, and verapamil. *Am Heart J* 1983; 106:1341–1347.
5. Dawson JR, Whitaker NHG, Sutton GC. Calcium antagonists in chronic stable angina. Comparison of verapamil and nifedipine. *Br Heart J* 1981; 46:508–512.
6. Midtbo K, Hals O, van der Meer J. Verpamil compared with nifedipine in the treatment of essential hypertension. *J Cardiovasc Pharmacol* 1982; 4(Suppl 3):363–368.
7. Sacks H, Kennelly BM. Verapamil in cardiac arrhythmias (letter). *Br Med J* 1972; 2:716.
8. Fleckenstein A. Specific inhibitors and promoters of calcium action in the excitation-contraction coupling of heart muscle and their role in the prevention or production of myocardial lesions. In: Harris P, Opie LH, eds. *Calcium and the Heart.* London: Academic Press, 1971;135–188.
9. Opie LH, White DA. Adverse interaction between nifedipine and beta-blockade. *Br Med J* 1980; 281:1462–1464.
10. Hugenholtz P, Verdouw PD, de Jong JW, et al. Nifedipine for angina and acute myocardial ischemia. In: Opie LH, ed. *Calcium Antagonists and Cardiovascular Disease.* New York: Raven Press, 1984;237–255.
11. Opie LH. *Drugs and the Heart.* London: Lancet, 1980;27–38.
12. Opie LH, Singh BN. Calcium channel antagonists (slow channel blockers). In: Opie LH, ed. *Drugs for the Heart Second Expanded Edition.* Orlando, Florida: Grune & Stratton, 1987;34–53
13. Norris RJ, Brooks SG. Pharmacokinetics of a sustained release formulation of verapamil in young and elderly adults. In: Raftery EB, ed. *Verapamil SR. Once-daily Calcium Blockade in Angina and Hypertension.* Langhorne: ADIS Press International, 1987;38–46.
14. Brodsky SJ, Cutler SS, Weiner DA, et al. Hepatotoxicity

due to treatment with verapamil. *Ann Intern Med* 1981; 94:490–491.

15. Terry RW. Nifedipine therapy in angina pectoris: Evaluation of safety and side effects. *Am Heart J* 1982; 104:681–689.

16. Leisten L, Kuhlmann J, Ebner F. Side effects and pharmacodynamic interactions. In: Krebs R, ed. *Treatment of Cardiovascular Diseases by Adalat^R (Nifedipine).* Stuttgart-New York: Schattauer, 1986;270–314.

17. Prida XE, Gelman JS, Feldman RL, et al. Comparison of diltiazem and nifedipine alone and in combination in patients with coronary artery spasm. *J Am Coll Cardiol* 1987; 9:412–419.

18. MacDonald JB. Muscle cramps during treatment with nifedipine (Letter). *Br Med J* 1982; 285:1744.

19. Jee LD, Opie LH. Nifedipine for hypertension and angina pectoris: Interactions during combination therapy. In: Opie LH, ed. *Calcium Antagonists and Cardiovascular Disease.* New York: Raven Press, 1984;339–346.

20. Jariwalla AG, Anderson EG. Production of ischaemic cardiac pain by nifedipine. *Br Med J* 1978; 1:1181–1182.

21. Sia STB, MacDonald PS, Triester B, et al. Aggravation of myocardial ischaemia by nifedipine. *Med J Aust* 1985; 142:48–50.

22. Bertel O, Conen D, Radu EW, et al. Nifedipine in hypertensive emergencies. *Br Med J* 1983; 286:19–21.

23. Opie LH. Fluid retention with nifedipine in antihypertensive therapy. *Lancet* 1986; ii:1456.

24. Marone C, Luisoli S, Bomio F, et al. Body sodium-blood volume state, aldosterone, and cardiovascular responsiveness after calcium entry blockade with nifedipine. *Kidney Int* 1985; 28:658–665.

25. Guazzi MD, De Cesare N, Galli C, et al. Calcium-channel blockade with nifedipine and angiotensin converting-enzyme inhibition with captopril in the therapy of patients with severe primary hypertension. *Hypertension* 1984; 70:279–284.

26. Gillmer DJ, Kark P: Pulmonary oedema precipitated by nifedipine. *Br Med J* 1980; 280:1420–1421.

27. Diamond JR, Cheung JY, Fang LST. Nifedipine-induced renal dysfunction. Alterations in renal hemodynamics. *Am J Med* 1984; 77:905–909.

28. Krebs R. Adverse reactions with calcium antagonists. *Hypertension* 1983; 5(Suppl II):II-125–II-129.

29. Bhatnager SK, Amin MMA, Al-Yusuf AR. Diabetogenic effects of nifedipine. *Br Med J* 1984; 289:19.

30. Murphy MB, Scriven AJI, Dollery CT. Role of nifedipine in treatment of hypertension. *Br Med J* 1983; 287:257–259.

31. Myers MG, Leenen FHH, Burns R, et al. Nifedipine tablet vs hydralazine in patients with persisting hypertension who receive combined diuretic and beta-blocker therapy. *Clin Pharmacol Ther* 1986; 39:409–413.

32. Sowers JR, Mohanty PK. Comparison of calcium-entry blockers and diuretics in the treatment of hypertensive patients. *Circulation* 75 (Suppl V):V170–V173.

33. Hossack KF, Pool PE, Steele P, et al. Efficacy of diltiazem in angina of effort: A multicenter trial. *Am J Cardiol* 1982; 49:567–572.

34. Lindenberg BS, Weiner DA, McCabe CH, et al. Efficacy and safety of incremental doses of diltiazem for the treatment of stable angina pectoris. *J Am Coll Cardiol* 1983; 2:1129–1133.

35. Moser M. Calcium entry blockers for systematic hypertension. *Am J Cardiol* 1987; 59:15A–121A.

36. Petru MA, Crawford MH, Sorenson SG, et al. Short- and long-term efficacy of high-dose oral diltiazem for angina due to coronary artery disease: A placebo-controlled, randomized, double-blind crossover study. *Circulation* 1983; 68:139-147.

37. Pool PE, Massie BM, Venkararaman K, et al. Diltiazem as monotherapy for systemic hypertension: A multicenter, randomized, placebo-controlled trial. *Am J Cardiol* 1986; 57:212-217.

38. Roth A, Harrison E, Mitani G, et al. Efficacy and safety of medium- and high-dose diltiazem alone and in combination with digoxin for control of heart rate at rest and during exercise in patients with chronic atrial fibrillation. *Circulation* 1986; 73:316-324.

39. Steinberg JS, Katz RJ, Bren GB, et al. Efficacy of oral diltiazem to control ventricular response in chronic atrial fibrillation at rest and during exercise. *J Am Coll Cardiol* 1987; 9:405-411.

40. Ishikawa T, Imamura T, Koiwaya Y, et al. Atrioventricular dissociation and sinus arrest induced by oral diltiazem. *New Engl J Med* 1983; 309:1124-1125.

41. Hung J, Lamb IH, Connolly SJ, et al. The effect of diltiazem and propranolol, alone and in combination, on exercise performance and left ventricular function in patients with stable effort angina: A double-blind, randomized, and placebo controlled study. *Circulation* 1983; 68:560-567.

42. Strauss WE, Egan T, McIntyre KM, et al. Combination therapy with diltiazem and propranolol: Precipitation of congestive heart failure. *Clin Cardiol* 1985; 8:363-366.

43. CMS Update. Annual review of yellow cards—1985. *Br Med J* 1986; 293:688.

44. Bardet J, Baudet M, Rigaud M, et al. Diltiazem, a new calcium antagonist, versus propranolol in treatment of spontaneous angina pectoris (abstr). *Am J Cardiol* 1979; 43:416.

45. Krikler DM, Curry VL. Torsade de pointes, an atypical ventricular tachycardia. *Br Heart J* 1976; 38:117-120.

46. Hanley SP, Hampton JR: Ventricular arrhythmias associated with lidoflazine: side-effects observed in a randomized trial. *Eur Heart J* 1983; 4:889-893.

47. Ferlinz J, Citron PD. Hemodynamics and myocardial performance characteristics after verapamil use in congestive heart failure. *Am J Cardiol* 1983; 51:1339-1345.

48. Piepho RW, Culbertson VL, Rhodes RS. Drug interactions with the calcium-entry blockers. *Circulation* 1987: 75(Suppl V):V-181-V-194.

49. Jee LD, Opie LH. Acute hypotensive response to nifedipine added to prazosin in treatment of hypertension. *Br Med J* 1983; 287:1514-1516.

50. Sluiter HE, Huysmans F Th M, Thien Th A, et al. The influence of alpha$_1$-adrenergic blockade on the acute antihypertensive effect of nifedipine. *Eur J Clin Pharmacol* 1985; 29:263-267.

51. Elliott HL, Pasanisi F, Meredith PA, et al. Acute hypotensive response to nifedipine added to prazosin. *Br Med J* 1984; 288:238.

52. Pasanisi F, Elliot HL, Meredith PA, et al. Combined alpha-adrenoceptor antagonism and calcium channel blockade in normal subjects. *Clin Pharmacol Ther* 1984; 36:716-723.

53. Menasche S, Elkik F, Cocco G, et al. Synergistic antihypertensive effect of diltiazem combined with the alpha-adrenoceptor blocker alfuzosine (abstr). Presentation to NY Acad Sci, Feb 1987.

54. Urthaler F, James TN. Experimental studies on the

pathogenesis of asystole after verapamil in the dog. *Am J Cardiol* 1979; 44:651–656.

55. Kieval J, Kirstein EB, Kessler KM, et al. The effects of intravenous verapamil on hemodynamic status of patients with coronary artery disease receiving propranolol. *Circulation* 1982; 65:653–659.

56. Packer M, Meller J, Medina N, et al. Hemodynamic consequences of combined beta-adrenergic and slow calcium channel blockade in man. *Circulation* 1982; 65:660–668.

57. Johnston DL, Lesoway R, Humen DP, et al. Clinical and hemodynamic evaluation of propranolol in combination with verapamil, nifedipine and diltiazem in extertional angina pectoris: A placebo-controlled, double-blind, randomized, crossover study. *Am J Cardiol* 1985; 55:680–687.

58. Winniford MD, Fulton KL, Corbett JR. et al. Propranolol-verapamil versus propranolol-nifedipine in severe angina pectoris of effort: A randomized, double-blind crossover study. *Am J Cardiol* 1985; 55:281–285.

59. McLean AJ, Knight R, Harrison PM, et al. Clearance based oral drug interaction between verapamil and metoprolol and comparison with atenolol. *Am J Cardiol* 1985; 55:1628–1629.

60. Pfisterer M, Muller-Brand J, Burkart F. Combined acebutolol/nifedipine therapy in patients with chronic coronary artery disease: Additional improvement of ischemia-induced left ventricular dysfunction. *Am J Cardiol* 1982; 49:1259–1266.

61. Millard RW, Lathrop DA, Grupp G, et al. Differential cardiovascular effects of calcium channel blocking agents: Potential mechanisms. *Am J Cardiol* 1982; 49:449–506.

62. Warltier DC, Zyvolski MG, Gross GJ, et al. Comparative actions of dihydropyridine slow channel calcium blocking agents in conscious dogs: systemic and coronary hemodynamics with and without combined beta adrenergic blockade. *J Pharmacol Exp Ther* 1984; 230:367–375.

63. Lynch P, Dargie H, Krikler S, et al. Objective assessment of antianginal and their combination. *Br Med J* 1980; 281:184–187.

64. Opie LH, Jee L, White D. Antihypertensive effects of nifedipine combined with cardioselective beta-adrenergic receptor antagonism by atenolol. *Am Heart J* 1982; 104:606–612.

65. Brooks N, Cattell M, Pidgeon J, et al. Unpredictable response to nifedipine in severe cardiac failure (letter). *Br Med J* 1980; 281:1324.

66. Hamann SR, Kaltenborn KE, McAllister RG. Nifedipine-propranolol interaction: Dependence of cardiovascular effects on plasma drug concentrations. *J Cardiovasc Pharmacol* 1987; 10:182–189.

67. Kleinbloesem CH, van Brummelen P, Sandberg THW, et al. Kinetic and haemodynamic interactions between nifedipine and propranolol in healthy subjects utilizing controlled rates of drug input. In: Kleinbloesem CH, ed. *Nifedipine: Clinical Pharmacokinetics and Haemodynamic Effects.* 's-Gravenhage: Drukkerij JH Pasmans BV, 1985; 151–165.

68. Rosenkranz B, Ledermann H, Frolich JC. Interaction between nifedipine atenolol: pharmacokinetics and pharmacodynamics in normotensive volunteers. *J Cardiovasc Pharmacol* 1986; 8:943–949.

69. Chaffman M, Brogden RN: Diltiazem: A review of its pharmacological properties and therapeutic efficacy. *Drugs* 1985; 29:387–454.

70. Tilmant PY, Lablanche JM, Thieuleux FA, et al. Detrimental effect of propranolol in patients with coronary arterial spasm countered by combination with diltiazem. *Am J Cardiol* 1983; 52:230-233.

71. Rocha P, Zannier D, Baron B, et al. Acute hemodynamic effects of intravenous nicardipine in patients treated chronically with propranolol for coronary artery disease. *Am J Cardiol* 1987; 59:775-781.

72. Culling W, Ruttley MSM, Sheridan DJ. Acute haemodynamic effects of delodipine during beta-blockade in patients with coronary artery disease. *Br Heart J* 1984; 52:431-434.

73. Duncker DJ, Hartog JM, Hugenholtz PG, et al. The effects of nisoldipine (Bay K 5552) on cardiovascular performance and regional blood flow in pentobarbital — anesthetized pigs with or without β-adrenoceptor blockade. *Br J Pharmacol* 1986; 88:9-18.

74. Kimura E, Kishida H: Treatment of variant angina with drugs: A survey of 11 cardiology institutes in Japan. *Circulation* 1981; 63:844-848.

75. Toyosaki N, Natsume T, Katsuki T, et al. Synergetic effects of nifedipine and diltiazem in effort angina pectoris (abstr). *Circulation* 1987; 76(Suppl IV):IV-92.

76. Lessem J, Bellinetto A. Interaction between digoxin and calcium antagonist (abstr). *Am J Cardiol* 1982; 49:1025.

77. Pedersen KE. Digoxin interactions. The influence of quinidine and verapamil on the pharmacokinetics and receptor binding of digitalis glycosides. *Acta Med Scand* 1985; (Suppl 697):12-40.

78. Schwartz JB, Raizner A, Akers S. The effect of nifedipine on serum digoxin concentrations in patients. *Am Heart J* 1984; 107:669-673.

79. Elkayam U, Parikh K, Torkan B, et al. Effect of diltiazem on renal clearance and serum concentration of digoxin in patients with cardiac disease. *Am J Cardiol* 1985; 55:1393-1395.

80. Oyama Y, Fujii S, Kanda K, et al. Digoxin-diltiazem interaction. *Am J Cardiol* 1984; 53: 1480-1481.

81. Kleinbloesem CH, van Brummelen P, Hillers J, et al. Interaction between digoxin and nifedipine at steady-state in patients with atrial fibrillation. In: Kleinbloesem CH, ed. *Nifedipine: Clinical Pharmacokinetics and Haemodynamic Effects.* 's-Gravenhage: Drukkerij JH Pasms BV, 1985; 167-173.

82. Kirch W. Dihydropyridine derivatives, influence on digoxin disposition and haemodynamics (abstr). Presentation to NY Acad Sci, Feb 1987.

83. Kirch W, Hutt HJ, Heidemann H, et al. Drug interactions with nitrendipine. *J Cardiovasc Pharmacol* 1984; 6(Suppl 7):S982-S985.

84. Cantelli I, Bracchetti D. Combined use of digoxin and nifedipine in the treatment of congestive heart failure. *Pract Cardiol* 1985; 11:75-87.

85. Maisel AS, Motulsky HJ, Insel PA. Hypotension after quinidine plus verapamil. *New Engl J Med* 1985; 312:167-171.

86. Lee JT, Davy J-M, Kates RE. Evaluation of combined administration of verapamil and disopyramide in dogs. *J Cardiovasc Pharmacol* 1985; 7:501-507.

87. MacPhee GJA, McInnes GT, Thompson GG, et al. Verapamil potentiates carbamazepine neurotoxicity: A clinically important inhibitory interaction. *Lancet* 1986; i:700-703.

88. Bassan MM, Weiler-Ravell D, Shalev O. Comparison of the antianginal effectiveness of nifedipine, verapamil and

isosorbide dinitrate in patients receiving propranolol: A double-blind study. *Circulation* 1983; 68:568-575.

89. Tolins M, Weir EK, Chesler E, et al. "Maximal" drug therapy is not necessarily optimal in chronic angina pectoris. *J Am Coll Cardiol* 1984; 3:1051-1057.

90. White HD, Polak JF, Wynne J, et al. Addition of nifedipine to maximal nitrate and beta-adrenoceptor blocker therapy in coronary artery disease. *Am J Cardiol* 1985; 55:1303-1307.

91. Singer DRJ, Markandu ND, Shore AC, et al. Captopril and nifedipine in combination for moderate to severe essential hypertension. *Hypertension* 1987; 9:629-633.

92. Muller FB, Bolli P, Linder L, et al. Calcium antagonists and the second drug for hypertensive therapy. *Am J Med* 1986; 81(Suppl 6A):25-29.

93. MacGregor GA: Hypertension. In: Krebs R, ed. *Treatment of Cardiovascular Diseases by Adalat^R (Nifedipine)*. Stuttgart: Schattauer, 1986; 231-258.

94. Daniels AR, Opie LH. Atenolol plus nifedipine for mild to moderate systemic hypertension after fixed doses of either agent alone. *Am J Cardiol* 1986; 57:965-970.

95. Smith SR, Kendall MJ, Lobo J, et al. Ranitidine and cimetidine: Drug interactions with single dose and steady-state nifedipine administration. *Br J Clin Pharmacol* 1987; 23:311-315.

96. Kirch W, Janisch HD, Heidmann H, et al. Effect of cimetidine and ranitidine on the pharmacokinetics and the antihypertensive action of nifedipine. *Dtsch Med Wochenschr* 1983; 108:1757-1761.

97. Lahiri A, Dasgupta P, Rodrigues EA, et al. Acute drug withdrawal in patients with stable angina on long-term treatment with verapamil. In: Raftery EB, ed. *Verapamil SR*. Langhorne: ADIS Press International, 1987;18-29.

98. Raftos J, Verapamil in the long-term treatment of angina pectoris. *Med J Aust* 1980; 2:78-80.

99. Stone PH. Calcium antagonists for Prinzmetal's variant angina, unstable angina and silent myocardial ischemia. Therapeutic tool and probe for identification of pathophysiologic mechanisms. *Am J Cardiol* 1983; 59:101B-115B.

100. Gottlieb SO, Ouyang P, Achuff SC, et al. Acute nifedipine withdrawal:Consequences of preoperative and late cessation of therapy in patients with prior unstable angina. *J Am Coll Cardiol* 1984; 4:383-388.

101. Sorkin EM, Clissold SP, Brogden RN. Nifedipine. A review of its pharmacodynamic and pharmacokinetic properties, and therapeutic efficacy, in ischemic heart disease, hypertension and related cardiovascular disorders. *Drugs* 1985; 30:182-274.

102. Frishman W, Zawada ET, Smith K, et al. Comparison of hydrochlorothiazide and sustained-release diltiazem for mild to moderate systemic hypertension. *Am J Cardiol* 1987; 59:615-623.

103. Schroeder JS, Walker SD, Skalland ML, et al. Absence of rebound from diltiazem therapy in Prinzmetal's variant angina. *J Am Coll Cardiol* 1985; 6:174-178.

104. Daniels AR, Opie LH. Monotherapy with the calcium channel antagonist nisoldipine for systemic hypertension and comparison with diuretic drugs. *Am J Cardiol* 1987; 60:703-707.

CALCIUM CHANNEL ANTAGONISTS: PART V: SECOND-GENERATION AGENTS

SUMMARY. Second-generation agents include new dihydropyridines, such as amlodipine, felodipine, isradipine, nicardipine, nimodipine, nisoldipine, and nitrendipine. Verapamil-like agents include tiapamil, gallopamil, and anipamil. Among the diphenylalkylamines, bepridil is of special interest. New preparations of existing agents include slow-release formulations of nifedipine, verapamil, and diltiazem. From all these agents will be selected those that are longer-acting and provide higher vascular selectivity.

Qualities of an Ideal Calcium Antagonist

For hypertension, the ideal calcium antagonist should be long-acting with once-a-day dosage, vascular selective, and yet free of the vasodilatory counter-regulatory side-effects such as baroreceptor activation, tachycardia, and increased plasma catecholamines. A mild sustained diuretic effect would probably also be of benefit. Side effects such as facial flushing, dizziness, and ankle edema should be minimal. Pharmaceutically, the agent should be water-soluble with minimal hepatic metabolism and with renal excretion (none of the agents, old or new, meet this requirement). For use in angina, the ideal calcium antagonist would be without any ischemia-provoking side effects such as tachycardia or catecholamine activation; an inhibitory effect on the sinus node and a mild negative inotropic effect would probably be of advantage. Effects on the atrio-ventricular (AV) node should be minimal.

The existing second-generation calcium antagonist agents will now be reviewed together with mention of some agents still in the early stages of development.

Dihydropyridines

New dihydropyridine calcium antagonists (Table V-1) have been designed and more are in the offing, with the aims of achieving greater vascular selectivity, a longer half-life, and less of a negative inotropic effect than

219

Table V-1. Properties of some new calcium antagonists

	Plasma Terminal Half-Life	Possible Dose	Possible Proposed Indications	Special Properties
Dihydropyridines*				
Amlodipine	36 hr	2.5–10 mg once daily	Hypertension, angina	Less lipid-soluble than nifedipine. Prolonged action.
Felodipine	10 hr^a	5–10 mg three times daily	Hypertension, angina, congestive heart failure	Highly vascular selective
Isradipine	7 hr	5–7.5 mg two to three times daily	Hypertension, angina	Longer-acting than nifedipine
Nicardipine	4–5 hr or less^b	5–30 mg three times daily	Hypertension, angina (congestive heart failure)	Water-soluble, light-insensitive, otherwise similar to nifedipine ? More vascular selective
Nimodipine	5 hr^c	0.35 mg/kg 4-hourly 30–40 mg three to four times daily	Cerebral spasm, subarachnoid hemorrhage, early stroke	? Cerebral vascular selective yet has effect on coronary arteries
Nisoldipine	2–12 hr^{d,e}	5–20 mg once or twice daily^f	Hypertension, angina	Highly specific for calcium current

Nitrendipine	8 hr	10–20 mg once or twice daily	Hypertension, angina	Doubles digoxin levels
Verapamil-like*				
Anipamil	36 hr	60–80 mg once daily	Hypertension	Little effect on AV node
Gallopamil	7hr^g	50 mg three times daily	Angina	Similar to verapamil but more potent
Bepridil	40 hr	200–400 mg once daily	Arrhythmias, angina	Problem of proarrhythmic effects; Q-T interval prolongation

^{a}[139].
^{b}[30].
^{c}[140].
^{d}[141].
^{e}[142].
^{f}May require 8-hourly doses for angina, see [62].
^{g}[143].

with the prototypical compound, nifedipine. New verapamil and diltiazem-like agents are likewise being tested for a longer half-life and less of an effect on the myocardium or AV node.

Amlodipine

The major specific points of this dihydropyridine are longer duration of action than nifedipine (elimination plasma half-life in humans: 36 hours [1]). It also has a slow onset of its effects, possibly because it is three to four times less lipid-soluble than nifedipine [2]. Although it binds to the dihydropyridine site, it also seems to have some cross-binding to the diltiazem site [3]. Theoretically, amlodipine may take longer to reach the dihydropyridine receptor sites on the vessel to explain the less sudden onset of action than nifedipine, so that amlodipine might be claimed to have fewer acute vasodilatory side effects. However, strict clinical trials comparing amlodipine with nifedipine are still awaited. Preliminary tests in angina pectoris show promising results for amlodipine 2.5 to 10 mg as a single daily dose [4] with an optimal dose of 10 mg daily [5]. In hypertension, as initial monotherapy, amlodipine 2.5 to 5 mg daily is very nearly as effective as 5 to 10 mg daily with, however, only half the patients becoming "normotensive," according to an abstract [6]. Amlodipine (10 mg daily) is more effective than placebo when added to captopril 125 mg twice daily, according to an abstract [7].

Felodipine

This agent has been developed to be more vascular selective than nifedipine. Using the ratio of activity on rat portal vein versus myocardium [8], nifedipine is 14:1 vascular selective, diltiazem 7:1, and verapamil 1.4:1; however, felodipine was much more selective with a ratio of 100:1. These data are claimed to show a high degree of vascular selectivity.

In *congestive heart failure,* felodipine has been particularly well tested. For example, it has hemodynamic benefits in congestive heart failure secondary to ischemic heart disease [9] or in congestive heart failure of other etiologies [10]. Its acute hemodynamic effect is maintained for at least 5 days to 4 weeks [10, 11]. The impaired baroreflex control of the circulation, found in patients with congestive heart failure, tends to normalize with felodipine treatment [12]. There are no strict comparisons with nifedipine in congestive heart failure. A problem recently raised is that felodipine (10 mg twice daily over 3 weeks) confers no subjective benefit in a double-blind study despite the hemodynamic improvements [13]. When combined with digoxin, the blood digoxin level can increase from 11% to 47% [14].

In *hypertension*, felodipine 5 to 10 mg three times daily seemed to be similar to nifedipine 10 to 20 mg three times daily with a similar side effect profile (flushing, pedal edema, tachycardia, headaches) with, however, a longer duration of action [15] so that felodipine can be given twice daily. As with nifedipine, a single dose is accompanied by elevation of heart rate, plasma catecholamines, renin, and angiotensin-II; during chronic therapy with felodipine 10 mg twice daily, heart rate reverted to normal while plasma norepinephrine and renin were still elevated [16]. Felodipine can be combined with a β-blocker [17] and is likely to have a similar profile of benefits, side-effects, and cotherapy with other antihypertensives as in the case of nifedipine.

In *angina*, the relative absence of either a negative inotropic or negative chronotropic effect (there may be a tachycardia as in the case of nifedipine) is likely to place felodipine in a category resembling that of nifedipine and nicardipine, where there is a direct anti-anginal benefit with an indirect disadvantage induced by the tachycardia. In pacing-induced angina, felo-dipine appeared to act chiefly by afterload reduction, although an effect on coronary blood flow could not be excluded [18]. Therefore, as in the case of nifedipine, combination with β-blockade may be an advantage [19, 20].

Isradipine (PN-200)

In *effort angina*, isradipine 2.5 to 7.5 mg three times daily was similar to nifedipine 10 to 30 mg daily [21]. The antianginal efficacy of isradipine 7.5 mg lasted for less than 9 hours, and the side effect profile over a 2-week period resembled that of other dihydropyridines, including ankle edema and facial flushing [22].

In *congestive heart failure*, hemodynamic benefits resemble those of other dihydropyridines [23]. Long-term benefit has been suggested in a small, open, un-controlled study [24].

In mild to moderate *hypertension*, isradipine 5 to 7.5 mg daily was effective in 70% to 80% percent of patients in one study [25]; however, such data clearly depend on the criteria used to define success and the dose given. It may be noted that dihydropyridines only work effectively in about 50 percent of patients if strict criteria are used (diastolic blood pressure [DBP] < 90 mmHg; see nitrendipine [26], or nisoldipine [27]). Ex-perimental antiatherogenic effects are claimed [28] which would put this compound in the same category as nifedipine and other calcium antagonists from this point of view. However, there may be fewer side effects with isradipine than with nifedipine (equianginal doses) according to a recent abstract [29].

Nicardipine

This dihydropyridine has many similarities to nifedipine including the proposed indications and the short duration of action [30]. It is also widely available in Europe including the United Kingdom. The dose range goes somewhat higher than that of nifedipine (5 to 40 mg nicardipine three times daily; bioavailability reduced when taken with food). Claimed advantages over nifedipine are 1) less of a negative inotropic effect, so that nicardipine may be more vascular specific, with 2) a relatively greater effect on coronary arteries [31], and 3) the physical properties with nicardipine being water soluble and not light sensitive, so that intravenous administration is easier. Visser and colleagues [32] recently found that intracoronary nicardipine gave less inhibition of systolic and diastolic function than did nifedipine in 12 patients with coronary artery disease, the doses being chosen to give an equal increase in coronary sinus outflow. Subjective side effects may be fewer than with nifedipine, without strict comparisons being available [33].

Angina pectoris. Nicardipine 30 to 40 mg three times daily is well tested in *effort angina* where symptoms and exercise capacity improve, although 4 of 58 patients had increased angina, reminiscent of the effects of nifedipine [34]. During pacing angina myocardial metabolism improves [35] using careful dose titration up to a maximum of 7.5 mg intravenously. However, the absolute benefits achieved in the study of Scheidt and coworkers [34] were modest. Exercise duration only increased from 6.3 to 6.8 minutes during a 6-week period; an increased heart rate could have offset the oxygen-sparing benefit resulting from a decreased afterload as the blood pressure fell. Besides the worsening of angina in four of the patients (already referred to), vasodilatory side effects were noted in 11 patients.

During prolonged therapy of chronic effort angina tested over 4 months in an open parallel design [36], nicardipine 40 mg three times daily improved exercise time from 7.7 to 11.2 minutes (+45%) which was, however less than that achieved by diltiazem (+95%, 360 mg daily) or verapamil (+79%, 360 mg daily). The tachycardia induced by nicardipine both at rest and during exercise could have offset the vasodilatory benefit because the peak rate-pressure product during exercise rose during nicardipine therapy (+ 27%; no change for diltiazem or verapamil vs. placebo). In *vasospastic angina,* nicardipine (20 mg three times daily up to 40 mg four times daily) was effective with a mean optimal dose of about 90 mg daily [37]. During percutaneous transluminal coronary angioplasty (PTCA), pretreatment with intracoronary nicardipine protects against ischemia [38]. In *angina combined with hypertension,* nicardipine in a dose of about 100 mg daily was the approximate equivalent of nifedipine about 60 mg daily with the exercise time increasing from 6.9 to 9.5 minutes for nicardipine [39].

Congestive heart failure. In congestive heart failure, nicardipine reduced peripheral vascular resistance and increased peripheral blood flow [40]. There was no obvious negative inotropic effect nor any rise in plasma norepinephrine levels [41]. (For general reservations about the use of calcium antagonists in congestive heart failure, see Part III.)

Hypertension. In hypertension, nicardipine is likely to be as effective as nifedipine without any compelling advantage for either agent in many patients. For mild to moderate hypertension, nicardipine 30 mg three times daily decreased supine blood pressure in 25 patients from approximately 165/105 mmHg to 145/90 mmHg without tachyardia [42] with, however, the chief side effec↓ being flushing (in 4 patients). The antihypertensive effect is dose-dependent on the DBP and accompanied by a tachycardia [43]. Nicardipine has an acute and may have a subacute (1-week) diuretic effect [44, 45]; the subacute effect has not been confirmed [46]. Longer-term observations would be of interest. Nicardipine may successfully be combined with atenolol [47] or propranolol [48]; nicardipine improves the depressed cardiac output after β-blockade, probably by reduction of systemic vascular resistance [48]. Thus a similar series of indications, contraindications, and beneficial drug combinations can be anticipated with nicardipine as with nifedipine; although possible differences between these two agents may exist with regard to the relative effects on the peripheral vessels and the myocardium [49]; such differences still need translation into clinical practice.

Nimodipine

Some experimental data suggest that nimodipine is more selective for cerebral than for other peripheral vessels [50] so that nimodipine has been well tested against the cerebral spasm associated with subarachnoid hemorrhage. In a dose of 0.35 mg/kg 4-hourly, nimodipine helped to prevent complications of subarachnoid hemorrhage [51] and was also effective in early stroke (dose 120 mg daily in three divided doses

[52]) apparently without side effects. In a recent double-blind placebo-controlled study not yet published in full, nimodipine 30 mg four times daily or placebo was added to standard therapy by 10% depolymerized dextran for 28 days. Nimodipine improved the level of consciousness and mortality ($p <$ 0.02) in these patients with stroke [53]. Thus nimodipine is coming to have a definite role in the therapy of early stroke and subarachnoid hemorrhage. What is not clear is whether nifedipine, much more widely available, would not have had similar benefits if tested. Experimentally, both nimodipine and nifedipine are effective coronary vasodilators, with nimodipine being the more powerful [54].

Nisoldipine

This dihydropyridine is highly specific for the slow calcium current [55, 56] and therefore has become one of the standard dihydropyridine agents in experimental pharmacology. It is claimed to be 24 times more specific a vasodilator than nifedipine [57], which may explain the greater rise of plasma renin and norepinephrine following nisoldipine than nifedipine [58]. However, in the blood-perfused dog myocardium, nisoldipine and nifedipine had nearly identical cardiovascular profiles [59]. Acutely 6 µg/kg IV given to patients with suspected coronary artery disease acts as a coronary and peripheral vasodilator without obvious negative inotropic effects because the left ventricular (LV) end-diastolic pressure did not change, although first derivative of the left ventricular pressure (LV dP/dt) fell [60]. Isovolumic indices of contractility such as cardiac action potential (V_{max}) increased probably due to reflex sympathetic stimulation.

In *effort angina*, efficacy has been shown for 5 to 20 mg twice daily [61]. In acute studies, 10 to 20 mg acutely improved effort tolerance within 1 hour, the higher dose being effective for 8 hours [62], despite an increase of the rate-pressure product at peak exercise. Several studies, not yet published in full, show the effectiveness of nisoldipine in a variety of ischemic syndromes varying from vasospastic to rest angina. However, specific comparisons with nifedipine are generally lacking. In a preliminary communication, Reicher-Reiss et al. [63] claim that nisoldipine 10 mg daily has a similar antianginal potency to nifedipine 10 mg three times daily. On the other hand, when added to atenolol in the therapy of patients with severe angina, it is suggested that nifedipine 20 mg three times daily is more effective than nisoldipine 20 mg once daily [64]. The tachycardia caused by this and almost all dihydropyridines may be a disadvantage in the therapy of angina.

In *hypertension*, nisoldipine 10 mg once daily was the equivalent of slow-release nifedipine 20 mg twice daily in a double-blind double-dummy study; in both, DBP was reduced better than systolic values [65]. Nisoldipine caused more of an acute rise of plasma noradrenaline and renin levels than did nifedipine [58]. Daniels and Opie [66] compared nisoldipine with hydrochlorothiazide in a double-blind crossover study. A significant number of patients dropped out of the trial during the run-in period because of nisoldipine-induced headaches. The latter side effect also limited the benefit of nisoldipine as monotherapy in an open-label prolonged study after the initial double-blind period (see Table V-1). Nonetheless, nisoldipine 10 mg one to two times daily was similar to hydrochlorothiazide-amiloride (25 mg, 5 mg respectively, 1/2 to 1 tablet Moduretic) in benefitting about half the patients. The combination nisoldipine-diuretic seemed particularly effective and free of side effects. Patients who did not respond well to monotherapy with one agent responded to the combination so that altogether 96% of the patients with mild to moderate hypertension responded in this series to nisoldipine, the diuretic, or the combination. However, this figure does not allow for the 25% of patients who dropped out of the trial in the initial period because of headaches. In another chronic study on hypertension, nisoldipine (mean dose 32 mg daily) reduced systemic vascular resistance and blood pressure over 1 year; heart rate and cardiac index only rose after acute administration and there were no reports of dropouts due to headaches [67]. However, in a clinical data pool study, 22% of patients treated for hypertension with nisoldipine experienced headaches [68].

In *congestive heart failure*, nisoldipine gave some good hemodynamic effects yet with neurohumoral activation, so that plasma renin and norepinephrine levels increased [69], with in the end seven of ten patients deteriorating after 2 months of follow-up. "The neurohumoral and renal effects of nisoldipine were particularly marked in the seven patients who eventually developed pulmonary edema" [69]. In contrast, Kiowski et al. [70] found that the hemodynamic benefits of nisoldipine were sustained over 4 weeks of follow-up, without any increase in plasma renin, epinephrine, or norepinephrine. It is difficult to understand the contradictory results of these studies; a clue may be that the systemic vascular resistance and plasma renin value of the patients of Kiowski et al. [70] seemed about 50% higher than those of Barjon and colleagues [69].

Nitrendipine

Among the first of the second-generation dihydro-pyridines extensively tested, nitrendipine was one of the first (see Table V-1). Because of its use as a reference standard in binding studies, nitrendipine is already well known to experimental pharmacologists. However, nitrendipine is not a pure calcium channel antagonist, but also has some agonist properties [71]. It is claimed to be six times more powerful than nifedipine as a vasodilator in normal men [57]. The clinical features distinguishing nitrendipine from nifedipine are as follows. First, nitrendipine has a longer duration of action so that in hypertension it can be given once daily [72], although a twice-daily dose is sometimes required. Besides vasodilation, other antihypertensive mechanisms include 1) inhibition of secretion of aldosterone [73], as in the case of other dihydropyridines. The pharmacologic half-life of nitrendipine is 7.9 hours in normal volunteers [74]. The first approved indication for nitrendipine will be *hypertension* with a dose of 10 to 20 mg one to two times daily. Yet nitrendipine is likely to be equally effective when coronary dilation is required as in coronary spasm or effort *angina*.

Comparative efficacy. Strict comparisons with nifedipine (the reference dihydropyridine) are still awaited; nitrendipine is likely to be about as effective as slow-release nifedipine (with nitredipine 20 mg approximately equal to slow-release nifedipine 40 mg [75]). In an open comparison, nitrendipine 20 to 40 mg once daily was about as effective as nifedipine (mean dose 47 mg daily) or verapamil (mean dose 427 mg daily) [72], when given to patients with mild to moderate hypertension. With both agents the goal DBP of 95 mmHg was reached in the majority of patients (39 of 51 with verapamil; 33 of 46 with nitrendipine [72, 76]). In black hypertensive patients, nitredipine 20 to 60 mg daily was more effectively hypotensive than was acebutolol 200 to 400 mg [77, 78]. The possibility that calcium antagonists are effective antihypertensive agents in the black population has already been raised in Part III of this series. In comparison with hydralazine 50 to 100 mg daily [79], nitrendipine 10 to 40 mg daily had similar potency with a similar incidence of headaches and yet with fewer patients dropping out from the nitrendipine group.

Combination therapy. Nitrendipine has successfully been combined with propranolol [80] or diuretic [80, 81] or angiotensin-converting enzyme (ACE) inhibitor therapy in the treatment of hypertension [82]. Nitrendipine has also been combined with β-blocker–diuretic therapy [80]. Drug interactions with nitrendipine are likely to be similar to those found with nifedipine except that there appears to be a more clear-cut effect on digoxin. Nitrendipine 20 mg daily almost doubles the digoxin level during chronic administration [83]. This interaction may be of importance in congestive heart failure, in which single oral doses of nitrendipine 10 to 20 mg daily reduced systemic vascular resistance and increased cardiac index without increasing heart rate [84]. However, general reservations have been expressed in relation to all calcium antagonists when used in patients with congestive heart failure (see Part III, section on Congestive Heart Failure).

Other Dihydropyridines

Many other dihydropyridines are under development and include azodipine, darodipine, flordipine, iodipine, mesudipine, niguldipine, niludipine, nivaldipine, oxodipine, riodipine, and ryosidine. All are likely to have the same therapeutic profile as nifedipine with, however, some pharmaceutical differences relating, e.g., to the duration of action that might benefit specific patient groups. There may be some advantages for certain agents from the point of view of regional vascular specificity. However, it seems unlikely that all these compounds will find a therapeutic niche in this highly overcrowded and competitive market. Among the differences, the most important might lie in the pharmacokinetic half-life.

New Preparations of Existing Compounds

Slow-release nifedipine is widely replacing standard nifedipine capsules in Europe, because of the slower onset of action and the impression of few acute vasodilatory side effects. The standard dose for hypertension is 20 to 40 mg once or twice daily. In a comparison of slow-release nifedipine 20 mg twice daily with atenolol 100 mg daily, atenolol achieved blood pressure control (DBP < 90 mmHg) in 40% to 50% and nifedipine in only about 10% to 20% of patients, with the combination working in most of those not responding to monotherapy with either of the agents [85]. However, in another study [86], slow-release nifedipine in the same doses compared well with acebutolol 400 mg daily [86]. Monotherapy by slow-release nifedipine for mild to moderate hypertension requires higher doses than might be expected, sometimes up to 80 mg daily total dose [87, 88]. As this agent does not have inherent long-acting pharmacokinetic properties, its future in hypertension therapy may be less auspicious than expected as new once-a-day agents with truly prolonged kinetic half-lives appear.

Continuous-release (GITS) nifedipine is under evaluation; once-daily doses are the antihypertensive equivalent of standard nifedipine with fewer side effects [89].

Slow-release verapamil. Several slow-release preparations are now being promoted including those made by Knoll, by Searle, and by Rorer (for the latter, see Raftery [90]). One slow-release verapamil preparation (Verapamil SR, 360 mg) seems effective in stable effort angina when given only once daily [91], although some effects on hemodynamic parameters seem to fade over 4 weeks of therapy. A lower dose of another slow-release preparation (240 mg daily) gave benefits on the electrocardiographic features of ischemia during exercise testing of anginal patients 3 to 8 hours after the tablet but not at 24 hours, nor was the exercise time prolonged at any time [92]. In hypertension, two to three times daily administration of slow-release verapamil (120 mg twice daily up to 240 mg three times daily) is effectively antihypertensive [93]. Studies with 24-hour ambulatory blood pressure monitoring suggest that one preparation of slow-release verapamil in a dose of 240 to 480 mg daily is potentially a true once-daily agent, although blood pressure levels at 24 hours were higher than at 6 hours [43]. Another preparation required twice-daily dosage [95]. It should be borne in mind that during chronic therapy ordinary verapamil by virtue of altered pharmacokinetics with formation of compounds such as norverapamil can be given on a twice-daily basis [96, 97]. Furthermore, clearance of both verapamil and its major metabolite norverapamil is decreased in elderly patients [98].

Of the various preparations, that made by Knoll (Isoptin Retard tablet) releases about 100% of its contents within 7 hours, while that made by Rorer (Verapamil-sustained-release [SR] capsule) releases about 80% of its contents within 12 hours and therefore may have a pharmacokinetic advantage [99]. Such differences may explain the apparently longer anti-anginal action of one preparation over the other (compare Brugmann [92] with Kohli et al. [91]); however, formal comparative studies are lacking. Blood levels with single doses of slow-release preparations are much higher than those of ordinary verapamil [98]. Thus what should be compared are the clinical effects and blood levels of both verapamil and norverapamil during chronic twice-daily administration of the ordinary preparation versus once-daily dosage of the slow-release preparation under evaluation. At present the data showing a true 24-hour effect of slow-release verapamil are good for some preparations but not for others.

Slow-release diltiazem.   This preparation, also under study, allows twice daily dosing of diltiazem. In the management of angina, Diltiazem SR was effective both at 240 mg (120 mg 12-hourly)and 360 mg (180 mg 12-hourly) daily doses; there were few differences in benefit or side effects [100].

Verapamil-like Agents

Tiapamil.

This very promising agent has had its commercial development blocked. Compared with verapamil, it 1) has more marked sodium blocking qualities [101] so that there is a definite antiarrhythmic effect against the standard type of ventricular arrhythmias (unlike verapamil which only benefits certain specific ventricular arrhythmias); and 2) reduces heart rate and peripherally dilates with apparently little negative inotropic effect [102]. From the latter point of view, this compound resembles diltiazem.

Gallopamil

This compound (D600) has for long been well tested pharmacologically and frequently used instead of verapamil. Clinical tests have been slower in appearing. In *angina pectoris*, gallopamil 150 mg was similar to propranolol 240 mg daily from the point of view of antianginal benefit. Whereas propranolol decreased rate-pressure product, gallopamil caused a small rise when the peak exercise systolic blood pressure increased, showing that the mechanism of the antianginal effects of gallopamil had to be different from that of propranolol. However, 1 of 20 patients developed cholestatic jaundice on gallopamil. The overall effects of gallopamil seem similar to those of verapamil except that gallopamil did not cause constipation [103]; however, in that study there was no direct comparison between the two agents. Strict comparisons between gallopamil and verapamil are awaited. In comparison with nifedipine (10 mg), gallopamil (50 mg) gave less ST segment depression at a given workload than did nifedipine, and the heart rates were lower [104]. It was proposed that gallopamil 50 mg had the same antianginal efficacy as nifedipine 20 mg and verapamil 320 mg. In *unstable angina pectoris,* gallopamil (infusion 30 µg/kg/min for 10 minutes followed by 0.3 to 1.2 µg/kg/min) was studied in five patients with the aim of defining pharmacokinetics

[105]; however, two of the five patients developed myocardial infarction so the study was inconclusive.

Anipamil

This agent is also well tested pharmacologically and has a very prolonged duration of action up to 36 hours [106]. The drug is claimed to have little effect on AV nodal tissue so that one of the chief therapeutic indications should be for hypertension. In rats pretreated for 5 days, ischemic-reperfusion injury was less [107]. In rabbits pretreated with anipamil for 3 days up to 12 hours before isolation of the heart for perfusion, anipamil protected against hypoxia and reperfusion [108].

Devapamil

Thus far devapamil is only in the early stages of testing which show that it is about 4 times more potent than gallopamil and 12 times more potent than verapamil in its effects on smooth muscle tone and labeled calcium uptake [109].

(−) Verapamil

Standard verapamil is racemic (±); the calcium antagonist property is largely concentrated in the (−) component, which is experimentally more effective against acute sudden death in rats with coronary occlusion [110], probably acting by inhibition of ventricular fibrillation [111]. Thus far (−) verapamil has not been commercially developed.

Diphenylalkylamines and Related Agents; "Internal" Calcium Blockers

Spedding [112] has divided calcium antagonists into three groups: 1) dihydropyridines; 2) verapamil and diltiazem; and 3) diphenylalkylamines and related compounds including cinnarizine, flunarizine, lidoflazine, bepridil, perhexiline, and prenylamine. The International Society of Cardiology (see Table I-2) further separated verapamil and diltiazem on the basis of their differential interaction with the dihydropyridine site. In general, Spedding's group III compounds are highly lipophilic and more likely to act as calmodulin antagonists [113]. The calcium channel agonist Bay-K-8644 completely protects K^+-depolarized smooth muscle from the inhibitory effects of dihydropridines, only partially protects from the effects of verapamil and diltiazem, and fails to protect from the effects of Spedding's group III agents [114], suggesting that the latter group has an important "internal" site of action independent of the calcium channel, such as calmodulin. Furthermore, there may be an effect on the outward potassium current [115]. If this quality is common to the group as a whole, it would explain why some members of the group such as bepridil and prenylamine have been found to prolong the Q-T interval with proarrhythmic consequences. Such possible effects on the calmodulin and the outward potassium channel are in addition to effects on the calcium channel in certain tissues such as some vascular beds but, at least in the case of cinnarizine and flunarizine, not in the myocardium. Although most of these compounds are not really strictly speaking "new" calcium antagonists, yet there is interest in their use in the broader aspects of cardiovascular medicine. Of these agents, that best studied from the cardiologic point of view is bepridil, with antiarrhythmic and antianginal properties.

Bepridil

This agent is a combined sodium-calcium channel blocker, currently still under evaluation, with complex electrophysiologic properties including inhibition of phase zero of the V_{max}; prolongation of the refractory period of atrial and ventricular muscle, shortening of the action potential duration of Purkinje fibers, and lengthening of the ventricular action potential [116]. It is a somewhat more potent calcium than sodium channel blocker [116]. The major problem is the proarrhythmic tendency [117].

Electrophysiologic properties and use in arrhythmias. The effect of bepridil on slow-channel activity in the AV node resembles that of verapamil or diltiazem. However, the marked prolongation of the atrial refractory period suggests that the drug may be specifically beneficial in the prevention and treatment of atrial flutter or fibrillation [116, 117]. Thus, intravenous bepridil (4 mg/kg) prevented electrophysiologic induction of sustained ventricular tachycardia in 3 of 5 patients and prolonged oral bepridil therapy (300 to 400 mg daily) prevented the induction of such arrhythmias in 6 of 12 patients [118]. Because of quinidinelike effects (sodium blockade) on the accessory pathway in patients with Wolff-Parkinson-White syndrome, bepridil may have an advantage over intravenous verapamil or diltiazem. The reason is that bepridil is unlikely to accelerate the ventricular response in patients with Wolff-Parkinson-White syndrome who develop atrial fibrillation [118]. However, direct comparisons between bepridil and verapamil are apparently not available.

For *angina pectoris*, the hemodynamic properties are important. Intravenous bepridil (2 to 4 mg/kg) causes short-term coronary and peripheral vasodilation, followed by late negative inotropic and chronotropic effects [119].

In the clinical treatment of angina pectoris, the optimal bepridil dose is probably 400 mg once daily [120] which increases exercise time and time to onset of angina [121]. Because the half-life is about 40 hours, once-daily dosing is adequate [122]. In a randomized double-blind crossover dose-titration trial on 24 patients with stable angina of effort [122], bepridil 200 to 400 mg daily was as effective an antianginal agent as was nadolol 120 to 240 mg daily. The mean daily doses were bepridil 367 mg and nadolol 215 mg. There were the following differences: with nadolol heart rate, peak systolic blood pressure, and exercise rate-pressure product were all lower, whereas with bepridil the Q-T interval was longer. These differences are typical for the comparison between calcium antagonists as a group and β-blockers as a group in the therapy of angina pectoris, except that bepridil also causes the prolongation of the Q-T-interval. Bepridil had no negative inotropic effect in the conditions of the study of Pflugfelder et al. [122], yet more careful evaluation is required in patients with compromised left ventricular function. Bepridil has been successfully combined with propranolol in the therapy of effort angina, where average bepridil doses of 273 mg daily were safely added to propranolol 131 mg daily [123]. Again, further evaluation in the presence of compromised left ventricular function is required.

Proarrhythmic effects. The major problem with bepridil is the proarrhythmic tendency, probably related to the prolonged *Q-T-interval* [124]. In the correct setting, especially when there is concomitant hypokalemia, a prolonged Q-T interval may predispose to torsades de pointes. In addition, other ventricular arrhythmias may be common [117]. Nonetheless, a prolonged Q-T interval may also have a "good" effect because it is a mechanism of antiarrhythmic benefit. The possibility that Q-T interval has both "good" and "bad" consequences makes it "difficult to judge when a prolonged QT-interval is good, bad or indifferent" [125]. Until the significance of the possible proarrhythmic effect is settled, it would be important to take the following *precautions* when bepridil is used: 1) cotherapy with thiazide diuretics should be avoided unless plasma K^+ is repetitively checked; 2) plasma magnesium should also be monitored; and 3) cotherapy with other drugs promoting torsades de pointes such as amiodarone, sotalol, quinidine, disopyramide, and tricyclic antidepressants, should all be avoided.

Lidoflazine

This agent has gone through several phases. Although an effective antianginal agent, it was previously criticized because of the fear that it would cause "coronary steal." Then lidoflazine came to be reinvestigated and its antianginal activity confirmed [126]. However, the more recent realization that lidoflazine significantly prolongs the Q-T interval and causes a proarrhythmic effect in about 20% of patients (5 of 24 patients, 1 died) means that this agent can no longer be recommended [127] when so many other antianginal agents are available. The clinical study by Hanley and Hampton [127] is likely to carry considerable weight, despite the consequent dog study which showed that lidolflazine did not precipitate digitalis arrhythmias [128].

Cinnarizine and Flunarizine

As pointed out in Part I of this book, these agents currently have no cardiovascular indications. Some projected areas of interest are as follows. In *migraine*, these agents appear to be at least as effective as more established drugs such as pizotifen (see Part I, section on New Indications, Migraine) without, however, proof that efficacy is specifically related to calcium channel blockade; e.g., an antihistaminic effect might be relevant. In *cerebral ischemia or hypoxia*, flunarizine is claimed to be as effective as the dihydropyridines in experimental protection, whereas verapamil and diltiazem are ineffective [129]. Nonetheless flunarizine failed to improve the neurologic outcome when given after the onset of complete cerebral ischemia in the dog [130]. At a cellular level flunarizine may have certain actions on vascular smooth muscle different from those of nifedipine [131].

Calmodulin Antagonists

Activation of calmodulin by calcium is an essential step in vascular smooth muscle contraction. Therefore a specific calmodulin antagonist should be able to achieve vascular smooth muscle relaxation. In general, the more lipophilic agents of Spedding's group III are more likely to be calmodulin antagonists than the less lipophilic agents such as nifedipine [113]. The classical calmodulin antagonists trifluoperazine and chlorpromazine are both vasodilators.

The combined effects of such agents on calmodulin and on inhibition of voltage-dependent calcium entry means that they should be more active on vascular smooth muscle than nifedipine, as shown in the case of Wy-46531 [132]. The role of calmodulin in myocardial contraction is not as well established as in vascular smooth muscle, which may explain the lesser negative inotropic properties of the compound used by Silver et al. [132] when compared with standard calcium antagonists.

Fendiline

This agent relaxes vascular smooth muscle even in the presence of a calcium channel agonist [133] and is thought to be a calmodulin antagonist with superior vasodilating ability to that of nifedipine [134]. Its hemodynamic properties in humans include, according to a preliminary investigation, reduction of blood pressure and left ventricular contractility but no electrophysiologic effects on the sinus or AV node [135]. According to another recent abstract, fendiline 100 mg twice daily was the approximate antianginal equivalent of nifedipine 10 mg three times daily in patients with effort angina [136].

Internal Calcium Cycle Blockers

Besides the calmodulin antagonists, another group of agents acts primarily on the sarcoplasmic reticulum to inhibit the cyclical uptake and release of calcium. The prototypical agents are ryanodine (an insecticide) and caffeine, both of which have an antiarrhythmic effect in the ischemic perfused rat heart [137]. A new compound, KT-362, is believed to cause vasodilation by inhibition of a process also sensitive to caffeine, suggesting that it interferes with the caffeine-sensitive release of calcium from the sarcoplasmic reticulum [138]. This compound is a modified benzothiazepine and, therefore, structurally related to diltiazem.

References

1. Faulkner JK, McGibney D, Chasseaud LF, et al. The pharmacokinetics of amlodipine in healthy volunteers after single intravenous and oral doses and after 14 repeated oral doses given once daily. *Br J Clin Pharmacol* 1986; 22:21–25.
2. Burges RA, Gardiner DG, Gwilt M, et al. Calcium channel blocking properties of amlodipine in vascular smooth muscle and cardiac muscle in vitro: Evidence for voltage modulation of vascular dihydropyridine receptors. *J Cardiovasc Pharmacol* 1987; 9:110–119.
3. Rigby JW, Greengrass PM, Gardiner DG, et al. Interaction of amlodipine with calcium channel binding sites (abstr). *Cardiovasc Drugs Ther* 1987; 1:281.

4. Lee P, Jackson NC, Cocco G, et al. A dose response study of amlodipine in stable angina (abstr). *Cardiovasc Drugs Ther* 1987; 1:261.

5. Kinnard DR, Harris M, Hossack KF. Endurance testing for evaluation of antianginal therapy with amlodipine, a calcium channel blocking agent. *J Am Coll Cardiol* 1988; 12:791–796.

6. Frick MH: Amlodipine once daily in the treatment of hypertension (abstr). *Cardiovasc Drugs Ther* 1987; 1:238.

7. Maclean D, Mitchell ET, Wilcox RG. A double-blind crossover comparison of amlodipine or placebo added to captopril in moderate to severe hypertension (abstr). *Cardiovasc Drugs Ther* 1987; 1:263.

8. Ljung B: Vascular selectivity of felodipine. *Drugs* 1985; 29(Suppl 2):46–58.

9. Tweddel AC, Hutton I. Felodipine in ventricular dysfunction. *Eur Heart J* 1986; 7:54–60.

10. Timmis AD, Smyth P, Kenny JF, et al. Effects of vasodilator treatment with felodipine on haemodynamic responses to treadmill exercise in congestive heart failure. *Br Heart J* 1984; 52:314–320.

11. Binetti G, Pancaldi, Giovanelli N, et al. Hemodynamic effects of felodipine in congestive heart failure. *Cardiovasc Drugs Ther* 1987; 1:161–167.

12. Kassis E, Amtorp O. Cardiovascular and neurohumoral postural responses and baroreceptor abnormalities during a course of adjunctive vasodilator therapy with felodipine for congestive heart failure. *Circulation* 1987; 75:1204–1213.

13. Tan LB, Murray RG, Littler WA. Felodipine in patients with chronic heart failure: Discrepant haemodynamic and clinical effects. *Br Heart J* 1987; 58:122–128.

14. Dunselman PHJM, Scaf AHJ, Kuntze CEE, et al. Interaction between felodipine and digoxin in patients with congestive heart failure (abstr). *Cardiovasc Drugs Ther* 1987; 1:231.

15. Aberg H, Lindsjo M, Morlin B. Comparative trial of felodipine and nifedipine in refractory hypertension. *Drugs* 1985; 29(Suppl 2):117–123.

16. Katzman PL, Hulthen UL, Hokfelt B: Catecholamines, renin-angiotensin-aldosterone, and cardiovascular response during exercise following acute and long-term calcium antagonism with felodipine in essential hypertension. *J Cardiovasc Pharmacol* 1987; 10:439–444.

17. Hansson BG, Lyngstam O, et al. Antihypertensive effect of felodipine combined with β-blockade. A comparison between 2 and 3 daily dosages. *Drugs* 1985; 29 (Suppl 2):131–136.

18. Emanuelsson H, Hjalmarson A, Holmberg S, et a;. Effects of felodipine on pacing-induced angina pectoris. *J Cardiovasc Pharmacol* 1986; 8:500–506.

19. Culling W, Ruttley MSM, Sheridan DJ. Acute haemodynamic effects of delodipine during beta-blockade in patients with coronary artery disease. *Br Heart J* 1984; 52:431–434.

20. Freeling R, Harvard Davis R, Goves JR, et al. Control of hypertension in elderly patients with felodipine and metopropol: A double-blind, placebo-controlled clinical trial. *Br J Clin Pharmacol* 1987; 24:459–464.

21. Taylor SH, Jackson NC, Allen J, et al. Efficacy of a new calcium antagonist PN 200-110 (Isradipine) in angina pectoris. *Am J Cardiol* 1987; 59:123B–129B.

22. Parker JO, Enjalbert M, Bernstein V. Efficacy of the calcium antagonist isradipine in angina pectoris. *Cardiovasc Drugs Ther* 1988; 1:661–664.

23. Greenberg B, Siemienczuk D, Broudy D. Hemodynamic effects of PN 200-110 (Isradipine) in congestive heart failure. *Am J Cardiol* 1987; 59:70B-74B.

24. Broudy DR, Greenberg BHm Siemienczuk D. Beneficial effects of the calcium antagonist PN 200-110 in patients with congestive heart failure. *J Cardiovasc Pharmacol* 1987; 10:190-195.

25. Davidov ME, Gonasun LA. Safety and efficacy of isradipine (PN 200-110), a new calcium antagonist in the treatment of essential hypertension (abstr). Presentation to NY Acad Sci, Feb 1987.

26. Ventura HO, Messerli FH, Oigman W, et al. Immediate hemodynamic effects of a new calcium-channel blocking agent (nitrendipine) in essential hypertension. *Am J Cardiol* 1983; 51:783-786.

27. Daniels AR, Opie LH. Effect of slow-release nifedipine on glucose tolerance. In: Lichtlen PR, ed. Sixth *International Adalat^R Symposium*. Amsterdam: Excerpta Medica, 1986; 495-496.

28. Weinstein DB, Heider JG: Antiatherogenic properties of calcium antagonists. *Am J Cardiol* 1987; 59:163B-172B.

29. Pool PE, Seagren SC, Salel AF. Isradipine in the treatment of angina pectoris. *Cardiovascular Rev Rep* 1987; Special Suppl:13.

30. Graham DJM, Dow RJ, Hall DJ, et al. The metabolism and pharmacokinetics of nicardipine hydrochloride in man. *Br J Clin Pharmacol* 1985; 20:23S-28S.

31. Takenaka T, Asano M, Shiono K, et al. Cardiovascular Pharmacology of nicardipine in animals. *Br J Clin Pharmacol* 1985; 20:7S-22S.

32. Visser CA, Koolen JJ, Van Wezel H, et al. Hemodynamics of nicardipine in coronary artery disease. *Am J Cardiol* 1987; 59:9J-12J.

33. Subramanian VB. Calcium antagonists in chronic stable angina pectoris. Amsterdam: Excerpta Medica, 1983, 97-116, 152-156, 217-229.

34. Scheidt S, LeWinter MM, Hermanovich J, et al. Efficacy and safety of nicardipine for chronic, stable angina pectoris: A multicenter randomized trial. *Am J Cardiol* 1986; 58:715-721.

35. Thomassen A, Bagger JP, Nielsen TT, et al. Metabolic and hemodynamic effects of nicardipine during pacing-induced angina pectoris. *Am J Cardiol* 1987; 59:219-224.

36. Khurmi NS, Raftery EB. Comparative effects of prolonged therapy with four calcium ion antagonists (diltiazem, nicardipine, tiapamil and verapamil) in patients with chronic stable angina pectoris. *Cardiovasc Drugs Ther* 1987; 1:81-87.

37. Gelman JS, Feldman RL, Scott E, et al. Nicardipine for angina pectoris at rest and coronary arterial spasm. *Am J Cardiol* 1985; 56:232-236.

38. Hanet C, Rousseau MF, Vincent M-F, et al. Myocardial protection by intracoronary nicardipine administration during percutaneous transluminal coronary angioplasty. *Am J Cardiol* 1987; 59:1035-1040.

39. Metra M, Nodari S, Nordio G, et al. Comparison of nicardipine and nifedipine in patients with both stable angina pectoris and systemic hypertension: A chronic study (abstr). Presentation to NY Acad Sci, Feb 1987.

40. Riew KD, Kubo SH, Cody RJ. The direct vasodilator effect of nicardipine and its relationship to basal sympathetic tone in patients with chronic congestive heart failure (abstr). Presentation to NY Acad Sci, Feb 1987.

41. Ryman KS, Kubo SH, Lystash J, et al. Effect of nicardipine

on rest and exercise hemodynamics in chronic congestive heart failure. *Am J Cardiol* 1986; 58:583-588.

42. Asplund J: Nicardipine hydrochloride in essential hypertension - a controlled study. *Br J Clin Pharmacol* 1985; 20:120S-124S.

43. Taylor SH, Silke B, Ahuja RC, et al. Influence of nicardipine on the blood pressure at rest and on the pressor responses to cold, isometric exertion, and dynamic exercise in hypertensive patients. *J Cardiovasc Pharmacol* 1982: 4:803-807.

44. Baba T, Boku A, Ishizaki T, et al. Renal effects of nicardipine in patients with mild to moderate essential hypertension. *Am Heart J* 1986; 111:552-557.

45. Van Schaick BAM, Van Nistelrooy AEJ, Geyskes GG. Antihypertensive and renal effects of nicardipine. *Br J Clin Pharmacol* 1984; 18:57-63.

46. Chaignon M, Bellet M, Lucsko M, et al. Acute and chronic effects of a new calcium inhibitor, nicardipine, on renal hemodynamics in hypertension. *J Cardiovasc Pharmacol* 1986; 8:892-897.

47. Kolloch R, Stumpe KO, Overlack A. Blood pressure, heart rate and A-V conduction responses to nicardipine in hypertensive patients receiving atenolol. *Br J Clin Pharmacol* 1985; 20:130S-134S.

48. Rousseau MF, Van Mechelen EH, Veriter C, et al. Hemodynamic and cardiac effects of nicardipine in patients with coronary artery disease. *J Cardiovasc Pharmacol* 1984; 6:833-839.

49. Sheridan DJ, Thomas P. Vascular versus myocardial selectivity of calcium antagonists. *J Cardiovasc Pharmacol* 1987; 10(Suppl 1):S165-S168.

50. Towart R. The selective inhibition of serotonin-induced contractions of rabbit cerebral vascular smooth muscle by calcium antagonistic dihydropyridines. An investigation of the mechanism of action of nimodipine. *Circ Res* 1981; 48:650-657.

51. Allen GS, Ahn HS, Preziosi TJ, et al. Cerebral arterial spasm—a controlled trial of nimodipine in patients with subarachnoid hemorrhage. *N Engl J Med* 1983; 308:619-624.

52. Gelmers HJ. The effects of nimodipine on the clinical course of patients with acute ischemic stroke. *Acta Neurol Scand* 1984; 69:232-239.

53. Gelmers HJ, Gorter K, et al. de Weerdt CJ, et al. New aspects in stroke therapy (abstr). Presentation to NY Acad Sci, Feb 1987.

54. Nyborg NCB, Mikkelsen EO. Comparison of the inhibitory effects of nifedipine and nimodipine on mechanical responses of isolated rat coronary small arteries. *J Cardiovasc Pharmacol* 1987; 9:519-524.

55. Kass RS. Nisodipine: A new more selective calcium current blocker in cardiac Purkinje fibers. *J Pharmacol Exp Ther* 1983; 223:446.

56. Knorr A: The pharmacology of nisoldipine. *Cardiovasc Drugs Ther* 1987; 1:393-402.

57. Graefe K-H, Ziegler R, Wingender W, et al. Cardiovascular effects of dihydropyridine calcium-channel antagonists and their relation to drug levels in plasma. *Ann NY Acad Sci* 1988; 522:628-629.

58. Laederach K, Weidmann P, Lauener F, et al. Comparative acute effects of the calcium channel blockers tiapamil, nisoldipine and nifedipine on blood pressure and some regulatory factors in normal and hypertensive subjects. *J Cardiovasc Phamacol* 1986; 8:294-302.

59. Taira N, Takahashi K: Cardiovascular profile of nisoldipine as compared to nifedipine in dogs. In: Hugenholtz PG, Meyer J, eds. *Nisoldipine 1987*. Berlin: Springer-Verlag, 1987;131–143.

60. Serruys PW, Suryapranata H, Planellas J, et al. Acute effects of intravenous nisoldipine on left ventricular function and coronary hemodynamics. *Am J Cardiol* 1985; 56:140–146.

61. Lopez LM, Rubin MR, Holland JP, et al. Improvement in exercise performance with nisoldipine, a new second generation calcium blocker in stable angina patients, clinical investigations. *Am Heart J* 1985; 110: 991–996.

62. Lam J, Chaitman BR, Crean P, et al. A dose-ranging, placebo-controlled, double-blind trial of nisoldipine in effort angina: Duration and extent of antianginal effects. *J Am Coll Cardiol* 1985; 6:447–452.

63. Reicher-Reiss H, Vered Z, Goldbourt H, et al. Efficacy of nisoldipine compared with nifedipine in chronic stable angina. In: Hugenholtz PG, Meyer J, eds. *Nisoldipine 1987*. Berlin: Springer-Verlag, 1987;233–237.

64. Pedersen TR, Kantor M: Nifedipine three times daily versus nisoldipine once daily in patients with severe effort angina pectoris pretreated with atenolol (abstr). *Cardiovasc Drugs Ther* 1987; 1:275.

65. Rosendorff C, Goodman C. Double-blind, double-dummy, cross-over study of the efficacy and safety of nisoldipine (BAY K-5552) versus nifedipine. *Curr Ther Res* 1985; 37:912–920.

66. Daniels AR, Opie LH. Monotherapy with the calcium channel antagonist nisoldipine for systemic hypertension and comparison with diuretic drugs. *Am J Cardiol* 1987; 60:703–707.

67. Lund-Johansen P, Omvik P: Central hemodynamic changes of calcium antagonists at rest and during exercise in essential hypertension. *J Cardiovasc Pharmacol* 1987;10 (Suppl 1):S139–S148.

68. Catagay M, Frost N, Weiss KH, et al. Assessment of long-term efficacy and tolerability of nisoldipine by the clinical data pool. In: Hugenholtz PG, Meyer J, eds. *Nisoldipine 1987*. Berlin: Springer-Verlag, 1987;201–210.

69. Barjon J-N, Rouleau J-L, Bichet D, et al. Chronic renal and neurohumoral effects of the calcium entry blocker nisoldipine in patients with congestive heart failure. *J Am Coll Cardiol* 1987; 9:622–630.

70. Kiowski W, Erne P, Pfisterer M, et al. Arterial vasodilator, systemic and coronary hemodynamic effects of nisoldipine in congestive heart failure secondary to ischemic or dilated cardiomyopathy. *Am J Cardiol* 1987; 59:1118–1125.

71. Hess P, Lansman JB, Tsien RW. Different modes of Ca channel gating behaviour favoured by dihydropyridine Ca agonists and antagonists. *Nature* 1984; 311:538–544.

72. Muller FB, Bolli P, Erne P, et al. Antihypertensive therapy with long-acting calcium antagonist nitrendipine. *J Cardiovasc Pharmacol* 1984; 6 (Suppl 7):S1073–S1076.

73. Scriabine A, Anderson CL, Janis RA, et al. Some recent pharmacological findings with nitrendipine. *J Cardiovasc Pharmacol* 1984; 6 (Suppl 7):S937–S943.

74. Kann J, Krol GJ, Raemsch KD, et al. Bioequivalence and metabolism of nitrendipine administered orally to healthy volunteers. *J Cardiovasc Pharmacol* 1984; 6 (Suppl 7): S968–973.

75. Franz IW, Wiewel D: Antihypertensive effects on blood pressure at rest and during exercise of calcium antagonists, β-receptor blockers, and their combination in hypertensive

patients. *J Cardiovasc Pharmacol* 1984; 6 (Suppl 7):S1037–S1042.

76. Muller FB, Bolli P, Erne P, et al. Calcium antagonism—a new concept for treating essential hypertension. *Am J Cardiol* 1986; 57:50D–53D.

77. M'Buyamba-Kabangu JR, Lepira B, Fagard R, et al. Relative potency of a beta-blocking and a calcium entry blocking agent as antihypertensive drugs in black patients. *Eur J Clin Pharmacol* 1986; 29:523–527.

78. M'Buyamba-Kabangu JR, Fagard R, Linjen P, et al. Calcium entry blockade or beta-blockade in long-term management of hypertension in blacks. *Clin Pharmacol Ther* 1987; 41:45–54.

79. Fagan TC, Sternleib C, Vlachakis N. Efficacy and safety comparison of nitrendipine and hydralazine as antihypertensive monotherapy. *J Cardiovasc Pharmacol* 1984; 6(Suppl 7):S1109–S1113.

80. Weber MA, Drayer JIM. The calcium channel blocker nitrendipine in single- and multiple-agent antihypertensive regimens: Preliminary report of a multicenter study. *J Cardiovasc Pharmacol* 1984; 6(Suppl 7):S1077–S1084.

81. Schoenberger JA, Glasser SP, Ram CVS, et al. Comparison of nitrendipine combined with low-dose hydrochlorothiazide to hydrochlorothiazide alone in mild to moderate essential hypertension. *J Cardiovasc Pharmacol* 1984; 6(Suppl 7):S1105–S1108.

82. Salzmann R, Bormann G, Herzig JW, et al. Pharmacological actions of APP 201-533, a novel cardiotonic agent. *J Cardiovasc Pharmacol* 1985; 7:588–596.

83. Kirch W, Hutt HJ, Heidmann H, et al. Drug interactions with nitrendipine. *J Cardiovasc Pharmacol* 1984; 6(Suppl 7):S982–S985.

84. Olivari MT, Levine TB, Weir EK, et al. Hemodynamic effects of nifedipine at rest and during exercise in primary pulmonary hypertension. *Chest* 1984; 86:14–19.

85. Daniels AR, Opie LH: Atenolol plus nifedipine for mild to moderate systemic hypertension after fixed doses of either agent alone. *Am J Cardiol* 1986; 57:965–970.

86. Singer DRJ, Markandu ND, Shore AC, et al. Nifedipine and acebutolol in combination for the treatment of moderate to severe essential hypertension. *J Hum Hypertens* 1987; 1:31–37.

87. Gould BA. Hornung RS, Mann S, et al. Slow channel inhibitors verapamil and nifedipine in the management of hypertension. *J Cardiovasc Pharmacol* 1982; 4(Suppl III):S369–S373.

88. MacGregor GA. Hypertension. In: Krebs R, ed. *Treatment of Cardiovascular Diseases by Adalat^R (Nifedipine)*. Stuttgart: Schattauer, 1986;231–258.

89. Vetrovec GW, Parker VE, Cole S, et al. Nifedipine gastrointestinal therapeutic system in stable angina pectoris. Results of a multicenter open-label crossover comparison with standard nifedipine. *Am J Med* 1987;83(Suppl 6B):24–29.

90. Raferty EB. *Verapamil SR. Once-Daily Calcium Blockade in Angina and Hypertension.* Langhorne: ADIS Press International, 1987.

91. Kohli RS, Rodrigues EA, Hughes LO, et al. Sustained release verapamil, a once daily preparation: Objective evaluation using exercise testing, ambulatory monitoring and blood levels in patients with stable angina. *J Am Coll Cardiol* 1987; 9:615–621.

92. Brugmann U. Calcium antagonists in hypertension and coronary heart disease. Results of a double-blind, randomized,

placebo-controlled study with sustained-release verapamil. In: Rosenthal J, ed. *Calcium Antagonists and Hypertension: Current Status.* Amsterdam: Excerpta Medica, 1986;209-219.

93. Buhler FR, Hulthen U, Kiowski W, et al. The place of the calcium antagonist verapamil in antihypertensive therapy. *J Cardiovasc Pharmacol* 1982; 4:S350-S357.

94. Taylor SH, Silke B. Continuous blood pressure control with sustained verapamil in essential hypertension. In: Raftery EB, ed. *Verapamil SR. Once-Daily Calcium Blockade in Angina and Hypertension.* Langhorne: ADIS Press International, 1987;57-62.

95. Midtbo K, Hals O, van der Meer J, et al. Instant and sustained-release verapamil in the treatment of essential hypertension. *Am J Cardiol* 1986; 57:59D-63D.

96. Schwartz JB, Keefe DL, Kirsten E, et al. Prolongation of verapamil elimination kinetics during chronic oral administration. *Am Heart J* 1982; 104:198-203.

97. Frishman W, Charlap S, Kimmel B, et al. Twice-daily administration of oral verapamil in the treatment of essential hypertension. *Arch Intern Med* 1986: 146:561-565.

98. Norris RJ, Brooks SG. Pharmacokinetics of a sustained release formulation of verapamil in young and elderly adults. In: Raftery EB, ed. *Verapamil SR. Once-Daily Calcium Blockade in Angina and Hypertension.* Langhorne: ADIS Press International, 1987;38-46.

99. Kellaway IW. The development and clinical implications of sustained release formulations. In: Raftery EB, ed. *Verapamil SR. Once-Daily Calcium Blockade in Angina and Hypertension.* Langhorne: ADIS Press International, 1987;30-37.

100. Weiner DA, Cutler SS, Klein MD. Efficacy and safety of sustained-released diltiazem in stable angina pectoris. *Am J Cardiol* 1986; 57:6-9.

101. Osterrieder W: Inhibition of the fast Na^+ inward current by the CA^{2+} channel blocker tiapamil. *J Cardiovasc Pharmacol* 1986; 8:1101-1106.

102. Eichler HG, Mabin TA, Commerford PJ, et al. Tiapamil, a new calcium antagonist: Hemodynamic effects in acute myocardial infarction. *Circulation* 1985; 71:770-786.

103. Khurmi NS, O'Hara MJ, Bowles MJ, et al. Randomized double-blind comparison of gallopamil and propranolol in stable angina pectoris. *Am J Cardiol* 1984; 53:684-688.

104. Hopf R, Drews H, Kaltenbach M. Anti-anginal effect of gallopamil as compared with nifedipine. In: Kaltenbach M, Hopf R, eds. *Gallopamil. Pharmacological and Clinical Profile of a Calcium Antagonist.* Berlin: Springer-Verlag, 1984;123-131.

105. Maddalena F, Casiglia E, Padrini R, et al. Gallopamil in unstable angina pectoris (abstr). Presentation to NY Acad Sci, Feb 1987.

106. Raschack M. Prolonged cardioprotective effects of anipamil, a new calcium antagonist (abstr), *Eur Heart J* 1984; 5:10.

107. Kirkels JH, Ruigrok TJ, Van Echteld CJ, Meijler FL. Protective effect of pretreatment with the calcium antagonist anipamil on the ischemic-reperfused rat myocardium: A phosphorus-31 nuclear magnetic resonance study. *J Am Coll Cardiol* 1988;11:1087-1093.

108. Ferrari R, Ceconi C, Curello S, et al, Long lasting protective effect of anipamil, a new calcium entry blocker, against myocardial ischemia and reperfusion damage (abstr), *Ann NY Acad Sci* 1988;522:522-524.

109. Nawrath H, Raschack M. (−)-Devapamil decreases tension and calcium-45 uptake in smooth muscle preparations from rat aorta (abstr). Presentation to NY Acad Sci, Feb 1987.

110. Au TLS, Curtis MJ, Walker MJA. Effects of (−), (+), and (+) verapamil on coronary occlusion-induced mortality and infarct size. *J Cardiovasc Pharmacol* 1987; 10:327-331.

111. Thandroyen FT, Higginson L, Opie LH, et al. The influence of verapamil and its isomers on vulnerability to ventricular fibrillation during acute myocardial ischemia and adrenergic stimulation in isolated rat heart. *J Mol Cell Cardiol* 1986; 18:645-649.

112. Spedding M. Calcium antagonist subgroups. *Trends Pharmaceut Sci* 1985; 6:109-114.

113. Spedding M. Activators and inactivators of Ca^{++} channels: New perspectives. *J Pharmacol* 1985; 16:319-343.

114. Spedding M, Berg C. Interactions between a "calcium channel agonist", Bay K 8644, and calcium antagonists differentiate calcium antagonist subgroups in K^+-depolarized smooth muscle. *Naunyn-Schmiedebergs Arch Pharmacol* 1984; 328:69-75.

115. Terada K, Ohya Y, Kitamura K, et al. Actions of flunarizine, a Ca^{2+} antagonist, on ionic currents in fragmented smooth muscle cells of the rabbit small intestine. *J Pharmacol Exp Ther* 1987; 240:978-983.

116. Kato R, Singh BN. Effects of bepridil on the electrophysiologic properties of isolated canine and rabbit myocardial fibers. *Am Heart J* 1986; 111:271-279.

117. Perelman MS, Mckenna WJ, Rowland E, et al. A comparison of bepridil with amiodarone in the treatment of established atrial fibrillation. *Br Heart J* 1987; 58:339-344.

118. Roy D, Montigny M, Klein GJ, et al. Electrophysical effects and long-term efficacy of bepridil for current supraventricular tachycardias. *Am J Cardiol* 1987; 59:89-92.

119. Remme WJ, van Hoofenhuyze DCA, Kraus XH, et al. Dose related coronary and systemic haemodynamic effects of intravenous bepridil in patients with coronary artery disease. *Eur Heart J* 1987; 8:130-140.

120. Shapiro W, DiBianco R, Thadani U, et al. Comparative efficacy of 200, 300 and 400 mg of bepridil for chronic stable angina pectoris. *Am J Cardiol* 1985; 55:36C-42C.

121. Hill JA, O'Brien JT, Scott E, et al. Effects of bepridil on exercise tolerance in chronic stable angina: A double-blind, randomized, placebo-controlled, crossover trial. *Am J Cardiol* 1984; 53:679-683.

122. Pflugfelder PW, Humen DP, O'Brien PA, et al. Comparison of bepridil with nadolol for angina pectoris. *Am J Cardiol* 1987; 59:1283-1288.

123. Frishman WH, Charlap S, Farnham DJ, et al. Combination propranolol and bepridil therapy in stable angina pectoris. *Am J Cardiol* 1985; 55:43C-49C.

124. Hill JA, Pepine CJ. Effects of bepridil on the resting electrocardiogram. *Int J Cardiol* 1984; 6:319-323.

125. Surawicz B, Knoebel SB. Long QT: Good, bad or indifferent? *J Am Coll Cardiol* 1984; 4:398-413.

126. Shapiro W, Narahara KA, Park J. The effects of lidoflazine on exercise performance and thallium stress scintigraphy in patients with stable angina pectoris. *Circulation* 1982; 65:1-43.

127. Hanley SP, Hampton JR. Ventricular arrhythmias associated with lidoflazine: Side-effects observed in a randomized trial. *Eur Heart J* 1983; 4:889-893.

128. Keren G, Tepper D, Butler B, et al. Studies on the possible mechanisms of lidoflazine arrhythmogenicity. *J Am Coll Cardiol* 1984; 4:742-747.

129. Wauquier A, Fransen J, Clincke G, et al. Calcium entry blockers as cerebral protecting agents. In: Godfraind T, et al., eds. *Calcium Entry Blockers and Tissue Protection.* New York: Raven Press, 1985;163-172.

130. Newberg LA, Steen PA, Milde JH, et al. Failure of flunarizine to improve cerebral blood flow or neurologic recovery in a canine model of complete cerebral ischemia. *Stroke* 1984; 15:666-671.

131. Itoh T, Satoh S, Ishimatsu T, et al. Mechanisms of flunarizine-induced vasodilation in the rabbit mesenteric artery. *Circ Res* 1987; 61:446-454.

132. Silver PJ, Sulkowski TS, Lappe RW, et al. Wy-46,300 and Wy-46,531: Vascular smooth muscle relaxant/antihypertensive agents with combined Ca^{2+} antagonist/myosin phosphorylation inhibitory mechanisms. *J Cardiovasc Pharmacol* 1986; 8:1168-1175.

133. Bayer R, Martini E, Heckelmann F. Calcium channel-independent action of fendiline in vascular smooth muscle (abstr). *J Mol Cell Cardiol* 1987; 19 (Suppl III):S4.

134. Marshall RJ, Winslow E, Relevance of intracellular actions of Ca^{++}-antagonists in the treatment of coronary heart disease (abstr). *J Mol Cell Cardiol* 1987; 19(Suppl III):S57.

135. Belz GG. Fendiline: Clinical pharmacological profile of a Ca^{++}-CaM-antagonist (abstr). *J Mol Cell Cardiol* 1987; 19(Suppl III):S5.

136. Erwes H. Fendiline in the treatment of coronary heart disease (abstr). *J Mol Cell Cardiol* 1987; 19 (Suppl III):S21.

137. Thandroyen FT, McCarthy J, Burton K, et al. Ryanodine and caffeine prevent ventricular arrhythmias during acute myocardial ischemia and reperfusion in rat heart. *Circ Res* 1988;62:306-314.

138. Shibata S, Wakabayashi S, Satake N, et al. Mode of vasorelaxing action of 5-[3][2−(3,4−dimethoxyphenyl)−ethyl]amino]−1−oxopropyl]−2,3,4,5−tetrahydro−1,5−benzothiazepine fumarate (KT-362), a new intracellular calcium antagonist. *J Pharmacol Exp Ther* 1987; 240:16-22.

139. Edgar B, Hoffman KJ, Lundborg P, et al. Absorption, distribution and elimination of felodipine in man. *Drugs* 1985; 29(Suppl 2):9-15.

140. Raemsch KD, Luecker PW, Wetzelsberger N. Pharmacokinetics of intravenously and orally administered nimodipine (abstr). *Clin Pharmacol Ther* 1987; 41:216.

141. Lasseter KC, Shamblen EC, Lettieri J, et al. Dose-proportional pharmacokinetics of nisoldipine in healthy volunteers (abstr). *Clin Pharmacol Ther* 1987; 41:234.

142. Pasanisi F, Meredith PA, Reid JL. The pharmacodynamics and pharmacokinetics of a new calcium antagonist nisoldipine in normotensive and hypertensive subjects. *Eur J Clin Pharmacol* 1985; 29:21-24.

143. Stieren B, Buhler V, Hege, et al. Pharmacokinetics and metabolism of gallopamil. In: Kaltenbach M, Hopf R, eds. *Gallopamil. Pharmacological and Clinical Profile of a Calcium Antagonist.* Berlin: Springer-Verlag, 1984;88-93.

CALCIUM CHANNEL ANTAGONISTS: PART VI: CLINICAL PHARMACOKINETICS OF FIRST AND SECOND-GENERATION AGENTS

SUMMARY. A survey of the pharmacokinetic properties of the three prototypical calcium antagonist agents shows that they have in common a very high rate of hepatic first-pass metabolism with, in the case of verapamil and diltiazem, the formation of an active metabolite that affects the dose during chronic therapy. Therefore, the major factor altering the pharmacokinetic properties and the dose of the drug required is the capacity of the liver to metabolize the drug, which in turn depends on the hepatic blood flow and the activity of the hepatic metabolizing systems. Hence liver disease, a low cardiac output, and coadministration of certain drugs inducing or inhibiting the hepatic enzymes, all indirectly affect the pharmacokinetic properties of the calcium antagonists. There are also other potential drug interactions of a kinetic or dynamic nature that may arise. In general, renal disease has little effect on the pharmacokinetics of calcium antagonists.

Patient Profiling for Drug Choice and Dose

Having made the decision to use a calcium antagonist the drug dosage needs to be matched to the patient. Here the art of patient profiling comes in. What is the influence of age, of concomitant left ventricular failure, of liver disease, and of renal failure? Does the chronic dose differ from the acute? To answer these questions needs an understanding of the pharmacokinetics of each calcium antagonist in normal patients and in those with conditions likely to alter the dosage. The pharmacokinetic properties of each of the major calcium antagonists need to be considered, including the influences of age and of major disease states. These data help to match the patient's unique physiological and pathological characteristics with the ideal dosage of the drug, so that patient profiling becomes an important component of the administration of calcium antagonists. First, the pharmacokinetics of the three prototypical agents, verapamil, nifedipine, and diltiazem, will be reviewed, followed in alphabetical order by those of the second-generation agents, which are almost all dihydropyridines.

245

Verapamil

Verapamil, the oldest of the calcium antagonists, has been best known for its antiarrhythmic effect on supraventricular tachycardias. More recently, the discoveries of German investigators in the late 1960s have come to be reapplied, so that the antianginal and antihypertensive qualities have now been confirmed. The hemodynamic effects (hypotension) of IV verapamil have a rapid onset, with a peak effect on blood pressure at 5 minutes. The peak depression of the AV node occurs at 10 to 15 minutes and lasts up to 6 hours. Oral verapamil starts to act within 1 to 2 hours, with a peak blood concentration at about the same time [1]. Because of the high rate of first-pass liver metabolism, the usual oral daily dose is 12 to 40 times the intravenous dose.

Pharmacokinetics

Absorption. Single-dose studies on normal volunteers show that after oral administration the drug is almost completely absorbed [2] and the plasma concentrations peak within 1 to 2 hours [1]. The bioavailability is, however, only about 10–35% [2, 3]. The discrepancy between low bioavailability and high absorption is explained by the fact that verapamil undergoes an extensive presystemic or first-pass extraction and metabolism.

Metabolism. Verapamil is metabolized in the liver through N-dealkylation (to norverapamil) and then 0-demethylation via the cytochrome P-450 metabolizing enzyme systems. *Norverapamil* appears rapidly in the plasma after oral administration of verapamil, and in concentrations similar to those of the parent compound; like verapamil, norverapamil undergoes delayed clearance during chronic dosing. Whereas norverapamil has 22% of the vasodilating activity of the parent compound [4], the 0-demethylated metabolite exhibits the same potency as the parent. Because, however, the latter compound is present as the glucuronide, which has no pharmacological activity, its presence in the blood is of no pharmacodynamic significance. When radiolabeled verapamil is administered to volunteers, about 70% of the dose is excreted in the urine and 15% in feces, with only about 3% recovered in the urine in the unchanged form.

Plasma levels. Therapeutic plasma levels (80 to 400 ng/ml = $2-8 \times 10^{-7}$ M) are seldom used in the assessment of drug doses for patients [5]. The calculated free verapamil concentration is about $2-8 \times 10^{-8}$ M. The extensive variation in plasma concentrations measured during long-term dosing may indicate that a steady state may be difficult to reach using verapamil; therefore, interpretation of plasma concentrations and the use of such data for monitoring the verapamil dose may be extremely difficult. Furthermore, there is, as yet, little evidence that verapamil plasma levels correlate with clinical efficacy. For example, the plasma concentrations required to produce PR prolongation are three to five times greater after oral than after IV administration; the proposed explanation is that verapamil has two stereoisomers and that the more potent L-isomer is preferentially metabolized by the liver [2].

Plasma protein binding. Plasma protein binding is high (84% to 93%) and is independent of plasma concentrations. The proteins to which verapamil bind are an α_1-acid glycoprotein and albumin. There are no known drug interactions with other drugs at the level of plasma proteins over a very wide verapamil concentration range of 35 to 1557 ng/ml [6].

Elimination, distribution, and clearance. Single-dose studies in healthy volunteers and patients with cardiovascular or hepatic disease indicate that the elimination half-lives range between 3 to 7 hours and 2 to 16 hours, respectively. The *volume of distribution* of verapamil is very high, varying from 1.8 to 6.8 l/kg in healthy volunteers, and is increased to 12.1 l/kg in hepatic cirrhosis [2]. The total systemic clearance nearly approximates the hepatic blood flow and is about 1 l/kg/hour (range 0.7–1.3) [2]. There is wide intersubject variation in the clearance values.

Dosage

Oral dose. The usual dose is 240 to 360 mg (split into two or three daily doses); top doses of 480 to 720 mg have also been used. Large differences of pharmacokinetics between individuals mean that dose titration is required. Lower or higher doses may therefore be needed; the highest reported daily dose is 960 mg [7], but such levels are rarely tolerated. During chronic oral dosing, the formation of norverapamil metabolites and altered rates of hepatic metabolism may mean that a lower total daily dose of verapamil is preferable; for example, if verapamil has been titrated upwards to a dose of 160 mg three times daily during chronic dosing, the "correct" dose could be 160 mg two times daily. Several *slow-release preparations* are now available in Europe and in the USA. The usual dose is one to two capsules daily (160 to 320 mg total daily dose).

Intravenous dose. IV verapamil should be used only in monitored patients. When used for *uncontrolled atrial fibrillation* combined with myocardial disease, verapamil is infused at a very low dose (0.0001 mg/kg/min) and titrated against the ventricular response, especially if the patient has already received β blockade or when digitalis toxicity is suspected. In the absence of these relative contraindications, verapamil may safely be started at a higher rate (0.005 mg/kg/min, increasing). For *paroxysmal supraventricular tachycardias,* when there is no myocardial depression, a bolus of 5 to 10 mg (0.07 to 0.15 mg/kg) can be given over 1 minute and repeated 10 minutes later if needed; the infusion rate after a successful bolus is 0.005 mg/kg/min for about 30 to 60 minutes decreasing thereafter [8]. For supraventricular tachycardias, when there is a risk of hypotension (prior β blockade, myocardial disease, disopyramide therapy), pretreatment with calcium gluconate (90 mg, see reference 9) should be tried before an infusion of verapamil (1 mg/min over 10 minutes). Another more complex regime, designed to maintain blood levels at about 150 ng/ml is: (1) a loading bolus of 10 mg over 2 minutes; (2) a rapid infusion of 0.375 mg/min for 30 minutes and then (3) a maintenance infusion of 0.125 mg/min [10].

Kinetics during chronic dosing. During chronic dosing, verapamil accumulation occurs, as shown by steady-state plasma concentrations two to three times higher than with acute dosing [11, 12]. There is also a considerable increase in the area under the concentration-time curve (AUC) of both verapamil and norverapamil during chronic dosing [3, 13]. The increased verapamil levels may be caused by saturation of the first-pass hepatic metabolism or by an actual prolongation of the half-life (controversial: compare references 11 and 12 with reference 2). There is also much interindividual variation in the bioavailability during chronic dosing. However, assuming a direct correlation between plasma concentrations and efficacy/side effects, the verapamil dose should be reduced to produce the desired plasma concentration and to minimize the occurrence of unwanted side effects.

Effects of age on dosage. In *pediatric patients,* long-term therapy at a daily dose of 0.4 to 2.9 mg/kg (mean, 1.36 mg/kg) can achieve clinical control of supraventricular tachycardia with mean plasma levels of 248 ng/ml and norverapamil levels of 64 ng/ml; elimination half-life is longer in younger than in older children [14].

In *elderly patients,* lower doses of verapamil are required [15], probably because hepatic blood flow is lower and hence the rate of metabolism of verapamil is less, with an increase in peak plasma verapamil concentrations by about 25% [16]. An important benefit in the elderly is the absence of any loss of memory, as has been found with β blockers and methyldopa [16].

In *pregnancy,* verapamil has been used (360–480 mg daily) against pregnancy hypertension [17]. Because about 20–25% of verapamil crosses the placenta, oral verapamil in a dose up to 480 mg daily can be used in the control of *intrauterine fetal tachycardias [18].*

Liver cirrhosis. When IV verapamil is given, the total plasma clearance is reduced, the volume of distribution is almost doubled, and the terminal half-life is prolonged about fourfold. Echizen and Eichelbaum [2] suggest that the dose should be reduced by about one half. In the case of oral verapamil, much higher blood levels are reached in patients with cirrhosis, the area under the curve is considerably greater, and the elimination time is much prolonged. Echizen and Eichelbaum [2] suggest that the dose should be reduced to about one fifth of that given to subjects with normal hepatic status.

Renal and other diseases. The kinetics of verapamil are unaltered in *renal disease,* both in the case of the IV and the oral preparations, so that no dose adjustment is required [19]. However, in very advanced renal disease, the excretion of active verapamil metabolites is reduced so that the dose of verapamil also needs to be less [15].

In *diabetes,* although there have been fears that calcium antagonists could precipitate diabetes, verapamil unexpectedly appears to have a mild hypoglycemic effect [20], so that it would be wise to check blood glucose values upon the addition of verapamil to oral hypoglycemic agents.

Lipid disorders. Thus far there has been no report that verapamil could alter blood lipid constituents.

Myocardial disease. A low cardiac output, by decreasing hepatic blood flow, will decrease the hepatic clearance of verapamil and thereby increase blood levels. Furthermore, there is a greater risk of added pharmacokinetic interaction with β blockers, quinidine, or disopyramide therapy so that a considerable negative inotropic effect could result.

Drug Interactions

The major pharmacokinetic drug interactions are with digoxin (verapamil considerably increases digoxin levels) and at the level of hepatic metabolism that is accelerated by cimetidine (controversial, see references 2 and 21). The enzyme inducers, phenobarbital, rifampin, phenytoin, and sulfinpyrazone, all tend to accelerate verapamil metabolism [21–23]. With rifampicin 600 mg daily, there is nearly total reduction in the bioavailability of oral verapamil (120 mg) but not of intravenous verapamil [23a]. Because of the high first-pass liver metabolism of verapamil, up to a doubling of the dose of verapamil may be required during the coadminstration of enzyme inducers [21]. Data concerning a possible phenytoin-verapamil interaction are scant; however, the trend should be in the same direction as with the other enzyme inducers. There are pharmacodynamic interactions between verapamil and β-blockers, alpha blockers, and the antiarrhythmic drugs quinidine and disopyramide (for further details, see Part IV of this series, Table IV-5).

Nifedipine

Dihydropyridines are, in general, powerful arteriolar vasodilators with relatively scant effects on the SA and AV nodes in clinical doses. The major direct negative inotropic effect of the prototypical drug nifedipine is usually outweighed by its arteriolar unloading effects in clinical practice. Thus the arterial unloading qualities of nifedipine have been used in the management of all grades of hypertension, acute pulmonary edema, and angina of effort. Vigorous vasodilatory qualities explain the use of nifedipine in Prinzmetal's variant angina and in Raynaud's phenomenon. In congestive heart failure (CHF), arterial vasodilation usually offsets the direct negative inotropic effect. Lacking a clinically significant action against the AV node, nifedipine is ineffective against supraventricular arrhythmias. Because of reflex sympathetic stimulation following vasodilation and the absence of direct clinical effects on the SA node, nifedipine tends to increase the heart rate. The latter change is lessened during chronic therapy as the baroreflexes become less sensitive to the effects of vasodilation.

Pharmacokinetics

Absorption. Nifedipine (capsule form) is almost fully absorbed after an oral dose, although only about 45% to 68% of the drug reaches the systemic circulation. This relatively low bioavailability is due to active first-pass hepatic metabolism. Peak blood values are reached within 20 to 45 minutes; nifedipine remains detectable in the blood for up to 6 hours. The hypotensive effect starts within 20 minutes of an oral dose and within 5 minutes of a sublingual or bite-and-swallow dose; the duration of action is 8 to 12 hours in some studies with an effect of only 4 to 6 hours in other studies.

Metabolism. Nifedipine undergoes almost complete (95%) hepatic oxidation to three pharmacologically inactive metabolites, which are then excreted in the urine.

Plasma levels. Considerable variations in peak plasma nifedipine concentrations after oral and sublingual administration, and the time required to reach these peaks, have been found. Presumably there are interindividual differences in the rate of drug absorption and/or in the extent of first-pass hepatic extraction and metabolism.

Despite the difficulties involved in establishing a direct relationship between nifedipine plasma concentrations and clinical effects, some studies have shown plasma nifedipine concentrations to correlate well with changes in blood pressure [24], heart rate, and lower esophageal sphincter pressure [25]. Kleinbloesem et al. [26] found that the minimal effect of nifedipine plasma concentration was about 15 mg/ml. In hypertrophic cardiomyopathy, optimal blood levels are 60–120 ng/ml; negative inotropic effects dominate at higher concentrations [26a]. The therapeutic concentration in humans is 15 to 200 mg/ml [27], ie.e., $0.3-4\times10^{-7}$M. The calculated free unbound plasma level is about $0.1-2\times10^{-8}$M.

Plasma protein binding. The protein binding of nifedipine to albumin is concentration-dependent and varies from 92% to 98%. Because the drug is so poorly soluble in water, little nifedipine is found free in the cerebrospinal fluid or plasma [27].

Elimination, distribution, and clearance. The elimination half-life of nifedipine is apparently dependent upon the dosage form in which it is administered, with half-lives of 3 hours, 5 to 11 hours, and 1.5 hours measured after oral capsule, oral tablet, and intravenous administration, respectively [2]. However, the slow-release preparation of nifedipine has a much lower absorption than elimination time and therefore the longer half-life really reflects a delayed rate of absorption, which is termed flip-flop kinetics [28]. The total systemic clearance of nifedipine from the plasma is about 0.5 l/kg/hour (range 0.4 to 0.6), which is primarily due to hepatic metabolism, and the volume of distribution about 0.6 to 1.4 l/kg, showing significant distribution to the tissues [2].

Dosage and route of administration

Nifedipine capsules. The usual dose for *angina* is 10 to 20 mg (one to two capsules) three times daily, going up to 20 mg four times daily [29]. In effort angina, dose titration is advisable to avoid precipitation of pain by nifedipine in some patients. In severe *hypertension*, 10 mg sublingually usually brings down the pressure within 20 to 60 minutes. In mild to moderate hypertension, the required dose as monotherapy may be up to 20 mg three times daily.

Sublingual vs. bite-and-swallow dosage. Although sublingual nifedipine is the standard route used when a very rapid action is required, recent data suggest that the bite-and-swallow method gives much higher blood levels more rapidly than true sublingual absorption [30, 31].

Nifedipine tablets (Adalat Retard^R). Nifedipine tablets cause blood levels to fall and rise more slowly, thus lessening some of the subjective side effects of nifedipine because the baroreflexes have a greater time to reset [32]. Nonetheless, it should be noted that this compound has an absorption time that exceeds the elimination time, so that the typical half-life is in fact dependent on the rate of absorption. As an approximation, the dose of nifedipine tablets may be about twice as high as that of nifedipine capsules.

GITS nifedipine. The gastrointestinal therapeutic system allows a slow controlled rate of release of nifedipine with sustained plasma levels 6 to 30 hours after administration [33]. The usual daily dose is similar to the total daily dose of capsules [34].

Intravenous dose. In Europe, a bolus of 15 µg/kg over 5 minutes followed by 0.9 mg/hour over 24 hours has been used in the treatment of acute myocardial infarction [35]. Nifedipine needs to be given through black polyethylene syringes and lines to prevent photodegradation [35]. Pharmacokinetic parameters included a steady-state level of 17 ng/ml, plasma clearance of 0.9 l/min, volume of distribution 3.9 l/kg, and elimination half-life of 3.6 hours.

Acute vs. chronic dosage of nifedipine. There is no suggestion of any difference in kinetics between the acute and chronic dosage as in the case of verapamil.

Effects of age on dosage. In *pediatric patients* with hypertensive emergencies, sublingual nifedipine 0.25 mg to 0.5 mg/kg has been used as a single dose [36]. In infants with hypertrophic cardiomyopathy with cardiac failure, nifedipine was started as 0.6 mg/kg/day in divided doses and then increased to 0.9 mg/kg/day [37].

In *elderly patients*, there is reduced first-pass metabolism so that the elimination half-life is almost double that of younger patients. This difference, together with the fear of abrupt peripheral vasodilation with cerebral underperfusion, suggests that the initial dose in elderly patients should be 5 mg and not 10 mg (the 5-mg capsule form is available in many countries, otherwise cut a 10-mg capsule in half). Using the slow-release preparation, the elimination half-life varies from about 4 to 6 hours in young patients to 7 to 9 hours in the elderly [28, 38]. In elderly patients, nifedipine slow release has been used in doses of 20 to 60 mg twice daily [39].

In *pregnant patients,* nifedipine is usually held to be contraindicated. However, nifedipine has successfully been used to treat severe pregnancy hypertension [40].

Liver cirrhosis. The elimination half-life of nifedipine is prolonged in liver cirrhosis, probably because hepatic blood flow is decreased and there is decreased activity of the drug-degrading liver enzymes. Furthermore, the free fraction of nifedipine is nearly doubled because of changes in plasma protein binding. For all these reasons [27], the dose of nifedipine should be reduced in liver cirrhosis.

Renal and other diseases. In *renal disease,* there is no difference in the clearance rates of nifedipine, even when there is severe renal impairment with creatinine clearance rates of below 10 ml/min [41]. The pharmacokinetics of nifedipine are also not altered during hemodialysis or peritoneal dialysis [42]. For these reasons, nifedipine appears to be a simple drug to use in renal failure.

Diabetes. In isolated case reports, nifedipine has been shown to impair glucose tolerance and occasionally to precipitate diabetes. Although these effects are not consistent and there are no such effects upon careful prospective testing [43, 44], in individial patients with diabetes or in a prediabetic state, it would be prudent to monitor blood glucose during nifedipine administration.

Lipid disorders. Thus far there is no evidence that nifedipine alters any of the blood lipid constituents.

Drug interactions

The major interactions are at the level of hepatic metabolism. There is a kinetic interaction with propranolol whereby nifedipine enhances propranolol availability (less propranolol first-pass metabolism) and proranolol likewise acts on nifedipine [45]. Nifedipine only modestly increases blood digoxin levels [46]. Cimetidine inhibits hepatic metabolism of nifedipine and increases blood levels [47]. Diltiazem also increases nifedipine levels [48]. Hepatic enzyme inducers such as phenytoin, phenobarbital, rifampin, and sulfinpyrazone have opposite effects. In the case of phenytoin, nifedipine increases phenytoin levels through an unknown mechanism, based on a single case report [49]. Cigarette smoking decreases the effects of nifedipine, but not through a pharmacokinetic interaction, because blood nifedipine levels are unchanged; presumably smoking is acting by vasoconstriction [50]. There are pharmacodynamic interactions with β-blockers and alpha-adrenergic blockers. (For details, see Part IV of this book, Table IV-5).

Diltiazem

The peripheral vasodilator properties of diltiazem explain its use in hypertension and Raynaud's phenomenon. Its antianginal mechanism is largely based on coronary and peripheral vasodilation, but other properties may also be important, including an effect on myocardial diastolic function during ischemia. The electrophysiological properties of diltiazem closely resemble those of verapamil, so that diltiazem is also used in supraventricular tachycardias and atrial fibrillation.

Pharmacokinetics

Absorption. Following oral administration, over 90% is absorbed, but bioavailability is about 45% due to high first-pass hepatic metabolism [51]. The onset of action is within 15 to 30 minutes (oral), with a peak at 1 to 2 hours.

Metabolism. Diltiazem is actively metabolized in the liver, chiefly to desacetyldiltiazem, which accumulates during chronic therapy and has about 40% of the activity of the parent compound [52]. Thereafter, the metabolites are excreted chiefly by the gastrointestinal tract (65%), and to a lesser degree by the kidneys (35%).

Plasma levels. The therapeutic plasma concentration ranges are seldom measured and are not accurately known. The approximate range is 50 to 300 ng/ml or about $1-7 \times 10^{-7}$ M. The molar plasma value, corrected for protein binding, is about $1-5 \times 10-8$ M.

Protein binding and distribution. The protein binding is 80% to 86%. The percentage binding is not affected by the presence of the active desacetyl metabolite. Thirty-five to 40% of the bound fraction binds to albumin, whereas the remainder binds to α_1-acid glycoprotein and various gammaglobulins.

Elimination, distribution, and clearance. Reported half-lives for the elimination phase of diltiazem in healthy volunteers have ranged from 2 to 7 hours (average about 4.5 hours). The mean volume of distribution following single doses of diltiazem has approximated 5.3 l/kg [53]. Mean total clearance estimations in healthy volunteers and patients undergoing cardiac catheterization have ranged from 11.5 to 21.3 ml/kg/min [53]. In dogs, the plasma clearance is directly related to the hepatic blood flow [51].

Dosage

For all varieties of angina, the dose of diltiazem is 120 to 360 mg, usually in four daily doses. Strict 6-hour dosing may be needed for severe angina. Yet a single 120-mg dose improves exercise tolerance for 8 hours and three times daily dosing may be effective even in unstable or variant angina [54]. For prophylaxis of supraventricular tachycardia, doses are similar. For hypertension, twice daily doses are usual. Slow-release diltiazem-SR permits twice daily doses even in angina. IV diltiazem, not yet available in the USA and United Kingdom, is given like verapamil with a dose of 0.15 to 0.25 mg/kg over 2 minutes with ECG and blood pressure control.

Acute vs. chronic dosage. Because of the accumulation of the active desacetyl metabolite during chronic dosage, it is logical to reduce the dose of diltiazem, especially because the steady-state levels are increased [55].

Effect of age and pregnancy on dosage. In *pediatric patients,* no formal recommendations on doses have been made.

In *elderly patients,* the drug reaches a higher peak level and the blood level stays elevated for longer than in younger patients. Although more studies are required, these data suggest a reduction in the drug dose in elderly patients [2]. These changes suggest that it would be prudent to reduce the dose of diltiazem in elderly subjects. A decrease in hepatic blood flow could be responsible for the change in pharmacokinetics.

There are insufficient data to indicate whether or not diltiazem is safe for *pregnant women* and their babies; therefore diltiazem should only be used if the indication is highly specific.

Liver cirrhosis. There appear to be no detailed studies concerning the effect of liver cirrhosis on diltiazem. However, because of the high rate of first-pass metabolism of diltiazem, it would be prudent to reduce the dose in patients with liver cirrhosis.

Renal and other diseases. Renal disease, even when severe, introduces few changes into the pharmacokinetic pattern of diltiazem because only a fraction of the hepatic metabolites of diltiazem are excreted by the kidney [56]. Therefore, in general, diltiazem dose need not be altered in severe renal disease nor during hemodialysis or peritoneal dialysis.

Myocardial failure. There appear to be no data on the use of diltiazem in myocardial failure. However, a decreased hepatic blood flow is likely to decrease the conversion of diltiazem to its metabolite and to increase the blood diltiazem level. Drug dosage would therefore appear to be indicated.

Diabetes. There is no indication that diltiazem interferes with diabetic control.

Lipid disorders. Diltiazem does not alter blood lipid patterns.

Drug interactions

Diltiazem has a less marked effect than verapamil on blood digoxin levels; otherwise interactions are similar. There is, however, less added negative inotropic effect when combined with quinidine, disopyramide, or β blockade. Cimetidine delays hepatic metabolism of diltiazem so that the diltiazem dose should be reduced by about one third [21]. Conversely, hepatic enzyme inducers such as phenobarbital, phenytoin, rifampin, and sulfinpyrazone should all decrease the dose of diltiazem required. However, the appropriate observations have not been made.

Amlodipine

The major difference from the other dihydropyridines is the much longer half-life and the slower onset of effects, possibly explained by the much lower lipid solubility than in the case of nifedipine [57].

Pharmacokinetics (Table VI-I)

Absorption. The absorption is slow, with peak blood levels being reached after 6 to 12 hours [58]. The bioavailability is about 60% to 65%.

Metabolism. There is hepatic metabolism to inactive metabolites, which are subsequently excreted in the urine.

Plasma levels. 2–12 ng/ml, 24 hours after doses of 2.5 to 10 mg orally [59]. The plasma levels increase during chronic dosage [58], probably because of the very long half-life of amlodipine. The approximate

Table VI-1. Amlodipine pharmacokinetics

Authors	Subjects	Dose	T_{max} (h)	$T_{1/2\beta}$ (h)	AUC (ng.h/ml)	Distribution volume (l/kg)	Conc max (nmol/l)	Clearance (l/min)	PPB (%)
Faulkner et al. [58]	Normal	2.5–10 mg p.o.	6–10	35–45	238	21	2–12	0.5	97.5
Elliott et al. [60]	males	5 mg p.o.	—	52	321	—	4–8	—	—

Abbreviations: T_{max} = time to reach maximum plasma concentrations; $T_{1/2\beta}$ = elimination half-life, β phase; AUC = area under the curve; Conc = concentration; PPB = plasma protein binding.

calculated free plasma concentration is $0.5-3 \times 10^{-10}$ M.

Plasma protein binding. This is 95.5%.

Elimination, distribution, and clearance. The elimination half-life is 35 to 45 hours, apparently increasing with chronic dosage. The volume of distribution is approximately 20 l/kg [58]. There is a low clearance rate of 7 ml/min/kg [58].

Dosage and interactions

Dosage. For hypertension, doses of 2.5 to 10 mg once daily are given [59]; similar doses are used for angina (see Section V of this book).

In the *elderly*, the clearance is reduced and the dose may need reduction [60, 61].

Liver cirrhosis. There appears to be no data on pharmacokinetics in hepatic cirrhosis; first principles would suggest that the dose should be reduced.

Renal disease. As with other dihydropyridine calcium antagonists, the dose is unchanged.

Drug interactions. These may not resemble the patterns found for nifedipine. For example, no effect on digoxin levels has been found during coadministration of amlodipine, nor is there any effect of cimetidine on amlodipine levels.

Felodipine

Pharmacokinetics

Absorption. Felodipine solution is rapidly absorbed, with a peak plasma level being reached within about 1 hour in healthy volunteers [62]. The relatively low bioavailability of about 15% is accounted for by the high rates of hepatic metabolism. The onset of action is within 15 to 45 minutes as judged by the hypotensive effect in the case of the oral solution or after IV administration [63–65]. However, the speed of onset of the oral solution is more rapid than that of the tablets, for which the hypotensive effect takes about 1 hour [66].

Metabolism. There are numerous, at least eight, metabolites formed by hepatic breakdown [62], some of which have longer half-lives. However, none of the metabolites have been shown to be pharmacologically active.

Plasma levels (Table VI-2). The maximal plasma levels are about 14 to 115 nmol/l (about 5 to 40 ng/ml) depending on the dose (5 to 40 mg in normal volunteers) [62]. In patients with hypertension already treated by β blockers and diuretics, the plasma concentrations are 12 to 21 nmol/l at the time of the hypotensive effect.

Plasma protein binding. Plasma protein binding is in excess of 99% [62] so that the true effective free concentration in the plasma would be about 0.05 μmol/l or 5×10^{-8} M (similar range as other calcium antagonists). This concentration is experimentally able to have a vascular dilating effect without any major myocardial depressant effects [67].

Elimination and clearance. The elimination half-life varies from 2.5 to 14 hours [62]. The clearance is about 1.2–1.6 l/min [62].

Dosage. The oral dose is 7.5 to 10 mg twice daily in the therapy of hypertension [68, 69]. For the therapy of angina, thrice daily doses (5 to 10 mg three times daily) may be required.

Liver cirrhosis. In view of the high rates of presystemic elimination, a decreased dose requirement is probable in liver cirrhosis.

Renal disease. As in the case of other calcium antagonists, high rates of liver metabolism suggest that felodipine doses are unchanged in all degrees of renal failure [70].

Drug interactions. The major drug interactions are likely to be with digoxin, other drugs interacting at the level of live metabolism, and pharmacodynamic interactions such as with a β blockade.

Gallopamil

Gallopamil is a verapamil-like agent. The oral absorption is high (about 90%) and rapid, with peak plasma levels obtained 1 to 2 hours after administration [71] and with peak concentrations up to about 25 ng/ml. Bioavailability is about 15% during acute administration but rises during chronic dosage to about 23% [71]. The terminal half-life of 4 to 5 hours does not change

Table VI-2. Felodipine pharmacokinetics

Authors	Subjects	Dose	T_{max} (h)	$T_{1/2\beta}$ (h)	AUC (nmol/l/h)	Distribution volume (l/kg)	Conc max (nmol/l)	Clearance (l/min)	PPB (%)
Edgar et al. [62]	Normal	5-40 mg p.o.	0.6	2.5-14	20-275	—	14-115	1.2-1.6	>99
		1-3 mg IV	—	up to 10	—	4-10	—	—	—

For abbreviations, see Table VI-1.

with chronic administration. Plasma protein binding is about 85% to 90%. Ultimately about half is excreted in the feces and half in the urine, but very little in the unchanged form because of active metabolism. The total clearance is about 1 l/min or approximately equal to liver blood flow, so that hepatic metabolism, by N-dealkylation, is the major pathway for breakdown. During steady-state administration, there appears to be a decreased rate of hepatic metabolism (and/or increased rate of formation of active metabolites) and the steady-state plasma concentration is increased to 70 ng/ml. In liver disease, the dose should be decreased; whereas in renal disease, the dose should be unchanged. In atrial fibrillation, the elimination half-life is prolonged, possibly the result of a greater distribution volume and/or altered liver blood flow. Drug interactions, although not yet well studied in detail, can be expected to resemble verapamil.

Isradipine

Pharmacokinetics

Absorption. The absorption of the capsule is rapid and nearly complete, with peak plasma levels reached at 1.6 hours at a peak plasma level of 10 ng/ml [72]. Bioavailability is about 20% [72].

Metabolism. There is a high first-pass hepatic metabolism to several metabolites [73], ultimately eliminated by urine and feces (ratio 2:1). These metabolites have no pharmacological activity [74].

Plasma levels (Table IV-3). Peak concentrations are up to 10 ng/ml [72]. The calculated free plasma concentration is about 10^{-9} M.

Plasma protein binding. The value of 96% is provided by the manufacturers.

Elimination, distribution, and clearance. The terminal half-life is about 8 hours, the volume of distribution is high (4 l/kg), and the clearance is relatively low (0.7 l/min).

Dosage and concurrent disease

Dosage. The dosage is 5 to 7 mg two to three times daily in angina [75] and 5 to 20 mg daily in hypertension [76, 77]. In congestive heart failure, an infusion of 0.1 mg/kg/min for 30 minutes has been followed by 0.3 μg/kg for 30 minutes [78].

In *elderly patients,* no major dose adjustments are required, at least in the "young elderly" with a mean

Table VI-3. Isradipine pharmacokinetics

Authors	Subjects	Dose	T_{max} (h)	$T_{1/2\beta}$ (h)	AUC (h.ng/ml)	Distribution volume (l/kg)	Conc max (ng/ml)	Clearance (l/min)	PPB (%)
Schran et al. [72]	Normal	10 mg	1.6	8	43	4.0	10	0.7	—
	Renal disease	10 mg	1.1–1.4	9–12	29–55	5.7	7–10	0.7	—
Chellingsworth et al. [79]	Hypertensive "young"	2.5–5.0 mg p.o.	0.9–1.9	—	23–33	—	8–9	—	—
	"elderly"	2.5–5.0 mg p.o.	1.1–1.6	—	37–51	—	10–11	—	—
Pinquier et al. [109]		—	—	—	—	—	—	—	96

For abbreviations, see Table VI-1. "young" = mean age 40; "elderly" = mean age 73 age of 66 to 72 years [77, 79]. Nonetheless, blood levels tend to be higher in the elderly [72], as might be expected from their lower cardiac output.

Liver disease. The peak concentrations are somewhat higher, but there are few major changes in pharmacokinetics [72].

Renal disease. In severe renal impairment, the bioavailability falls [72].

Nicardipine

Pharmacokinetics

Absorption. After oral administration, nicardipine is rapidly and completely absorbed, and peak plasma concentrations are found between 20 minutes and 2 hours [80–82]. Arterial dilation, as manifest by an increased brachial artery blood flow, lasts for 2 to 6 hours following ingestion [80]. As in the case of most other dihydropyridines, there is a low systemic bioavailability (7% to 30%, depending on the dose [83]). Eating reduces the bioavailability to nicardipine, presumably by delaying absorption, decreasing portal blood concentrations, and hence increasing the percentage of hepatic metabolism [82].

Metabolism. Nicardipine is extensively metabolized to inactive metabolites so that very little of the parent drug is recovered in the urine [80].

Plasma levels (Table VI-4). These are 30 to 110 ng/ml, and the calculated free unbound plasma concentration is approximately 10^{-9} M.

Plasma protein binding. Plasma protein binding is 98% to 99.5% [84] at concentrations of 100 ng/ml.

Elimination and clearance. The plasma elimination half-life is short, being 4 to 5 hours [82], or even down to 35 to 110 minutes [85]. Intravenous nicardipine clearance rates are 0.4 to 1.2 l/min [83, 85, 86], with lower rates being found in patients with coronary artery disease [86]. Decreases in clearance rates with increasing doses of nicardipine suggest saturation of the hepatic mechanisms for the removal of the drug.

Dosage and concurrent disease

Dosage. The usual dosage is 5 to 30 mg three times daily. In chronic stable angina, a nicardipine dose of 90

Table VI-4. Nicardipine pharmacokinetics

Authors	Subjects	Dose	T_{max} (h)	$T_{1/2\beta}$ (h)	AUC (h.ng/ml)	Distribution volume (l/kg)	Conc max (ng/ml)	Clearance (l/min)	PPB (%)
Campbell et al. [85]	Normal	10–160 µg IV	—	<60 min	—	62.6	—	1.2	—
Graham et al. [82]	Normal	1. 5 mg/hour IV	—	4h 45 min	100–150	—	—	0.6	—
		2. 10–40 mg 8-hourly for 3 days	1	—	—	—	8–150	—	—
		3. 20 mg orally	1	—	—	—	50	—	—
		4. 20 mg orally postprandial	1	—	—	—	35	—	—
Thuillez et al. [80]	Normal	20 mg 3 times daily	1	—	371	—	30–60	—	—
Forette et al. [88]	Hypertensives	90 mg daily for 1 wk	1.4	—	—	—	107	—	—
	Elderly hypertensives	90 mg daily for 1 wk	1.2	—	—	—	291	—	—
Urien et al. [84]	Isolated tissues	In vitro	—	—	—	—	—	—	98–99.5

For abbreviations, see Table VI-1.

mg daily gave very similar results to nifedipine 30 mg daily [87]. Because it is water soluble and light insensitive, intravenous administration should be possible. In the *elderly*, higher plasma concentrations are found, probably due to decreased first-pass hepatic metabolism in the really elderly (mean age 84 years [88]), so that the dose should be reduced. In the younger elderly (mean age 70 years [89]), there are no changes and no dose reduction is needed.

Chronic dosing. Plasma concentrations do not increase during prolonged periods of administration [83].

Liver cirrhosis. No pharmacokinetic data are available in liver cirrhosis, but first principles would suggest that the drug should be given in decreasing doses.

Renal disease. Because nicardipine is eventually excreted mainly as metabolites through bile and feces, the drug may be used with relative safety, even in severe renal failure [81].

Nimodipine

Like other dihydropyridines, this agent has a high rate of liver metabolism. The oral absorption is rapid, with peak levels, of 80 ng/ml about 0.7 hours after oral administration [90]. The time of onset of action is within 1 hour, as judged by the hypotensive effect [90]. The dosage is 0.35 mg/kg 4-hourly or 30 to 40 mg three to four times daily. The elimination half-life is 2.8 hours [91]. In liver disease, the time to peak plasma level is delayed to about 2 to 3 hours, and the hypotensive effect prolonged [90]. Therefore, a dose reduction is required in liver cirrhosis. In renal disease, the area under the curve is prolonged and the terminal half-life extended to a mean of 22 hours [91]. Because less than 0.1% of nimodipine given orally is excreted unchanged in the urine [90], it is likely that the effects of renal disease on nimodipine kinetics can be explained by delayed excretion of active hepatic metabolites.

Nisoldipine

Pharmacokinetics

Absorption. The oral tablet is rapidly absorbed with, however, a very low bioavailability of only 4% to 8% [92]. Maximal plasma levels are raised within about 1.5 hours [93]. The time of onset of the oral tablet is about 30 minutes, judging by the hypotensive response [93].

Table VI-5. Nisoldipine pharmacokinetics

Authors	Subjects	Dose	T_{max} (h)	$T_{1/2\beta}$ (h)	AUC (h.ng/ml)	Distribution volume (l/kg)	Conc max (ng/ml)	Clearance (l/min)	PPB (%)
Ahr et al. [95]	Normal	20 mg p.o.	1–2	8–11*	—	2.7	3.5–5.5	—	99.7
Pasanisi et al. [93]	Normal	10 mg p.o.	1.7	2.1	—	—	1.8	—	—
Van Harten et al.	Normal	20 mg p.o.	—	13.1	—	—	4.5	0.9	—
[99]	Cirrhotics	5 mg p.o.	—	19.0	—	—	3.5	0.5	—
	Normal	0.3 mg IV	—	9.7	—	4.1	4.7	—	—
	Cirrhotics	0.37 mg IV	—	16.6	—	6.4	5.2	—	—

For abbreviations, see Table VI-1.
*Redistribution from the tissue.

Metabolism. Nisoldipine undergoes extensive hepatic metabolism to at least five metabolites [94]. The rate of biotransformation probably depends on the liver blood flow [92].

Plasma levels (Table VI-5). The peak plasma level is about 1 to 4 ng/ml [93–95]. The approximate free unbound plasma levels can be calculated at $1-3 \times 10^{-10}$ M.

Plasma protein binding. Because the unbound fraction of the drug is only 0.3% [95], the percentage protein binding is 99.7%—possibly one of the highest among the calcium antagonists.

Elimination and clearance. The elimination half-life is very variable, as in the case of some of the other calcium antagonists. Values from 2 to 13 hours are reported [92]. Although it is claimed that the longer times reflect better methodology (gas chromatography with electron capture), that technique also gave a half-life of only 2 hours in the study of Pasanisi et al. [93]. Probably the most accurate value is 11 hours [95a]. The absorption of nisoldipine is actually slower than the elimination (flip-flop model) [95].

The systemic *clearance* is about 0.9 l/min [92].

Dosage and interactions

Dosage. For hypertension, the dose is 5 to 20 mg once or twice daily. Despite the short half-life, monotherapy with 24-hour action can be achieved, however, with relatively high doses [96]. For angina, 8-hour therapy may be needed [97].

Liver cirrhosis. In cirrhosis, the oral clearance is decreased, and the terminal half-life is increased [98, 99]. As expected, the longest half-lives are associated with the lowest clearance rates and more severe degrees of liver disease [100].

Renal disease. Kinetics are unaltered in chronic renal disease [101], as expected for a drug with hepatic metabolism as a prime fate.

Drug interactions. Nisoldipine increases blood *digoxin* levels by about 16% to 20% [102]. Nisoldipine increases bioavailability of *propranolol,* presumably by increasing splanchnic blood flow and decreasing the rate of first-pass metabolism of propranolol [103]. Cimetidine and nisoldipine can be expected to interact in such a way that bioavailability of each should be increased [99], although in practice the effect is not marked. Other drug interactions can be expected to be

Table VI-6. Nitrendipine pharmacokinetics

Authors	Subjects	Dose	T_{max} (h)	$T_{1/2\beta}$ (h)	AUC (h.ng/ml)	Distribution volume (l/kg)	Conc max (ng/ml)	Clearance (l/min)	PPB (%)
Dylewicz et al. [107]	Normal	5 mg IV	—	2.2	62	13.4	—	1.3	98
	Cirrhosis	-do-	—	7.8*	128*	65.3*	—	0.9*	97
	Normal	20 mg p.o × 6 days	2.3	—	95*	—	19	1.4	—
	Cirrhosis	-do-	2.4	—	309*	—	30	0.7*	—
Kann et al. [104]	Normal	20 mg p.o.	1.6	6.8	30	—	9	—	—
Andren et al. [110]	Hyper- tension	20 mg p.o. × 21 days	—	11.4	70	—	—	1.4	—
	Normal	40 mg p.o. × 21 days	—	8.1	144	—	—	1.4	—
Lesseter et al. [106]	Normal	10 mg	2.0	15.3	29	—	5	—	—
	Cirrhosis	10 mg	4.5	19.6	120*	—	5	—	—
	Normal	10 mg b.d. × 5 days	2.5	20.3	48	—	9	—	—
	Cirrhosis	10 mg b.d. × 5 days	2.2	23.8	166*	—	27*	—	—
Aronoff [108]	Normal	20 mg p.o.	2.0	5.9	51	—	11	—	—
	Chronic renal failure								
	Anuric	20 mg p.o.	2.1	5.2	123	—	27	—	—
	dialyzed	20 mg p.o.	1.5	3.3	57	—	19	—	—

For abbreviations, see Table VI-1.

similar to those of nifedipine (see Part IV of this book).

Nitrendipine

Pharmacokinetics

Absorption. The oral tablet is relatively well absorbed, with a bioavailability of 60% to 70% [104]. Peak plasma levels are reached within about 2 hours (see Table VI-6). The time of onset of action of the oral preparation is about 1 hour, judging by an increased heart rate [105].

Metabolism. Metabolism is by hepatic oxidative breakdown to four inactive metabolites [104], which are excreted chiefly in the feces (60%) and in the urine (30%).

Plasma levels. The plasma levels are very variable (see Table VI-6). Values of 9 to 42 ng/ml are obtained during chronic dosing, with trough levels of about 2.1 ng/ml [106]. Approximate free plasma levels are about $1-5 \times 10^{-9}$ M.

Plasma protein binding. Plasma protein binding is very high, being about 98% [107].

Elimination and clearance. The elimination half-life $(T_{1/2\beta})$ is also very variable (Table VI-6), including values of 2, 6, 7, and 15 hours in normal subjects, with, possibly, an average of 7 to 8 hours. The clearance is about 1.3 l/min.

Dosage and interactions

Dosage. The standard dose is 10 to 20 mg one to two times daily. In view of the variable elimination half-life, once daily administration cannot be guaranteed to sustain adequate blood levels.

Liver cirrhosis. In liver cirrhosis, there is an increased area under the curve, and a prolonged half-life [107], as well as an increased maximum plasma concentration [106]. Although the studies of Dylewicz et al. [107] do not fully accord with those of Lasseter et al. [106], the message is that in chronic liver disease oxidative breakdown of nitrendipine will be decreased, the are under the curve will be increased, and the dose should be reduced.

Renal disease. In *chronic renal disease,* there are no major changes in anuric individuals, whereas in chronic renal failure, the area under the curve and the plasma levels are increased, although statistical significance was not achieved [108]. Logically, chronic renal disease should have no effect on the kinetics of nitrendipine because of the very high rate of liver metabolism.

Drug interactions. The major drug interaction is the doubling of the digoxin dose during administration of nitrendipine. When β blockers are coadministered, the area under the curve and the plasma concentration of nitrendipine tends to rise, presumably because of reduced hepatic blood flow. Unexpectedly, cimetidine and ranitidine had no effects on nitrendipine kinetics (Table VI-7).

Patient Profiling—The Influence of Pre-existing Disease on Drug Dosage

The pharmacokinetic patterns of the three prototypical calcium antagonists are, therefore, relatively simple. They are all highly lipid-soluble, all are highly protein bound, and all undergo substantial first-pass hepatic metabolism. In the case of nifedipine, the parent compound is broken down to inactive metabolites. In the case of verapamil and diltiazem, among the major metabolites are those (one in each case) that have pharmacologic activity. Thus in the case of verapamil and diltiazem, chronic dosage may require a reduction in the overall dose used. In the case of nifedipine, drug usage stays constant.

Two major factors altering the pharmacokinetics are going to be a) the activity of the liver enzymes breaking down the calcium antagonist compounds and b) the hepatic blood flow that delivers the compounds to the liver. In effect, the major conditions altering drug dosage are going to be chronic liver disease and cardiac failure, as well as any other low cardiac-output state, including chronic β blockade. In general, renal failure is not going to be a major factor governing the dose of calcium antagonists, because verapamil, nifedipine, and diltiazem all undergo major metabolism in the liver. (An exception is nimodipine, which appears to produce active metabolites excreted by the kidney.) In the case of diltiazem, metabolite excretion is largely by the gut. In the case of verapamil, the formation of an active metabolite in the liver that is ultimately excreted in the kidney means that in very severe renal failure the dose should be reduced. Thus, apart from liver cirrhosis and conditions altering liver blood flow, the calcium antagonists as a group are remarkably easy to match to the patient. A further

Table VI-7. Nitrendipine drug interactions

Authors	Subjects	Dose	T_{max} (h)	AUC (h.ng/ml)	Conc max (ng/ml)	Clearance (l/min)
Kirch et al. [111]	Normal	20 mg p.o. × 7 days	2.0	132	42	1.3
	Normal	+ digoxin*	1.3	101	32	1.5
	Normal	+ metoprolol	1.1	141	24	1.2
	Normal	+ atenolol	1.8	224	54	0.7
	Normal	+ cimetidine	2.0	143	44	1.1
	Normal	+ ranitidine	1.1	207	33	0.9

For abbreviations, see Table VI-1.

*N.B. digoxin level doubled from 0.96 to 1.98 ng/ml (p < 0.01).

question is whether the use of calcium antagonists is likely to exaggerate any pre-existing disease or precipitate any disease states.

Will Calcium Antagonists Precipitate any Disease States?

Whereas β-blockers may exaggerate bronchospasm, cause heart failure, increase the severity of active peripheral vascular disease, interfere with insulin dosage in diabetes, and, speculatively, accelerate atherogenesis, none of these changes occur during the use of calcium antagonists. In particular, respiratory function is not impaired, diabetic control undergoes no change (with the possible exception of a lessened need for oral hypoglycemic agents during verapamil therapy), and, if anything, the atherogenic process should be inhibited by calcium antagonists. Therefore, again, calcium antagonists are relatively simple drugs to use and do not bring in their wake chronic unwanted medical complications.

Drug Interactions— The Major Complexities

Drug interactions of calcium antagonists occur with other cardiovascular agents such as alpha-adrenergic blockers, β-adrenergic blockers, digoxin, quinidine, and disopyramide (see Part IV of this book). Some of the most marked interactions are those of verapamil with digoxin, additive effects on the conduction system achieved by verapamil or diltiazem combined with β-blockers, added hypotensive effects when combined with alpha-adrenergic blockers, and added negative inotropic effects when verapamil is combined with quinidine or disopyramide. Drugs that inhibit the hepatic enzyme systems metabolizing the calcium antagonists, such as cimetidine, increase the activity of any given dose of the calcium antagonists. Conversely, enzyme-inducing drugs, such as rifampin and sulfinpyrazone, decrease the plasma levels of verapamil. Data concerning the effect of enzyme inducers on nifedipine and diltiazem are scant, but first principles suggest similar effects to those found with verapamil.

References

1. Eichelbaum M, Somogyi A. Inter- and intra-subject variations in the first-pass elimination of highly cleared drugs during chronic dosing. Studies with deuterated verapamil. *Eur J Clin Pharmacol* 1984;26:47–53.

2. Echizen H, Eichelbaum M. Clinical pharmacokinetics of verapamil, nifedipine and diltiazem. *Clin Pharmacokinetics* 1986;11:425–449.
3. Freedman SB, Richmond DR, Ashley JJ, et al. Verapamil kinetics in normal subjects and patients with coronary artery spasm. *Clin Pharmacol Ther* 1981;30:644–652.
4. Neugebauer G. Comparative cardiovascular actions of verapamil and its major metabolites in the anesthetised dog. *Cardiovasc Res* 1978;12:247–254.
5. Frishman W, Kirsten E, Klein M, et al. Clinical relevance of verapamil plasma levels in stable angina pectoris. *Am J Cardiol* 1982;50:1180–1184.
6. Keefe DL, Yee Y-G, Kates RE. Verapamil protein binding in patients and in normal subjects. *Clin Pharmacol Ther* 1981;29:21–26.
7. Woelfel A, Foster JR, McAllister RG, et al. Efficacy of verapamil in exercise-induced ventricular tachycardia. *Am J Cardiol* 1985;56;292–297.
8. Talano JV, Tommaso C. Slow channel calcium antagonists in the treatment of supraventricular tachycardia. *Prog Cardiovasc Dis* 1982;25:141–156.
9. Weiss AT, Lewis BS, Halon DA, et al. The use of calcium with verapamil in the management of supraventricular tachyarrhythmias. *Int J Cardiol* 1983;4:275–280.
10. Reiter MJ, Shand DG, Aanonsen LM, et al. Pharmacokinetics of verpamil: Experience with a sustained intravenous infusion regimen. *Am J Cardiol* 1982;50:716–721.
11. Schwartz JB, Keefe DL, Kirsten E, et al. Prolongation of verapamil elimination kinetics during chronic oral administration. *Am Heart J* 1982;104:198–203.
12. Schwartz JB, Abernethy DR, Taylor AA, et al. An investigation of the cause of accumulation of verapamil during regular dosing in patients. *Br J Clin Pharmacol* 1985;19:512–516.
13. Shand DG, Hammill SC, Aanonsen L, et al. Reduced verapamil clearance during long-term oral administration. *Clin Pharmacol Ther* 1981;30:701–703.
14. Hesslein P, Gow R, D'Souza J, et al. Age-dependent verapamil kinetics affect pediatric oral dose requirements (abstr). *Cardiovascular Pharmacotherapy International Symposium, Geneva, April 1985;*584.
15. Storstein L, Larsen A, Midtbo K, et al. Pharmacokinetics of calcium blockers in patients with renal insufficiency and in geriatric patients. *Acta Med Scand* 1983;(Suppl 681):25–30.
16. Cox JP, O'Boyle CA, Mee F, et al. The antihypertensive efficacy of verapamil in the elderly evaluated by ambulatory blood pressure measurement. *J Human Hypertens* 1988;2:41–47.
17. Orlandi C, Marlettini MG, Cassani A, et al. Treatment of hypertension during pregnancy with the calcium antagonist verapamil. *Curr Therap Res* 1986;39:884–893.
18. Maxwell DJ, Crawford DC, Curry PVM, et al. Obstetric importance, diagnosis and management of fetal tachycardias. *Br Med J* 1988;297:107–110.
19. Mooy J, Shols M, van Baak M, et al. Pharmacokinetics of verapamil in patients with renal failure. *Eur J Clin Pharmacol* 1985;28:405–410.
20. Marone C, Luisoli S, Bomio F, et al. Body sodium-blood volume state, aldosterone, and cardiovascular responsiveness after calcium entry blockade with nifedipine. *Kidney Int* 1985;28:658–665.
21. Piepho RW, Culbertson VL, Rhodes RS. Drug interactions with the calcium-entry blockers. *Circulation* 1987;75 (Suppl V):V181–V194

22. Rahn KH, Mooy J, Bohm R, et al. Reduction of bioavailability of verapamil by rifampin. *N Engl J Med* 1985;312:920-921.

23. Wing LMH, Miners JO, Lillywhite KJ. Verapamil disposition—effects of sulfinpyrazone and cimetidine. *Br J Clin Pharmacol* 1985;19:385-391.

23A. Barbarash RA, Bauman JL, Fischer JH, et al. Near-total reduction in verapamil bioavailability by rifampin. *Chest* 1988;94:954-959.

24. Taburet AM, Singlas E, Colin J-N, et al. Pharmacokinetic studies of nifedipine tablet. Correlation with antihypertensive effects. *Hypertension* 1985;5(Suppl II):II29-II33.

25. Hongo M, Traube M, McAllister RG, et al. Effects of nifedipine on esophageal motor function in humans: Correlation with plasma nifedipine concentration. *Gastroenterology* 1984;86:8-12.

26. Kleinbloesem CH, Van Brummelen P, Faber H, et al. Variability in nifedipine pharmacokinetics and dynamics: A new oxidation polymorphism in man. *Biochem Pharmacol* 1984;33:3721-3724.

26A. Betocchi S, Bonow RO, Cannon RO, et al. Relations between serum nifedipine concentration and hemodynamic effects in non-obstructive hypertrophic cardiomyopathy. *Am J Cardiol* 1988;61:830-835.

27. Kuhlmann J, Graefe K-H, Ramsch K-D, et al. Clinical pharmacology. In: Krebs R, ed. *Treatment of Cardiovascular Diseases by Adalat^R (Nifedipine)*. Stuttgart: Schattauer, 1986;93-144.

28. Scott M, Castledon CM, Adam HK, et al. The effect of ageing on the disposition of nifedipine and atenolol. *Br J Clin Pharmacol* 1988;25:289-296.

29. Endo M, Kanda I, Hosoda S, et al. Prinzmetal's variant form of angina pectoris. Re-evaluation of mechanisms. *Circulation* 1975;52:33-37.

30. Van Harten J, Burggraaf K, Danhof M, et al. Negligible sublingual absorption of nifedipine. *Lancet* 1987;2:1363-1365.

31. McAllister RG. Kinetics and dynamics of nifedipine after oral and sublingual doses. *Am J Med* 1986;81(Suppl 6A):2-5.

32. Kleinbloesem CH, Van Brummelen P, Van de Linde JA, et al. Nifedipine: Kinetics and dynamics in healthy subjects. *Clin Pharmacol Ther* 1984;35:742-749.

33. Chung M, Reitberg DP, Gaffney M, et al. Clinical pharmacokinetics of nifedipine gastrointestinal therapeutic system. A controlled-release formulation of nifedipine. *Am J Med* 1987;83(Suppl 6B):10-14.

34. Vetrovec GW, Parker VE, Cole S, et al. Nifedippine gastrointestinal therapeutic system in stable angina pectoris. Results of a multicenter open-label crossover comparison with standard nifedipine. *Am J Med* 1987;83(Suppl 6B):24-29.

35. Walley TJ, Heagerty AM, Woods KL, et al. Nifedipine infusion in acute myocardial infarction: Experience in 12 patients. *Clin Cardiol* 1987;10:800-803.

36. Dilmen U, Calgar MK, Senses DA, et al. Nifedipine in hypertensive emergencies (letter). *Br Med J* 1983;286:889.

37. Dickinson DF, Wilson N, Curry P. Use of nifedipine in hypertrophic cardiomyopathy in infants. A report of two cases. *Int J Cardiol* 1985;2:159-160.

38. Robertson DRC, Waller DG, Renwick AG, et al. Age-related changes in the pharmacokinetics and pharmacodynamics of nifedipine. *Br J Clin Pharmacol* 1988:25:297-305.

39. Gilchrist NL, Nicholls MG, Ewer TC, et al. A comparison of long-acting nifedipine and enalapril in elderly hypertensives: A randomised, single-blind, cross-over study. *J Human Hypertens* 1988;2:33-39.

40. Walters BNJ, Redman CWG. Treatment of severe pregnancy associated hypertension with the calcium antagonist, nifedipine. *Br J Obstet Gynaecol* 1984;91:330-336.

41. Bogaert MG, Rosseel MT, Joos R, et al. Plasma concentrations of nifedipine in patients with renal failure. *Arzneimittel-Forschung* 1984;34:307-308.

42. Martre HR, Sari AM, Taburet C, et al. Haemodialysis does not affect the pharmacokinetics of nifedipine. *Br J Clin Pharmacol* 1985;20:155-158.

43. Ravens KG. Effect of nifedipine on glucose tolerance in man. In: Lichtlen PR, ed. *6th International Adalat Symposium.* Amsterdam: Excerpta Medica, 1986;367-371.

44. Daniels AR, Opie LH. Effect of slow-release nifedipine on glucose tolerance. In: Lichtlen PR, ed. *6th Internatioal Adalat Symposium.* Amsterdam: Excerpta Medica, 1986;495-496.

45. Kleinbloesem CH, Van Brummelen P, Sandberg THW, et al. Kinetic and haemodynamic interactions between nifedipine and propranolol in healthy subjects utilizing controlled rates of drug input. In: Kleinbloesem CH, ed. *Nifedipine Clinical Pharmacokinetics and Haemodynamic Effects.* 's-Gravenhage: Drukkerij JH Pasmans BV, 1985;151-165.

46. Schwartz JB, Raizner A, Akers S. The effect of nifedipine on serum digoxin concentrations in patients. *Am Heart J* 1984;107:669-673.

47. Smith SR, Kendall MJ, Lobo J, et al. Ranitidine and cimetidine: Drug interactions with single dose and steady-state nifedipine administration. *Br J Clin Pharmacol* 1987;23:331-315.

48. Toyosaki N, Toyo-Oka T, Natsume T, et al. Combination therapy with diltiazem and nifedipine in patients with effort angina pectoris. *Circulation* 1988;77:1370-1375.

49. Ahmad S. Nifedipine-phenytoin interaction (letter). *J Am Coll Cardiol* 1984;3:1581-1582.

50. Deanfield J, Wright C, Krikler S, et al. Cigarette smoking and the treatment of angina with propranolol, atenolol and nifedipine. *N Engl J Med* 1984;310:951-954.

51. Piepho RW, Bloedow DC, Lacz JP, et al. Pharmacokinetics of diltiazem in selected animal species and human beings. *Am J Cardiol* 1982;49:525-528.

52. Rovei V, Gomeni R, Mitchard M, et al. Pharmacokinetics and metabolism of diltiazem in man. *Acta Cardiologica* 1980;35:35-45.

53. Chaffman M, Brogden RN. Diltiazem. A review of its pharmacological properties and therapeutic efficacy. *Drugs* 1985;29:387-454.

54. Fifer MA, Colucci WS, Lorell BH, et al. Inotropic, vascular and neuroendocrine effects of nifedipine in heart failure: Comparison with nitroprusside. *J Am Coll Cardiol* 1985;5:731-737.

55. Rovei V, Mitchard M, Morselli PL. Simple, sensitive, and specific gas chromatographic method for the quantification of diltiazem in human body fluids. *J Chromatography* 1977;138:391-398.

56. Pozet N, Brazier JL, Aissa AH, et al. Pharmacokinetics of diltiazem in severe renal failure. *Eur J Clin Pharmacol* 1983;24:635-638.

57. Burges RA, Gardiner DG, Gwilt M, et al. Calcium channel

blocking properties of amlodipine in vascular smooth muscle and cardiac muscle in vitro: Evidence for voltage modulation of vascular dihydropyrinidine receptors. *J Cardiovasc Pharmacol* 1987;9:110–119.

58. Faulkner JK, McGibney D, Chasseaud LF, et al. The pharmacokinetics of amlodipine in healthy volunteers after single intravenous and oral doses and after 14 repeated oral doses given once daily. *Br J Clin Pharmacol* 1986;22:21–25.

59. Webster J, Robb OJ, Jeffers TA, et al. Once daily amlodipine in the treatment of mild to moderate hypertension. *Br J Clin Pharmacol* 1987;24:713–719.

60. Elliott HL, Meredith PA, Faulkner JK, et al. A comparative evaluation of the disposition of amlodipine in young and elderly subjects (abstr). In: *Calcium Antagonists in Hypertension.* 25th Anniversary International Symposium, Basel, Switzerland, February 1988.

61. Abernethy DR, Lambert MD. Amlodipine dynamics and disposition in young and elderly hypertensive patients (abstr). In: *Calcium Antagonists in Hypertension.* 25th Anniversary International Symposium, Basel, Switzerland, February 1988.

62. Edgar B, Hoffmann KJ, Lundborg P, et al. Absorption, distribution and elimination of felodipine in man. *Drugs* 1985;29(Suppl 2):9–15.

63. Sluiter HE, Huysmans FTM, Thien TA, et al. Haemodynamic, hormonal, and diuretic effects of felodipine in healthy normotensive volunteers. *Drugs* 1985;29(Suppl 2):26–35.

64. Agner E, Rehling M, Trap-Jensen J. Haemodynamic effects of single-dose felodipine in normal man. *Drugs* 1985;29(Suppl 2):36–40.

65. Andersson OK, Granerus G, Hedner T. Felodipine. A calcium-inhibiting vasodilator in refractory hypertension. *Drugs* 1985;29(Suppl 2):102–108.

66. Elmfeldt D, Hedner T. Antihypertensive effects of felodipine compared with placebo. *Drugs* 1985;29(Suppl 2):109–116.

67. Ljung B. Vascular selectivity of felodipine. *Drugs* 1985; 29(Suppl 2):46–58.

68. Hansson BG, Lyngstam G, Lyngstam L, et al. Antihypertensive effect of felodipine combined with β-blockade. *Drugs* 1985;29(Suppl 2):131–136.

69. Katzman PL, Hulthen UL, Hokfelt B. Catecholamines, renin-angiotensin-aldosterone, and cardiovascular response during exercise following acute and long-term calcium antagonism with felodipine in essential hypertension. *J Cardiovasc Pharmacol* 1987;10:439–444.

70. Herlitz H, Aurell M, Bjorck S, et al. Renal effects of felodipine in hypertensive patients with reduced renal function. *Drugs* 1985;29(Suppl 2):192–197.

71. Stieren B, Buhler V, Hege HG, et al. Pharmacokinetics and metabolism of gallopamil. In: Kaltenbach M, Hopf R, eds. *Gallopamil. Pharmacological and Clinical Profile of a Calcium Antagonist.* Berlin: Springer-Verlag 1984;88–93.

72. Schran HF, Jaffe JM, Gonasun LM. Clinical pharmacokinetics of isradipine. *Am J Med* 1988;84(Suppl 3B):80–89.

73. Schran HF, Jaffe JM, Gonasun LL. The pharmacokinetics and metabolism of isradipine (abstr). *Cardiovasc Rev Rep* 1987;Special Supplement 3:7.

74. Hof RP, Ruegg UT. Pharmacology of the new calcium antagonist isradipine and its metabolites. *Am J Med* 1988;84(Suppl 3B):13–17.

75. Parker JO, Fnialbert M, Bernstein V. Efficacy of the

calcium antagonist isradipine in angina pectoris. *Cardiovasc Drugs Ther* 1988;1:657-660.

76. Kirkendall WM. Comparative assessment of first-line agents for treatment of hypertension. In: Expanding Role of Calcium Antagonists in Cardiovascular Therapy. *Cardiovasc Rev Rep* Special Supplement 1987;3:9.

77. Rowe JW. Approach to the treatment of hypertension in older patients. Preliminary results with isradipine. *Am J Med* 1988;84(Suppl 3B):46-50.

78. Van den Toren EW, Van Bruggen A, Ruegg PC, et al. Hemodynamic effects of an intravenous infusion of isradipine in patients with congestive heart failure. *Am J Med* 1988;84(Suppl 3B):97-101.

79. Chellingsworth MC, Willis JV, Broadfoot D, et al. Pharmacokinetics and pharmacodynamics of isradipine (PN 200-110) in young and elderly patients. *Am J Med* 1988;84(Suppl 3B):72-79.

80. Thuillez C, Guerret M, Duhaze P, et al. Nicardipine: Pharmacokinetics and effects on carotid and brachial blood flows in normal volunteers. *Br J Clin Pharmacol* 1984;18:838-847.

81. Clair F, Bellet M, Guerret M, et al. Hypotensive effect and pharmacokinetics of nicardipine in patients with severe renal failure. *Curr Therap Res* 1985;38:74-82.

82. Graham DJM, Dow RJ, Hall DJ, et al. The metabolism and pharmacokinetics of nicardipine hydrochloride in man. *Br J Clin Pharmacol* 1985;20(Suppl 1):23S-28S.

83. Sorkin EM, Clissold SP. Nicardipine. A review of its pharmacodynamic and pharmacokinetic properties, and therapeutic efficacy, in the treatment of angina pectoris, hypertension and related cardiovascular disorders. *Drugs* 1987;33:296-345.

84. Urien S, Albengres E, Comte A, et al. Plasma protein binding and erythrocyte partitioning of nicardipine in vitro. *J Cardiovasc Pharmacol* 1985;7:891-898.

85. Campbell BC, Kelman AW, Hillis WS. Noninvasive assessment of the haemodynamic effects of nicardipine in normotensive subjects. *Br J Clin Pharmacol* 1985;20(Suppl 1):55S-61S.

86. Silke P, Graham DJM, Verma SP, et al. Pharmacokinetic, haemodynamic and radionuclide studies with nicardipine in coronary artery disease. *Eur J Clin Pharmacol* 1986;29:651-657.

87. Bowles MJ, Khurmi NS, O'Hara MJ, et al. Randomized double-blind placebo-controlled comparison of nicardipine and nifedipine in patients with chronic stable angina pectoris. *Chest* 1986;89:260-265.

88. Forette F, Bellet M, Henry JF, et al. Effect of nicardipine in elderly hypertensive patients. *Br J Clin Pharmacol* 1985;20(Suppl 1):125S-129S.

89. Brown ST, Freedman D, DeVault GA, et al. Elderly Multicenter Study Group. Safety, efficacy and pharmacokinetics of nicardipine in elderly hypertensive patients. *Br J Clin Pharmacol* 1985;22(Suppl):289S-295S.

90. Gengo FM, Fagan SC, Krol G, et al. Nimodipine disposition and haemodynamic effect in patients with cirrhosis and age-matched controls. *Br J Clin Pharmacol* 1987;3:47-53.

91. Kirch W, Raemsch KD, Duehrsen U, et al. Clinical pharmacokinetics of nimodipine in normal and impaired renal function. *Int J Clin Pharm Res* 1984;4:381-384.

92. Friedel HA, Sorkin EM. Nisoldipine. A preliminary review of its pharmacodynamic and pharmacokinetic properties, and therapeutic efficacy in the treatment of angina pectoris, hypertension and related cardiovascular disorders. *Drugs* 1988;in press.

93. Pasanisi F, Meredith PA, Reid JL. The pharmacodynamics and pharmacokinetics of a new calcium antagonist nisoldipine in normotensive and hypertensive subjects. *Eur J Clin Pharmacol* 1985;29:21-24.

94. Lasseter KC, Shamblen EC, Lettieri J, et al. Dose-proportional pharmacokinetics of nisoldipine in healthy volunteers. *Clin Pharmacol Ther* 1987;41:234.

95. Ahr G, Wingender W, Kuhlmann J. Pharmacokinetics of nisoldipine. In: Hugenholtz PG, Meyer J, eds. *Nisoldipine.* Heidelberg: Springer-Verlag, 1987;59-66.

95A. Van Harten J, Van Brummelen P, Zeegers RRECM, et al. The influence of infusion rate on the pharmacokinetics and haemodynamic effects of nisoldipine in man. *Br J Clin Pharmacol* 1988; 25:709-717

96. Daniels AR, Opie LH. Monotherapy with the calcium channel antagonist nisoldipine for systemic hypertension and comparison with diuretic drugs. *Am J Cardiol* 1987;60:703-707.

97. Lam J, Chaitman BR, Crean P, et al. A dose-ranging placebo-controlled, double-blind trial of nisoldipine in effort angina: Duration and extent of antianginal effects. *J Am Coll Cardiol* 1985;6:447-452.

98. Breimer DD, Lodewijks MTM, Van Brummelen P, et al. Pharmacokinetics and haemodynamic effects of nisoldipine in patients with liver cirrhosis. *Br J Pharmacol* 1986; 89(Suppl):482.

99. Van Harten J, van Brummelen P, Wilson JHP, et al. Pharmacokinetics and haemodynamic effects of nisoldipine in patients with liver cirrhosis. In: Hugenholtz PG, Meyer J, eds. *Nisoldipine.* Heidelberg: Springer-Verlag, 1987;76-79.

100. Joeres R, Ahr G, Hofsetter G, et al. Steady-state pharmacokinetics of nisoldipine in patients with liver disease. In: Hugenholtz PG, Meyer J eds. *Nisoldipine.* Heidelberg: Springer-Verlag, 1987;80-84.

101. Boelaert J, Valcke Y, Dammekens H, et al. Nisoldipine pharmacokinetics in renal dysfunction. *Acta Pharmacol Toxicol* 1986;59(Suppl 5):175.

102. Kirch W, Stenzel J, Dylewicz P, et al. Influence of nisoldipine on haemodynamic effects and plasma levels of digoxin. *Br J Clin Pharmacol* 1986;22:155-159.

103. Levine MAH, Ogilvie RI, Leenen FHH. Pharmacokinetic and pharmacodynamic interactions between nisoldipine and propranolol. *Clin Pharmacol Ther* 1988;43:39-48.

104. Kann J, Krol GJ, Raemsch KD, et al. Bioequivalence and metabolism of nitrendipine administered orally to healthy volunteers. *J Cardiovasc Pharmacol* 1984;6:S968-S973.

105. Jain AK, McMahon FG, Ryan JR, et al. Efficacy and safety of nitrendipine in patients with severe hypertension: A multiclinic study. *J Cardiovasc Pharmacol* 1984;6:S1053-S1059.

106. Lasseter KC, Shamblem EC, Murdoch AA, et al. Steady-state pharmacokinetics of nitrendipine in hepatic insufficiency. *J Cardiovasc Pharmacol* 1984;6:S977-S981.

107. Dylewicz P, Kirch W, Santos SR, et al. Bioavailability and elimination of nitrendipine in liver disease. *Eur J Clin Pharmacol* 1987;32:563-568.

108. Aronoff G. Pharmacokinetics of nitrendipine in patients with renal failure: Comparison to normal subjects. *J Cardiovasc Pharmacol* 1984;6:S974-S976.

109. Pinquier JL, Urien S, Lemaire M, et al. Comparative binding of two closely related dihydropyridines (isradipine and darodipine) to serum proteins and erythrocytes. *Pharmacology* 1988;36:305-312.

110. Andren L, Hansson L, Oro L, et al. Experience with nitrendipine—a new calcium antagonist—in hypertension. *J Cardiovasc Pharmacol* 1982;4:S387-S391.
111. Kirch W, Hutt HJ, Heidemann H, et al. Drug interactions with nitrendipine. *J Cardiovasc Pharmacol* 1984;6:S982-S985.

CALCIUM CHANNEL ANTAGONISTS
PART VII
SUMMARY TABLES

SUMMARY. This part summarizes in tabular form the information already presented in detail in the previous six parts.

Table VII-1 contains the indications and dosage of calcium antagonists, including the second generation agents.

Table VII-2 tabulates the pharmacokinetics of calcium antagonists.

Table VII-3 concerns the side-effects.

Table VII-4 lays out the contraindications, precautions, and drug interactions.

Table VII-5 gives the trade names of those calcium antagonists presently available and those due soon to become available in the USA, Federal Republic of Germany, or United Kingdom.

Table VII-1. Calcium antagonists: Indications and dosage

Agent	Indications or proposed indications	Dose
Verapamil	Supraventricular tachycardia (SVT) narrow QRS complexes	1. IV bolus 5–10 mg repeated after 10 min then 0.005 mg/kg/min if needed 2. IV infusion 1 mg/min to total of 10 mg 3. If myocardial disease, work up from 0.0001 mg/kg/min, titrating against heart rate
	Atrial flutter/fibrillation (control of ventricular rate)	Intravenous infusion, if needed (3) above; or 80–120 mg 3× daily increasing to 80–120 mg 4× daily.
	"Prophylaxis" of SVT	Orally 80–120 mg 3× daily added to digoxin (watch digoxin levels)
	Angina of effort, angina at rest	Orally 80–120 mg 3× daily
	Prinzmetal's angina and hypertrophic cardiomyopathy	Orally 80–120 mg 3× daily increasing to 80–120 mg 4× daily (rarely higher doses). Later reduce dose to 2× daily.
	Hypertension, mild to moderate	As for angina
	Hypertension, severe	Oral: as for angina IV: 25 mg over 10 min; adjust dose according to BP
	Hypertrophic cardiomyopathy	As for angina

(continued)

Table VII-1 (continued)

Agent	Indications or proposed indications	Dose
Nifedipine	Angina of effort	Capsules 30–80 mg/day in 3 or 4 doses
	Angina at rest and Prinzmetal's angina	Capsules 10 mg 3× daily up to 20 mg every 4 hr
	Acute left ventricular failure (pulmonary edema) in the setting of acute ischemia or severe hypertension	10 mg bite-and-swallow 6-hourly
	Hypertension, mild to moderate	Capsules 10 mg 2-4× daily. Tablets 20-40 mg 2× daily
	Hypertension, severe or refractory	10 mg bite-and-swallow; repeat hourly to 40 mg; start with 5 mg in elderly patient
Diltiazem	Supraventricular tachycardia narrow QRS complexes	To abort attack: 120 mg plus propanolol 160 mg
	Atrial flutter/fibrillation (control of ventricular rate)	Oral diltiazem added to digoxin
	Angina of effort and angina at rest including Prinzmetal	Oral 60–90 mg 3× daily increasing to 4× daily as indicated
	"Prophylaxis" of SVT	As for angina
	Hypertension, mild to moderate	As for angina
	Hypertrophic cardiomyopathy	As for angina

New dihydropyridines		
Amlodipine	Hypertension (angina)	2.5–10 mg once daily
Felodipine	Hypertension (angina)	5–10 mg 3× daily
Isradipine	Hypertension (angina)	5–7.5 mg 2–3× daily
Nicardipine	Hypertension, angina	5–40 mg 3× daily
Nimodipine	Subarachnoid hemorrhage, early stroke	0.35 mg/kg 4-hourly; 30–40 mg 3–4× daily
Nisoldipine	Hypertension, angina	5–20 mg once or twice daily
Nitrendipine	Hypertension (angina)	10–20 mg once or twice daily
Verapamil-like agents		
Anipamil	Hypertension	60–80 mg once daily
Gallopamil	Angina	50 mg 3× daily

Sodium-calcium channel blocker Angina; arrythmias including 200–400 mg once daily
SVT of WPW syndrome

SVT = supraventricular tachycardia
IV = intravenous
WPW = Wolff-Parkinson-White

Table VII-2. Pharmacokinetics of calcium antagonists

Drug	Bioavailability and absorption	Metabolism	Plasma level (ng/ml)	Protein binding (%)
Verapamil	Rapid absorption BA 10–20%	Hepatic. Norverapamil (active)	80–400	84–93
Nifedipine	Rapid absorption BA 45–68%	Hepatic. Inactive metabolites	15–200	92–98
Diltiazem	Rapid absorption BA 45%	Hepatic. Desacetyldiltiazem (active)	50–300	80–86
Amlodipine	Slow absorption. Peak blood levels only reached after 6–12h BA 60–65%	Hepatic. Inactive metabolites	2–12 Higher with repeated doses	97.5

Felodipine	Rapid absorption BA 15%	Hepatic. Inactive metabolites	5–40	99
Gallopamil	Rapid absorption BA 13–27%	Hepatic. Inactive metabolites	Up to 70 (chronic)	85–90
Isradipine	Rapid absorption BA 20%	Hepatic. Inactive metabolites	About 10	96
Nicardipine	Rapid absorption BA 7–30%	Hepatic. Inactive metabolites	30–60	98–99.5
Nimodipine	Rapid absorption BA 12%	Hepatic. Active metabolites	Up to 80	High
Nisoldipine	Rapid absorption BA 4–8%	Hepatic. Inactive metabolites	1–4	99.7
Nitrendipine	Rapid absorption BA 60–70%	Hepatic. Inactive metabolites	10–40	98

(continued)

Table VII-2. Continued

Drug	Calculated free plasma concentration	Elimination half-life	Elderly	Liver disease	Renal disease
Verapamil	$2-8 \times 10^{-8}M$	3-7h Prolonged with chronic therapy	Reduce dose	Reduce dose considerably	Dose unchanged unless GFR very low
Nifedipine	$0.1-2 \times 10^{-9}M$	Capsules 3h Tablets 5-11h	Reduce dose	Reduce dose	Dose unchanged
Diltiazem	$1-5 \times 10^{-8}M$	2-7h	Reduce dose	Reduce dose	Dose unchanged
Amlodipine	$0.5-3 \times 10^{-10}M$ or more	35-45h	Unchanged or reduce dose	No data; probably reduce dose	Dose unchanged

Felodipine	$5 \times 10^{-8}M$	3–14h	Reduce dose	Dose unchanged
Gallopamil	$10^{-8}M$	4–5h. May be longer if chronic therapy	Reduce dose	Dose unchanged
Isradipine	$10^{-9}M$	8h	Reduce dose	Dose unchanged
Nicardipine	$10^{-9}M$	4–5h	Reduce dose	Dose unchanged
Nimodipine	Unknown	3h	Reduce dose	Reduce dose
Nisoldipine	$1–3 \times 10^{-10}M$	2–13h	Reduce dose	Dose unchanged
Nitrendipine	$1–5 \times 10^{-9}M$	7–8h	Consider decreased dose	Dose unchanged

Table VII-3. Calcium antagonists: Side-effects

Agent	Side-effects
Verapamil	*Minor:* Constipation (frequent), headaches, dizziness, facial flushing. *Serious:* IV verapamil as a bolus given to patients with sick sinus syndrome or AV nodal disease or digitalis poisoning or excess β-blockade can be fatal. Hypotension, especially if LV failure.
Nifedipine	*Minor:* Headache, tachycardia, facial flushing, ankle edema. *Serious:* Provocation of angina; rarely cerebral ischemia, renal failure.
Diltiazem	*Minor:* (high dose) headaches, ankle edema, constipation, bradycardia. *Serious:* Rare skin rash. Adverse effects on sinus or AV node or myocardium can be expected in predisposed patients (see verapamil).
New dihydropyridines Amlodipine Felodipine Isradipine Nicardipine Nimodipine Nisoldipine Nitrendipine	See nifedipine. Agents or preparations with slower onset of action should have fewer vasodilatory side-effects. Some agents may have less cardiodepressive effects than nifedipine (e.g. felodipine, isradipine, nicardipine and nisoldipine).
Verapamil-like agents Anipamil Gallopamil	See verapamil.
Sodium-calcium channel blocker	Gastrointestinal and neurologic. Prolonged QT interval. Risk of torsades de pointes.

Table VII-4. Calcium antagonists: Contraindications, precautions and drug interactions

Agent	Contraindications, precautions and drug interactions
Verapamil	*C/T:* Sick sinus syndrome, digitalis toxicity, excess β-blockade, Wolff-Parkinson-White syndrome with antegrade conduction, myocardial failure. *Caution:* Combination with β-blockade. *Drug interactions:* Digoxin levels increased; enhanced hypotensive effect with prazosin, nitrates, quinidine and disopyramide; excess nodal inhibition or hypertension with β-blockade. Cimetidine increases half-life.
Nifedipine	*C/T:* Severe aortic stenosis, hypertrophic cardiomyopathy. *Cautions:* Myocardial failure; unstable angina with threatened infarction. *Drug interactions:* Digoxin (small elevation); excess hypotension with prazosin or nitrates, quinidine levels reduced. Cimetidine increases half-life and hypotensive effect. Diltiazem increases plasma levels.
Diltiazem	*C/I:* As for verapamil. *Caution:* Combination with β-blockade. *Drug interactions:* Digoxin (small elevation); interactions with nitrates, quinidine, disopyramide, β-blockade and cimetidine as for verapamil.

(continued)

Table VII-4 (continued)

Agent	Contraindications, precautions and drug interactions
New dihydropyridines	
Amlodipine	*C/I:* See nifedipine.
	Drug interactions: None with digoxin or cimetidine.
Felodipine	*C/I:* See nifedipine.
	Drug interactions: Check digoxin levels. Cimetidine may increase half-life.
Isradipine	*C/I:* See nifedipine.
	Drug interactions: Check digoxin levels. Cimetidine may increase half-life.
Nicardipine	*C/I:* See nifedipine.
	Drug interactions: Check digoxin levels. Cimetidine may increase half-life.
Nimodipine	*C/I:* See nifedipine.
	Drug interactions: Check digoxin levels. Cimetidine may increase half-life.
Nisoldipine	*C/I:* See nifedipine.
	Drug interactions: Check digoxin levels. Cimetidine may increase half-life.
Nitrendipine	*C/I:* See nifedipine.
	Drug interactions: Doubles digoxin dose. Cimetidine increases half-life.
Verapamil-like agents	
Anipamil	*C/I:* See verapamil.
Gallopamil	*C/I:* See verapamil.
Sodium-calcium channel blocker	*C/I:* Hypokalemia; co administration of drugs prolonging action potential duration; AV block; caution with diuretic therapy, bradycardia.

Table VII-5. Generic and trade names of first and second generation calcium antagonists

First generation agents	Trade name(s)
Verapamil	Isoptin, Calan
Nifedipine	Procardia, Adalat
Diltiazem	Cardizem, Tildiem

Second generation agents	Trade name(s)
Amlodipine	Norvasc
Felodipine	Plendil
Isradipine	DynaCirc
Nicardipine	Cardene
Nimodipine	Nimotop
Nisoldipine	Syscor*
Nitrendipine	Baypress

*thus far not registered in Germany, USA or United Kingdom

CALCIUM CHANNEL ANTAGONISTS: PART VIII: EPILOGUE. WHERE DO WE GO FROM HERE?

First Generation Agents

Only twenty years ago, calcium antagonists were laboratory curiosities. Not until the dramatic effects of verapamil were discovered by Schamroth [1], and reported in an article rejected in disbelief by a premier American journal, did any of these agents come to be widely used. Soon thereafter followed the 1st International Nifedipine 'Adalat' Symposium in Tokyo in 1973, the publication from which eventually persuaded clinicians to take seriously the antianginal properties of calcium antagonists. As in the case of β-blockers, the antihypertensive effects were discovered almost by chance and ignored by the manufacturers until in 1982 when at a meeting held in Berlin (and subsequently published as the 5th International Adalat Symposium), the antihypertensive properties of nifedipine were acknowledged. Diltiazem likewise was first introduced as an antianginal agent and only later were the antihypertensive properties established. Yet when one considers that the main action of all calcium antagonists is inhibition of vascular smooth muscle contraction, it is surprising that the antihypertensive effect has been so well disguised for so long. Probably this delay has been in part because the dominant role of the increased peripheral vascular resistance in hypertension has not been appreciated until recently.

Today calcium antagonists are well established treatment for hypertension and angina, and, in the case of verapamil and diltiazem, also for supraventricular arrhythmias. Their side-effect profile is satisfactory and their use precipitates no serious diseases or disorders. Contraindications are relatively few. Hence the spectacular success of these first generation agents. Their chief limitation is that none of them is inherently genuinely long-acting, although such preparations are becoming available. Secondly, the inherent negative inotropic effect, which all first generation agents have and is clinically manifest in the order $V>D>N$, is unwanted in the therapy of hypertension as is the inhibitory effect on the sinoatrial and atrioventricular nodes (verapamil and diltiazem). Hence the search for long-acting vascular selective agents. It should, however, be clear that some degree of negative inotropic effect, clinically most marked in the case of verapamil, may have an advantage in the therapy of angina pectoris which may explain why the second generation dihydropyridines are widely being registered for use in hypertension but only one of them for use in angina.

Second Generation Agents

The first generation agents have been called the 'patriarchs' (or matriarchs) of the calcium antagonist by Braunwald (see Foreword). Their progeny, the second generation calcium antagonists, are largely dihydropyridines or 'sons' of nifedipine. A major step has been the prolonged duration of action of some preparations and compounds. Amlodipine and GITS nifedipine have sustained plasma levels for 24 hours or more, whereas a number of dihydropyridines with shorter half-lives have a sufficiently prolonged biological action to allow twice daily dosing, at least in hypertension (felodipine, isradipine, nisoldipine, nitrendipine).

Vascular selectivity, a major aim of the second generation agents, has also been claimed. A lesser negative inotropic effect should be particularly attractive for use in patients with congestive heart failure, especially when due to ischemic heart disease. For example, felodipine has been particularly well tested in heart failure, though not yet registered for this indication anywhere. Isradipine, nicardipine and nisoldipine are likewise thought to have increased vascular selectivity and to be relatively non-cardiodepressant. However, the obvious benefit of less cardiodepression in hypertension may be offset by the disadvantages of the lack of negative inotropic effect in angina.

Hypertension

Hypertension is the major clinical indication common to all of the 'sons' of nifedipine. The chief mode of action is peripheral vasodilation and reduction of the systemic vascular resistance; an ancillary mode is probably by intermittent diuresis. The chief problem has been the absence of true once-daily preparations (now being remedied) and a relatively high incidence of side-effects which are irritating rather than being serious (headache, flushing, dizziness, tachycardia and pedal edema). Recent work has shown that a slow rise of blood levels (for example, comparing slow versus fast infusions of nisoldipine [2]) is less prone to acute vasodilatory side-effects, giving a theoretical advantage for those agents reaching the maximum plasma concentration rather slowly (for example, amlodipine).

Combination Therapy with ACE Inhibitors for Hypertension

Unfortunately all dihydropyridines of both generations activate the adrenergic-renin-angiotensin-aldosterone axis. Activation of the adrenergic-angiotensin-renin-aldosterone system is likely to increase peripheral vasoconstriction and therefore is a disadvantage. As an example, during the therapy of congestive heart failure by nisoldipine [3], those patients with increasing plasma catecholamine levels did worse. In hypertension, such baroreflex-mediated compensatory mechanisms act as a counter-regulatory response so that the acute hypotensive effect may be blunted. There are several approaches to this problem of adrenergic-renin activation. First, it is likely that all dihydropyridines inhibit the release of aldosterone from the adrenals so that true fluid retention is not seen with these compounds. The pedal edema is probably the result of local microvascular changes [4] and is probably an unavoidable and common side-effect even with the second generation dihydropyridines (see, for example, isradipine). Nonetheless, pedal edema is countered by co-therapy with captopril [5]. Furthermore, ACE inhibitor co-therapy should antagonize activation of the renin-angiotensin system, as shown experimentally [6]. Because angiotensin-II facilitates release of norepinephrine from terminal adrenergic neurons, co-therapy with ACE inhibition means that there will be blunting of the adrenergic response during acute vasodilation [6]. Furthermore, ACE inhibition may redirect blood flow to the liver and pancreas, otherwise relatively deprived during vasodilation induced by dihydropyridines [7]. The combination dihydropyridine-ACE inhibitor particularly improves renal blood flow as each of these agents has that effect [8]. For these reasons, based chiefly on animal experiments, the combination of an ACE inhibitor and a calcium antagonist, also well tested clinically, is increasingly in use.

Combination Therapy with β-blockers

Another favorable combination is that of dihydropyridines with β-blockers. Added hypotensive benefit may be achieved with lessened side-effects. Whereas there are still theoretical objections to the combination β-blocker-verapamil or diltiazem (because of the inhibitory effects on the sinus and AV nodes; and added negative inotropic effects particularly in the combination verapamil-β-blocker), it is much easier to combine β-blocker with a dihydropyridine. In hypertensive patients, even those with a low ejection fraction can have nifedipine added to pre-existing β-blocker therapy with improved systolic function [9]. The combination also appears to lessen some side-effects of dihydropyridines, such as flushing, sweating and tachycardia [10]. It is more than likely that combinations of all new dihydropyridines and β-blockers will be as well tolerated as nifedipine-atenolol; furthermore, the relatively non-cardiodepressant agents (felodipine, isradipine, nicardipine) have an added safety margin which should avoid the occasional cardiac catastrophy probably caused by excess negative inotropic effects of the nifedipine-β-blocker combination in patients with severely depressed left ventricular function.

New Calcium Antagonists for Effort Angina

In effort angina, all dihydropyridines should be equieffective, however only nicardipine is so far licensed for use in angina in the USA and the United Kingdom. The basic problem with nifedipine therapy in effort angina is that the reflex tachycardia may offset some of the benefits of afterload reduction. During prolonged therapy with the dihydropyridines, the initial tachycardia resulting from the acute administration disappears [11,12], at least when given for hypertension, presumably because of baroreflex resetting. In angina, even during chronic therapy there still seems to be a tachycardia at least with some dihydropyridines, for unknown reasons [13]. It would therefore make better sense to use either a combination of dihydropyridine-β-blocker or another calcium antagonist with an inherent negative inotropic effect such as verapamil, when selecting the ideal agent for angina pectoris.

In contrast, in vasospastic angina all dihydropyridines should be highly effective.

New Antiarrhythmic Calcium Antagonists

Of the new agents for angina pectoris, bepridil is very promising. It is a combined sodium-calcium channel blocker and also prolongs the action potential duration. It therefore has multi-antiarrhythmic effects, with some properties of Class I, Class III and Class IV agents, which may explain its wide spectrum of antiarrhythmic activity. Bepridil has excellent antianginal properties, including negative inotropic activity [14].

Its prolonged half-life means that once daily dosage is adequate. A defect of bepridil is QT-prolongation, so that hypokalemia and combination therapy with other agents prolonging the action potential duration must be avoided. For supraventricular arrhythmias, it is possible that bepridil could become the calcium antagonist of choice.

Cerebral Hemorrhage

Cerebral hemorrhage including early stroke and subarachnoid hemorrhage may be new indications for one of the second generation agents, namely nimodipine. This agent is well tested and apparently effective in man; whether it has special cerebroselective qualities or whether the benefit in subarachnoid hemorrhage and early stroke would be a property common to all dihydropyridines is not known.

Congestive Heart Failure

In congestive heart failure, felodipine is best tested without having achieved 'breakthrough' status. There still is a general feeling of reserve about the use of all calcium antagonists, including the highly vascular selective ones, in congestive heart failure.

Hypertrophic Cardiomyopathy

In hypertrophic cardiomyopathy (non-obstructive), new dihydropyridines have not been well studied. In principle, an important recent finding with nifedipine is likely to be applicable to all dihydropyridines, namely that beneficial vasodilatory properties dominate at lower doses with medium blood levels of the drug, whereas at high blood levels harmful negative inotropic effects come into play, so that the ejection fraction falls [15].

Summary

A major benefit of the second generation agents has been the more thorough testing, the better understanding of all the pharmacodynamic and pharmacokinetic effects, the careful assessment of the incidence of side-effects and the increasing realisation of the benefits of combination treatment with ACE inhibitor or β-blocker. However, there has been no 'gene jump' from the first to the second generation agents, nor is there a true generation gap between them. The major difference is going to lie in the duration of action.

References

1. Schamroth L. Immediate effects of intravenous verapamil on atrial fibrillation. *Cardiovasc Res* 1971;5:419-424.
2. Van Harten J, Van Brummelen P, Zeegers RRECM, et al. The influence of infusion rate on the pharmacokinetics and haemodynamic effects of nisoldipine in man. *Br J Clin Pharmacol* 1988;25:709-717.
3. Barjon J-N, Rouleau J-L, Bichet D, et al. Chronic renal and neurohumoral effects of the calcium entry blocker nisoldipine in patients with congestive heart failure. *J Am Coll Cardiol* 1987;9:622-630.
4. Gustafsson D, Grande P-O, Borgstrom P, Lindberg L. Effects of calcium antagonists on myogenic and neurogenic control of resistance and capacitance vessels in cat skeletal muscle. *J Cardiovasc Pharmacol* 1988;12:413-422.
5. Guazzi MD, De Cesare N, Galli C, et al. Calcium-channel blockade with nifedipine and angiotensin converting enzyme inhibition with captopril in the therapy of patients with severe primary hypertension. *Hypertension* 1984;70:279-284.
6. Bellet M, Sassano P, Guyenne P, et al. Converting-enzyme inhibition buffers the counter-regulatory response to acute administration of nicardipine. *Br J Clin Pharmacol* 1987;24:465-472.
7. Hof RP, Hof A. The renin-angiotensin system modulates the peripheral vascular effects of the calcium antagonist isradipine in anesthetized rabbits. *J Cardiovasc Pharmacol* 1988;12:233-238.
8. Clozel J-P. Effects of nitrendipine and cilazapril alone or in combination on hemodynamics and regional blood flows in conscious spontaneously hypertensive rats. *J Cardiovasc Pharmacol* 1988;12:600-607.
9. Jennings AA, Jee LD, Smith JA, et al. Acute effect of nifedipine on blood pressure and left ventricular ejection fraction in severely hypertensive outpatients: Predictive effects of acute therapy and prolonged efficacy when added to existing therapy. *Am Heart J* 1986;111:557-563.
10. Stanley NN, Thirkettle JL, Varma MPS, et al. The efficacy and tolerability of atenolol, nifedipine, and their combination in the management of hypertension. *Eur J Clin Pharmacol* 1988;34:543-548.
11. Omvik P, Lund-Johansen P, Haugland H. Nisoldipine. Central haemodynamics at rest and during exercise in essential hypertension: acute and chronic studies. *J Hypertens* 1988;6:95-103.
12. Grossman E, Oren S, Garavaglia GE, et al. Systemic and regional hemodynamic and humoral effects of nitrendipine in essential hypertension. *Circulation* 1988:78:1394-1400.
13. Khurmi NS, Raftery EB. Comparative effects of prolonged therapy with four calcium ion antagonists (diltiazem, nicardipine, tiapamil and verapamil) in patients with chronic stable angina pectoris. *Cardiovasc Drugs Ther* 1987;1:81-87.
14. Sharma MK, Voyles W, Prasad R, et al. Long-term bepridil monotherapy for angina pectoris. *Am J Cardiol* 1988;61:1210-1213.
15. Betocchi S, Bonow RO, Cannon RO, et al. Relation between serum nifedipine concentration and hemodynamic effects in non-obstructive hypertrophic cardiomyopathy. *Am J Cardiol* 1988;61:830-835.

INDEX

298